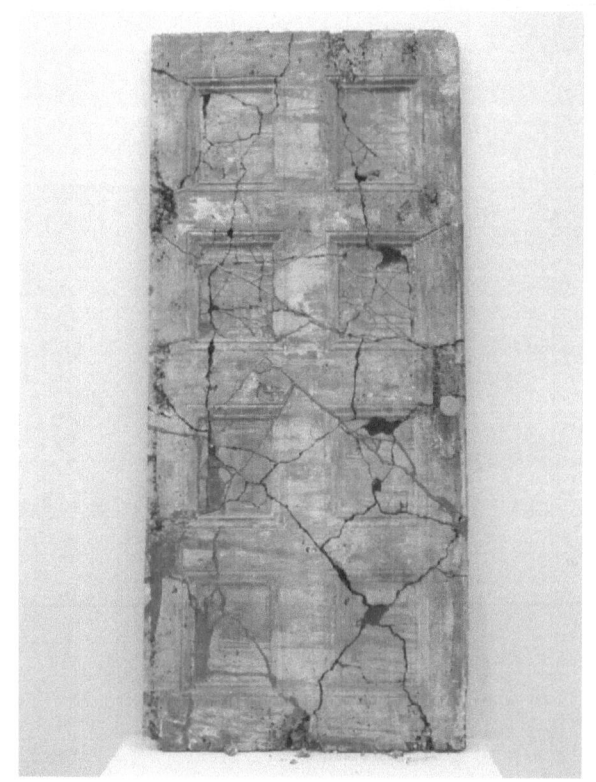

(タイトル・クレジット表記　日/英)

≪修復のモニュメント「ドア」≫
渡辺 篤
2016–2020年
写真: 井上圭佑
© Atsushi Watanabe 2020

MONUMENT OF RECOVERY "The Door"
Atsushi Watanabe
Photo by Keisuke Inoue
© Atsushi Watanabe 2020

Mental Health and Social Withdrawal in Contemporary Japan

This book examines the phenomenon of social withdrawal in Japan, which ranges from school nonattendance to extreme forms of isolation and confinement, known as *hikikomori*. Based on extensive original research, including interview research with a range of practitioners involved in dealing with the phenomenon, the book outlines how *hikikomori* expresses itself, how it is treated and dealt with, and how it has been perceived and regarded in Japan over time. The author, a clinical psychologist with extensive experience of practice, argues that the phenomenon although socially unacceptable is not homogenous and can be viewed not as a mental disorder, but as an idiom of distress, a passive and effective way of resisting the many great pressures of Japanese schooling and society more widely.

Nicolas Tajan is a program-specific associate professor in the Graduate School of Human and Environmental Studies at Kyoto University, Japan.

Mental Health and Social Withdrawal in Contemporary Japan

Beyond the *Hikikomori* Spectrum

Nicolas Tajan

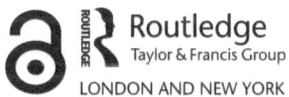

Routledge
Taylor & Francis Group

LONDON AND NEW YORK

First published 2021
by Routledge
2 Park Square, Milton Park, Abingdon, Oxon OX14 4RN

and by Routledge
52 Vanderbilt Avenue, New York, NY 10017

*Routledge is an imprint of the Taylor & Francis Group, an informa
business*

British Library Cataloguing-in-Publication Data
A catalog record for this book is available from the British Library

Library of Congress Cataloging-in-Publication Data
A catalog record has been requested for this book

ISBN: 978-0-8153-6574-7 (hbk)
ISBN: 978-0-367-64572-4 (pbk)
ISBN: 978-1-351-26080-0 (ebk)

Typeset in Times New Roman by
KnowledgeWorks Global Ltd.

Contents

Preface

"*Hikikomori* phenomenon, far from being homogeneous, begins to appear as it really is: the history of a myriad of singular subjects who, despite themselves, draw attention to their absence while making social renunciation an idiom that is deeply subjective and eminently social." This quotation encapsulates some of the central issues of this fascinating and important work. Nicolas Tajan is not an anthropologist but a clinical psychologist who was brought by his topic of inquiry to act and proceed in his research more and more like an anthropologist. As the above mentioned sentence indicates *hikikomori* is not a psychiatric category – showing this is one of the central aims of the book – the term refers to "the history of myriad singular subjects" rather than to an ailment with clear characteristic traits. The point is not merely that this failure at being a homogeneous set of individuals or psychological characteristics reflects the difference between the method of the psychiatrist, who sees instances of particular diseases and categorizes them as depression or bipolar disorder, and that of the anthropologist, who seeks to encounter others as they are in their diversity, rather than to categorize them. The point rather is that the reason why *hikikomori* escapes psychiatric categorization is neither because these categories do not constitute knowledge nor because it is true that all medical categories subsume under a single term myriad singular subjects, but because *hikikomori* fails to become an object of psychiatric knowledge. It is not a mental disease but a psychosocial phenomenon.

The *hikikomori* does not ask anything from the psychiatrist, or the medical profession in general, or from any others in particular actually, hiding, shut in a room in a house that he or she rarely leaves. There is a paradox here in viewing these persons as "patients." How do you meet someone who does not want to meet anyone? What if you succeed, is the person you met a *hikikomori* or not *hikikomori* anymore? This desire for isolation and loneliness, which Tajan describes as an "idiom of distress," is eminently social and challenges the health professions. Here are persons who do not ask for help, do not come forward with their complaints, and therefore are only made into "patients" by others. Which happens only sometimes, when they are not hidden from view by the family from (and within) which they are hiding. In either case, they do not seek help, for whatever reason they have renounced asking.

The clinic has always been about responding to the patient's demand, even if in many cases, this meant reinterpreting it in a different way. Medical and psychiatric categories are tools that help the specialist endowed with knowledge, called upon because of that knowledge, to respond to the patient's demands. Hence the need for a different method and approach when the person's way to 'address' others is silence, isolation, social renunciation; one that is not, or at least that is less, predicated on a hierarchical relation of knowledge and thus closer to that of anthropologists. Clinical psychologists interested in *hikikomori* have to do fieldwork. They cannot remain in their office waiting for the patients to come. They must go to them. This profoundly changes the relationship and indicates that these individuals in distress are not like those who can be analyzed, and disciplined through the use of psychiatric categories. In what ways are they different? This is what this book describes with finesse and attention and tries to interpret in a larger social and historical context.

The *hikikomori* phenomenon, according to Tajan, makes visible an ongoing process of social transformations of which it is part. One that is particularly visible in Japan, but that is also present in many places across the world. It concerns the place of medical professions in contemporary postmodern societies, the way individuals attempt to make themselves into subjects, their refusal of current mental health practices; and it questions the place and role of anthropological knowledge in this changing world.

Paul Dumouchel

Acknowledgements

Before beginning this book, I had the privilege of completing my Ph.D. in psychopathology at the University of Toulouse in 2014 under the exceptional supervision of Marie-Jean Sauret and Pierre-Henri Castel. In France, most of those who are interested in Lacanian psychoanalysis know Marie-Jean Sauret for his unique style that combines kindness, humor, firmness, and a sincere involvement in political matters. It is still a surprise for both of us that his legacy continues in Japan where I work now as an associate professor and a psychoanalyst. And, I honestly do not have enough words to say how privileged I feel to have met one of the most prolific thinkers in contemporary France: Pierre-Henri Castel. Since our first contact in September 2009, I owe him the freedom I took to allow myself to adopt an approach that is at the crossroads of Lacanian psychoanalysis, clinical psychopathology, history of psychiatry, and the anthropology of mental health.

I would also like to express my gratitude to Tsuiki Kosuke for allowing me to work from April of 2011 to March of 2017 in the Institute for Research in Humanities at Kyoto University. He was also immensely helpful in answering my questions about the Japanese language, culture, history, and society.

I am very thankful for all the people from the NPOs supporting *hikikomori* and *nīto* who agreed to welcome me and answer my questions, in particular the members of the NPO M. and the NPOs of the G. and H. prefectures, namely, Messrs. Arai, Nomura, Yamamoto, Murata, Sano, Wada, and Taniguchi, as well as Ueyama Kazuki, with whom I spoke at length. Within the professionals of H. prefecture supporting young truants and their parents, Ms. Otsuka, Mr. Sakurai, and Dr. Matsuda graciously contributed toward helping me better understand the Japanese health and medico-social fields. I would also like to thank Prof. Kubo along with Misaki and her parents.

For the rereadings and the remarks concerning the early versions of my work, I would like to thank Sophie Moulard, Aline Henninger, Natacha Vellut, Rodrigo Drozak, Philippe Lavergne, Jeanne Gaillard, Marc-Henri Deroche, and Miwaki Yasuo. Regarding the verification of kanji, romanizations, and their remarks on translations, I would like to thank Ueo Masamichi, Nobutomo Kenji, Horikawa Satoshi, Fukuda Daisuke, Yamaguchi Takeshi, Inoue Haruko, and Isomura Dai. For the last versions, my gratitude goes to Eyal Ben Ari, Hamasaki Yukiko, Nancy Pionnié-Dax, Shiozawa Meiko, James Coates; Ichida Yoshihiko, Koizumi Yoshiyuki, Hirose Jun, Ohji Kenta, and members of the Foucauldian Studies Research Seminar (Kyoto University, Institute for Research in Humanities); and Paul Dumouchel, Matsumoto Takuya, and Joan Jastram.

I thank my parents Monique and Jean-Jacques Tajan, and my wife Maiko Tajan, along with the rest of my family for all of their support.

Finally, I would like to thank the following institutions for granting me the funding that enabled me to carry out this research:

Japan Foundation [2010]

The Japanese Society for the Promotion of Science (JSPS) [*Post-Doctoral Fellowship (short-term) for North American and European Researchers, through a Nominative Authority* (CNRS), 2012]

Canon Foundation in Europe [*Canon Foundation in Europe Fellowship,* 2014]

The Japanese Society for the Promotion of Science (JSPS) [*Post-Doctoral Fellowship (standard) for North American and European Researchers,* 2015]

This work was supported by JSPS KAKENHI Grant Numbers 19K12975, 18H00999, and 18KK0068. Any opinions, findings, and conclusions or recommendations expressed in this material are those of the author and do not necessarily reflect the views of the author's organization, JSPS or MEXT.

All information that could reveal the identities of the people that have been questioned has been changed, and the names of the associations in which I have investigated have been anonymized, with the exception of Mr. Ueyama's testimony and various information available on the Internet (e.g., the testimonies Mr. Maruyama and Ms. Hayashi, Newstart, and KHJ websites).

Some portions of the current book have been published in their earlier versions in French, Japanese, or English publications listed here.

Tajan, Nicolas. 2015a. "Adolescents' School Non-Attendance and the Spread of Psychological Counselling in Japan." *Asia Pacific Journal of Counselling and Psychotherapy* 6 (1/2): 58–69.

Tajan, Nicolas. 2015b. "Social Withdrawal and Psychiatry: A Comprehensive Review of Hikikomori." *Neuropsychiatrie de l'Enfance et de l'Adolescence* 63 (5): 324–331.

Tajan, Nicolas. 2015c. "Japanese Post-Modern Social Renouncers: An Exploratory Study of the Narratives of Hikikomori Subjects." *Subjectivity* 8: 283–304.

Tajan, Nicolas. 2017a. *Génération hikikomori.* Paris: L'Harmattan (Collection Japon).

Tajan, Nicolas. 2017b. "Traumatic Dimensions of Hikikomori: A Foucauldian Note." *Asian Journal of Psychiatry* 27: 121–122.

Tajan, Nicolas, Yukiko Hamasaki, and Nancy Pionnié-Dax. 2017. "Hikikomori: The Japanese Cabinet Office's 2016 Survey of Acute Social Withdrawal." *The Asia-Pacific Journal* 15 (1): 1–11.

Tajan Nicolas, and Meiko Shiozawa. 2020. "Hikikomori wo saikōsuru – kaigai, tokuni furansu no jirei 「ひきこもり」を再考する—海外、特にフランスの事例" (Rethinking Hikikomori – Examples from France and Abroad), *Kyōku to Igaku* 教育と医学. 3/4: 54–61.

Introduction

Step aside, intersections, minor roads

"Trust the author you are studying. But what does it mean to 'trust an author'? It means the same thing as groping, proceeding with a kind of groping. Before you fully understand the problems someone poses (...) you have to silence the voices of objection at all costs. The voices of objection are those which would say too quickly: 'Oh, but look here, there is something wrong'. And to trust the author is to say, let's not talk too quickly (...) you have to let him speak."

Gilles Deleuze *Cours sur Michel Foucault* October 22, 1985

Defining *hikikomori*

Shakaiteki hikikomori designates a phenomenon of social withdrawal and the individuals concerned, i.e., shut-ins. *Shakaiteki* means "social" and the word *hikikomori* is composed of *hiku* (to pull, draw, retreat) and *komoru* (to shut oneself up, stay inside). *Hikikomori* has long been difficult to define; however, recently, a consensus appears to have been reached among psychiatrists. "*Hikikomori* is a form of pathological social withdrawal or social isolation whose essential feature is physical isolation in one's home. The person must meet the following criteria: a) marked social isolation in one's home; b) duration of continuous social isolation of at least 6 months; c) significant functional impairment or distress associated with the social isolation" (Kato, Kanba, and Teo 2020: 117).

This consensus represents marked progress from previous definitions. However, I have some reservations about the statement that it is a "pathological" form or that it must require "significant functional impairment or distress associated with the social isolation." It is not a criticism of colleagues, who I appreciate as individuals and scholars. It is simply that psychiatrists determine pathologies and are trained to treat what they call "disorders." I must say that I myself am passionate about the history of psychiatry and the way in which psychiatrists create psychiatric categories. I also find the new formulation of Kato, Kanba, and Teo (2020) interesting: "Individuals who occasionally leave their home (2–3 days/week), rarely leave their home (1 day/week or less), or rarely leave a single room may be characterized as mild, moderate or severe, respectively," (p. 117) while those who leave their room 4 or more days a week are excluded from the *hikikomori* category. In addition to their recognition that *hikikomori* co-occurs with other mental disorders, their contribution is an important step compared to previous works. That being said, my approach is very different because I am questioning the very fact that *hikikomori* is a pathology, including the modalities of assessing the impairment or distress of the persons concerned. More precisely, I question the basic assumptions of psychiatric categories from a standpoint where the history and anthropology of mental health, clinical psychopathology, and Lacanian psychoanalysis intersect. This point of view features in Japanese academic categories as "intellectual history" (*shisō shi*): I address the very notion of loneliness while simultaneously combining theories and methods of the history and anthropology of mental health, clinical psychopathology, and Lacanian psychoanalysis.

This book is about social withdrawal (from school nonattendance to acute social withdrawal called *hikikomori*) and psychological clinics in contemporary Japan. The volume builds on my ethnographic research on mental health practices in contemporary Japan (Tajan 2014, 2015a-c; Tajan and Shiozawa 2020), and its perspectives encompass aspects related to the meaning and experience of distress, illness, mental health, and support; the cultural, historical, clinical, and linguistic context of support practices and access to care; and the cultural influences on individual's and the population's mental health and expression of distress. Overall, the book aims at contributing to anthropological inquiry while making arguments relevant to the interdisciplinary study of subjectivity. More precisely, my goal is to stimulate the development of important theory, methods, and debates in the anthropology of mental health and to explore the links with neighboring fields in the humanities, social sciences, and mental health–related disciplines.

This study is an investigation of a hidden population, which is, by definition, difficult to encounter, and as a result authentic voices have rarely been heard. Philological, clinical, and ethnographic methods have been used. The philological methodology is crucial here because the study of texts (and interviews) in their original language (Japanese) ensures that the translation does not mislead the reader and that it respects the subjects' points of view. The clinical methodology is widely used in medicine and psychology, and originated from being at a patient's bedside, observing their symptoms. Given my training as a clinical psychologist and my psychoanalytical clinical practice, I conducted and interpreted sources and interviews with a clinical perspective and sensibility, using ethnographic methods. I used ethnographic methods and techniques such as participant observation and field interviews, which are often employed in cultural anthropology, when collecting the narratives of *hikikomori* subjects.

Anthropology matters for clinicians

I am not an anthropologist, yet I thought of this work as a volume that would follow on from *Encounters with Aging* by Lock (1995) and *Depression in Japan* by Kitanaka (2012). To me, these two books are required reading for anyone interested in mental health issues in contemporary Japan.

As I write this introduction and finalize this book in Spring 2020, our societies are experiencing unprecedented confinement due to the COVID-19 epidemic. I have been a program-specific associate professor at Kyoto University since February 2019, where Associate Professor Matsumoto Takuya and I contribute to the Laboratory of Psychopathology and Psychoanalysis and its Kyoto University International Mental Health Seminar. I also officiate as vice president of the International Mental Health Professionals Japan.

I am not a lover of Japan, but I like living here in Kyoto and its surroundings and suspect that I will stay here for a long time, maybe forever. It is perhaps the only place in the world that allows me to be immersed in three languages – Japanese, English, and French – on a daily basis, and it truly contributes to very simple feelings of happiness. However, a decade ago, I was far from imagining the direction my life would take. At the time, around 2009, I was in the Bordeaux area, where I worked full time in a guidance center offering psychotherapy to children, adolescents, and their families. I do not want to hide anything here: I loved my job; the team was amazing; and we were able to successfully support a number of children and families in distress.

To tell the truth, as soon as I finished my master's degree in psychology in 2005, I wanted to enroll in a Ph.D. program, but I also had a deep desire to invest myself in clinical practice, which for me continues to be, even today and hopefully for a long time, an invaluable source of teachings. Around 2009, I decided that it was time to embark on a Ph.D. At the same time, I wanted to live a year abroad, an opportunity I did not have before. Japan had started to interest me, though very gradually in recent years: its food, gardens, language, culture, and arts. Also, there was Jacques Lacan's idea that the Japanese were unanalyzable (Lacan 2005: 126), which intrigued me.

I planned my first trip to Japan in the summer of 2009, during which I had the opportunity to meet several psychoanalysts and psychiatrists, to whom I asked a simple question: currently, what is the most important issue in youth mental health? Their response was unanimous: *hikikomori* and the increase in autism and developmental disorders. Back in France, I had written a project on these themes, accepted a few months later by the Japan Foundation. During my Ph.D., I had to narrow the spectrum of my research to the study of *hikikomori*, but my interest in autism has remained alive and is one of the topics in my current research pipeline.

Since April of 2011, I have lived continuously in Kyoto, Japan. Here, I met my future wife, did my Ph.D. and postdoctoral research, got married, had two children, and started a psychoanalytic consulting room. Now, my life is in Japan, in the Kansai area.

I discovered what really interested me about Japan as a scholar and clinician, via *Encounters with Aging* by Margaret Lock and a Ph.D. thesis on *Depression in Japan* by Junko Kitanaka, with whom I first corresponded in January of 2010. Reading and studying these two volumes was a tipping point for me. I encountered an approach with which I had never been presented before during my training in France. I can say it now: in 1999, once I had obtained my baccalaureate, I wanted to enroll in an anthropology program, but this was impossible. In Bordeaux, anthropology was only accessible in the third year of a bachelor's degree, and we had to choose between enrolling for the first 2 years in psychology or sociology. It turns out that I was more interested in psychology. Another aspect that made me stay in psychology was that in 2001, I started my own psychoanalysis, which lasted 10 years. Those who have experienced living in France can attest to the highly stimulating atmosphere of psychoanalytical schools such as the *Ecole de la Cause Freudienne*, the *Ecole de Psychanalyse des Forums du Champ Lacanien*, or psychoanalytical associations such as *Espace Analytique* and *Le Pari de Lacan*, of which I am a member. Seminars and internships are held on an almost daily basis in every city, enabling participation in the French intellectual and clinical scene. In parallel with my involvement in psychoanalysis, I attended, as much as possible, anthropology classes and seminars in France and seminars in Japan at Kyoto University (with Prof. Tanaka Masakazu) and Ritsumeikan University (with Ass. Prof. Andrea de Antoni). The idea even came to my mind that I could perhaps become an anthropologist, though it never came to fruition.

What happened was the verification that my own psychoanalysis had produced a psychoanalyst, and that it was impossible for me to be both an anthropologist and a psychoanalyst at the same time. The reasons are difficult to explain because I would need to introduce the aspects of Lacanian theory and practice, which are, unfortunately, heavily misunderstood and misrepresented in the English-speaking world. At the very least, I can mention one reason pertaining to the Lacanian logic of discourse: psychoanalytic discourse implies that the object cause of desire (object a) is placed as the agent of the discourse, a style of agency that hardly corresponds to the type of discourse in which the anthropologist participates. (On this point and the former, the reader will forgive me for not going into further detail here.)

So I am not an anthropologist, but my desire is for my work to be anthropologically relevant. It is a humble goal, but achieving it would be enough for me. I know that my book does not have the academic breadth of the aforementioned volumes. For instance, some critics might point to my insistence on reviewing the work of other colleagues, but I saw this as necessary to give a broad picture of the phenomenon. Also, I am aware that

I have not produced a complete portrait of the works of Kawai Hayao or Saitō Tamaki and that a history and anthropology of school nonattendance in Japan still needs to be written. Let me be very clear here: the history and anthropology of mental health in Japan are under-investigated, and there is a great need for works published in the English language on many issues. Although some will read what comes off as an excuse, I must underline the reasons why a work on *hikikomori* has never been published by a scholar until now and why it was so difficult for me to achieve. Margaret Lock is an anthropologist, and her 1995 book focuses on a well-defined medical object: menopause. The same goes for Junko Kitanaka with depression, Karen Nakamura (2013) with schizophrenia, Chikako Ozawa de Silva (2006) with *Naikan*, and Carol Stevens (2014) with disability. I cannot help it: I am not an anthropologist; I am a psychoanalyst, a function that is not even recognized as legitimate in today's academic world. Psychoanalysts have been globally excluded from psychology departments (except in a number of French and Latin American universities); and universities never train psychoanalysts, although they train anthropologists. Moreover, compared to menopause, depression, schizophrenia, and disability, which are well-defined medical objects, *hikikomori* is neither medical nor well defined. This peculiarity of *hikikomori* as a contested and ill-defined medical object, despite its pervasiveness, made it extremely difficult to produce a consistent monograph on the subject: with the very specific countertransference it produces, this explains why this book – if we except the translation of Saitō Tamaki's 1998 *Adolescence without End* (Saitō 2013) – is the first volume available in English on the subject.

Relating to this particularity of the object is the second difficulty linked to my psychoanalytic orientation. Indeed, the greatest authors of *nihonjinron*, discourses on Japanese identity, are known as psychoanalysts: Doi Takeo and Kawai Hayao. Here again, anthropology was decisive for me in the presence of Harumi Befu's famous 2001 achievement. Coupled with the great classic *Orientalism* by Edward Said (1980), these works are for me other prerequisites, before even making the slightest statement on psychology and psychoanalysis in Japan or what Japanese subjects might feel and experience. The references to these authors also contribute toward situating my position not only in the psychoanalytical arena in the strict sense but also in intellectual history, as detailed previously.

In other words, in the Japanese field, no psychoanalysis is possible without anthropology, and simultaneously, psychoanalytic discourse is not the discourse that the anthropologist joins (in the Lacanian sense). Of course, the anthropologist can use psychoanalytic terms and speak of psychoanalysis, but in doing so, he most often joins the university discourse, the discourse of the master, or of the hysteric. From this point of view, one of the contributions of this work lies in the tension between historical, anthropological, psychopathological, and psychoanalytic approaches, regarded as a tension between discourses.

Reclusion exposed

In Japan, the *hikikomori* phenomenon affects hundreds of thousands of individuals: between 696,000 and 541,000 individuals aged 15–39 and 613,000 aged 40–64 (Cabinet Office 2010, 2016, 2019). In 2020, the *hikikomori* population aged 15–64 is roughly estimated to be around 1,154,000 individuals nationwide. Social withdrawal situations gradually increased in the 1990s, until they became a "social problem" (*shakai mondai*) in the early 2000s and a global issue in the 2010s.

In 1997, Ishida Ira published a novel *Ikebukuro West Gate Park* (*IWGP*), in which he introduced a *hikikomori* character. It is the first successful novel featuring a *hikikomori* character. His six volumes were extremely popular, adapted to a TV drama, a *manga*, and an anime in 2020. Following is an extract from the original novel.

> *Kazunori was first in the class when we were in the third year of college. A super good student, who had attended an excellent private high school. I am sure that he would have been a good college student today.* [Kazunori's mother] "Not only did he drop out of high school, but … It's very difficult to say, but here it is: he never leaves his room." *According to her, he hadn't been out of his house for the past three years. She would drop his meals off at the door of his room. He managed to go to the bathroom or to shower without meeting anyone in the family. He had added an interior lock to his door. A perfect recluse. [...]* [Kazunori's mother] "You are the first friend to come to visit him in three years. Today, he was not ready, and he was in a bad mood, but please don't let that deter you, come back. Try to be his friend, please. I beg you, she repeated three times. Head down, she was crying. Tears that melted on the surface of his lemon-cleared tea. From a distance, a waitress looked at us with undisguised curiosity. The star of our class was now living in his own room, which had been transformed into an isolation cell."
>
> *(Ishida cited by Giard 2017)*

The following year, a psychiatrist (Saitō 1998) played an important role in triggering media coverage of this phenomenon that was then relayed through countless television documentaries and newspaper articles. Abroad, journalists have progressively produced articles and reports from the 2000s to the present and have helped shape the image of *hikikomori*. For example, in 2002, a BBC report wondered about "the mystery of the missing million," million designating the *hikikomori* population. Films in the humanities and sciences (FHS 1999, 2003) also contributed two documentaries on the phenomenon. A 2004 report by the Dutch television BNN focused on this phenomenon and introduced the Newstart association to the general public. Next came the publication of the popularized work of an American journalist who attempted to describe, through *hikikomori*, how Japan created its lost generation (Zielenziger 2007).

The year 2008 saw the production of the medium-length film *Shaking Tokyo* directed by Bong Joon Ho and broadcasted with two other medium-length films (*Interior Design* by Michel Gondry and *Merde* by Leos Carax) under the title *Tokyo!* The same year, a movie on *hikikomori* was produced, entitled *Tobira no-mukō* (Thrush 2008), a title meaning "behind the door." A BBC World program aired on July 5, 2013, directed by Claudia Hammond. It was devoted to *hikikomori* in Japan (this is the sixth episode in a series called "The Truth About Mental Health"). The *New York Times* even featured an article by Tomoko Rich in 2019.

Novels on this phenomenon have been written in several languages. In French, there are novels entitled *Je suis un hikikomori* (Aubry 2010) and *Hikikomori* (Marcotte 2014). In English, there are *The Haunted Hikikomori* (Pearce 2013) and *Hikikomori and the Rental Sister* (Backhaus 2013a) translated into French under the title *Hikikomori* (Backhaus 2013b). Other novels entitled *Hikikomori* are available in Catalan (Faura 2008), Polish (Przewoźnik 2011), and German (Kuhn 2014).

On the artistic level, there was a performance in the West Space gallery in Melbourne, Australia, from March 22 to 29, 2012, under the title "Stay Home Sakoku." In this performance, Eugenia Lim locked herself up for a week in a 25-square meter room, continuously filmed, communicating with no one, and on a water-only diet. She was fed, via a flap, by visitors. An Internet portal was created especially for the occasion. In the fall of 2020, dancer Eric Minh Cuong Castaing and Scenographer Anne-Sophie Turion will be in residence at Villa Kujoyama, Kyoto, to produce a work dedicated to *hikikomori*.

Theater plays have also been performed in Mexico and Spain. In France, a play by Satake Yoji, inspired by this phenomenon, entitled *Le grenier* was performed in Paris in 2009.

Overview of the seven chapters

In the first chapter, I describe how clinical psychologists, through a system of school counselors, became crucial in treating school absentees and their parents. I present elements of Japanese psychology's history, showing how clinical psychology emerged at the very end of the 20th century. I introduce (in a descriptive and critical fashion) a charismatic character: Kawai Hayao. A scholar and man of authority, he contributed to the spread of clinical psychology and a large system of school counselors in charge of treating school nonattendance. Here, I study *Yungu shinrigaku to bukkyō* (Jungian Psychology and Buddhism), avoiding misrepresentations related to its previous American translation (Kawai 1995, 1996). I describe important elements of the Japanese educational system and question the place of school counseling between clinical psychologists and teachers. I underline a crucial transition: the shift from a stigmatizing medicalization of school refusal (*tōkō kyohi*) to a benevolent worry toward school nonattendance (*futōkō*).

In the second chapter, I relate four interviews leading me to consider the previous chapter's data from a different perspective. I limited my focus to H. prefecture, and, to grasp all the elements necessary to understand the management of school nonattendance, I successively question Ms. Otsuka, a school counselor; Mr. Sakurai, the manager of guidance center X.; Dr. Matsuda, a child and adolescent psychiatrist of guidance center J.; and Prof. Kubo, associate professor in a university of H. prefecture. These interviews contribute to describing the support provided to children with difficulties in H. city. In addition, they allow us to better grasp the contemporary emergence of professions such as clinical psychologists and child and adolescent psychiatrists. As surprising as it may seem, these professions only emerged at the beginning of the 21st century. Simultaneously, one observes the dramatic increase in developmental disorders (*hattatsu shōgai*), autism (*jiheishō*), and school nonattendance. Another unexpected result is discovered. Stereotypes of Japanese students crushed under the weight of entrance exams (junior high and high school, college), or exhausted by an inhumane amount of school pressure, are pervasive. Yet, they must be nuanced, and sometimes refuted. As we will see, even as junior high school students are effectively the object of intense surveillance, struggling high school students are abandoned by others.

In the third chapter, I give an overview of social withdrawal in premodern, modern, and contemporary periods. I analyze the book of a psychiatrist who pioneered *hikikomori* studies: the book is entitled *Shakaiteki hikikomori: owaranai shishunki* (*Hikikomori*: Adolescence Without End) (Saitō 1998). Then, I ask whether *hikikomori* could be considered a Japanese "culture-bound syndrome." Responding to this question requires a confrontation with *taijin kyōfushō*, defined as a Japanese interpersonal fear disorder in the DSM-5® (American Psychiatric Association 2013). I show that psychiatrists since Saitō Tamaki have systematically led their investigations relying on a process called "typification," and that they only meet a subcategory of shut-ins and their families.

In the fourth chapter, I detail epidemiological data in Japan and relate the psychological investigations in and outside Japan. One of the most interesting features of this chapter is the synthesis of the Cabinet Office surveys dedicated to the two generations of *hikikomori*: shut-ins aged 15–39 (2016) and shut-ins aged 40–64 (2019).

In the fifth chapter, I describe the first sociological and anthropological approaches, recounting investigations by Ogino (2004), Kaneko Sachiko (Kaneko 2006), Toivonen (2008), Miller and Toivonen (2010). Then, I detail my study of the support systems I investigated: nonprofit organizations (NPOs)—for instance, NPOs related to local communities and Buddhist schools and an NPO of H. city. I give evidence of my encounter with Mr. Yamamoto, a former member of the national association of *hikikomori*'s parents (*KHJ zenkoku hikikomori oya no kai*). Also, I describe another type of NPO, related to anti-capitalist movements: *Newstart*, NPO M., and their initiative of Japanese–Korean *hikikomori* university of the People. I conclude by discussing and showing the perspectives implicated by these systems for *hikikomori* and *nīto* youths.

In the sixth chapter, after having related some cases of *hikikomori* individuals who appeared in the media, I recount my meetings with persons struggling with acute social withdrawal. First is Mr. Ueyama (2001), the second person to publicly testify of his *hikikomori* experience in a book. I present my comment on his book's extract, a video-recorded interview, our correspondence, and our meetings. Then, I evoke several generations of *hikikomori* by examining an interview with Mr. Maruyama Yasuhiko and Ms. Hayashi Kyoko; a written account, collected in H. city NPO (Mr. Onishi); and a research interview with Mr. Arai, met in G. prefecture. I conclude by reflecting on subjectivity and social bonds in contemporary Japan.

In the seventh chapter, I start by detailing the globalization of social isolation, arguing that *hikikomori* is not limited to Japan and not solely related to Japanese culture. Second, I provide a brief overview of French *hikikomori* studies, including accounts by a mother and a 25-year-old male. Third, I present a case study of a binational *hikikomori*, Misaki, and her parents, using the most recent and stringent methodological tools of transcultural research: the Cultural Formulation Interview (CFI)–informant version (American Psychiatric Association 2016) as well as the McGill Illness Narrative Interview (MINI) (Groleau, Young, and Kirmayer 2006). It leads me to make recommendations and propose ways of rethinking social isolation. I conclude with 20 lessons on *hikikomori*.

Since the life stories of *hikikomori* adults often include an episode of truancy in which psychologists intervene, I will discuss these themes in the first two chapters and then devote myself to the study of the *hikikomori* phenomenon.

References

American Psychiatric Association. 2013. *Diagnostic and Statistical Manual of Mental Disorders, 5th Edition: DSM-5 [Paperback]*. Washington, DC: American Psychiatric Publishing.

———. 2016. *DSM-5 Handbook on the Cultural Formulation Interview*, edited by Lewis-Fernández, et al. [Paperback]. Washington, DC: American Psychiatric Publishing.

Aubry, Florence. 2010. *Je suis un hikikomori*. Namur: Mijade.

Backhaus, Jeff. 2013a. *Hikikomori*. Editions Anne Carrière.

———. 2013b. *Hikikomori and the Rental Sister: A Novel*. Algonquin Books.

Befu, Harumi. 2001. *Hegemony of Homogeneity: An Anthropological Analysis of Nihonjinron*. Melbourne: Trans Pacific Press.

Cabinet Office of the Government of Japan (Director-General for Policy on Cohesive Society) 内閣府政策統括官 (共生社会政策担当). 2016. *Wakamono no seikatsu ni kansuru chōsa hōkokusho* 若者の生活に関する調査 報告書 (Research Survey on Youth's life). https://www8.cao.go.jp/youth/kenkyu/hikikomori/h27/pdf-index.html

———. 2019. *Seikatsu Jōkyō ni Kansuru Chōsa* 生活状況に関する調査 (Survey on Living Conditions). https://www8.cao.go.jp/youth/kenkyu/life/h30/pdf-index.html

Faura, Jordi. 2008. *Hikikomori (L'era del buit)*. Alcira: Edicions Bromera.

Films in the Humanities and Sciences (FHS). 1999. *Japan, the Taboo of Failure*. Videorecording. Films-for-the-Humanities-and-Sciences.

———. 2003. *Japanese Education in Crisis*. Videorecording. Films-for-the-Humanities-and-Sciences.

Giard, Agnès. 2017. "On a tous en soi une pièce condamnée" In *Génération hikikomori*. Paris: L'Harmattan, collection "Japon, études du fait japonais".

Groleau, Danielle, Allan Young, and Laurence J. Kirmayer. 2006. "The McGill Illness Narrative Interview (MINI): An Interview Schedule to Elicit Meanings and Modes of Reasoning Related to Illness Experience." *Transcultural Psychiatry* 43 (4): 671–691.

Kaneko, Sachiko. 2006. "Japan's 'Socially Withdrawn Youths' and Time Constraints in Japanese Society: Management and Conceptualization of Time in a Support Group for Hikikomori." *Time & Society* 15 (2/3): 233–249.

Kato, Takahiro, Shigenobu Kanba, and Alan R. Teo. 2020. "Defining pathological social withdrawal: proposed diagnostic criteria for hikikomori" *World Psychiatry* 19 (1): 116–117.

Kawai, Hayao 河合隼雄. 1995. *Yungu shinrigaku to bukkyō* ユング心理学と仏教 (Jungian Psychology and Bouddhism). Tōkyō: Iwanami Shoten.

———. 1996. *Buddhism and the Art of Psychotherapy* (translation of *Yungu shinrigaku to bukkyō*). Texas A&M University Press.

Kitanaka, Junko. 2012. *Depression in Japan, Psychiatric Cures for a Society in Distress*. Princeton, NJ: Princeton University Press.

Kuhn, Kevin. 2014. *Hikikomori*. Berliner Taschenbuch Verl.

Lacan, Jacques. 2005. *Le Séminaire livre XXIII: Le Sinthome (1975–1976)*. Paris: Seuil.

Lock, Margaret. 1995. *Encounters with Aging. Mythologies of Menopause in Japan and North America*. Berkeley, CA: University of California Press.

Marcotte, Josée. 2014. *Hikikomori*. L'instant même.

Miller, Aaron L., and Tuukka Toivonen. 2010. "To Discipline or Accommodate? On the Rehabilitation of Japanese 'Problem Youth.'" *The Asia-Pacific Journal: Japan Focus*. http://www.japanfocus.org/-aaron-miller/3368.

Nakamura, Karen. 2013. *A Disability of the Soul: An Ethnography of Schizophrenia and Mental Illness in Contemporary Japan*. Ithaca: Cornell University Press.

Ogino, Tatsushi. 2004. "Managing Categorization and Social Withdrawal in Japan: Rehabilitation Process in a Private Support Group for Hikikomorians." *International Journal of Japanese Sociology* 13: 120–133.

Ozawa-de Silva, Chikako. 2006. *Psychotherapy and Religion in Japan: The Japanese Introspection Practice of Naikan*. Oxon, New York: Routledge.

Pearce, Lawrence. 2013. *The Haunted Hikikomori*. CreateSpace Independent Publishing Platform.

Przewoźnik, Tomasz. 2011. *Hikikomori*. http://hikikomori.eu/.

Rich, Tomoko. 2019. "Japan's Extreme Recluses Already Faced Stigma. Now, After Knifings, They're Feared." *The New York Times*, June 6, 2019.

Saitō, Tamaki 斎藤環. 1998. *Shakaiteki hikikomori — owaranai shishunki* 社会的 ひきこもり—終わらない思春期 (Social Hikikomori – Adolescence without End). Tōkyō: PHP Shinsho.

———. 2013. *Hikikomori: Adolescence without End*. Translated by Jeffrey Angles. Minnesota University Press.

Stevens, Carolyn S. 2014. *Disability in Japan*. Oxon, New York: Routledge, Japan Anthropology Workshop Series.

Tajan, Nicolas. 2014. "Le retrait social au Japon: Enquête sur le *hikikomori* et l'absentéisme scolaire (*futōkō*)." PhD diss., Toulouse University.

———. 2015a. "Adolescents' School Non-Attendance and the Spread of Psychological Counselling in Japan." *Asia Pacific Journal of Counselling and Psychotherapy* 6 (1/2): 58–69.

———. 2015b. "Social Withdrawal and Psychiatry: A Comprehensive Review of Hikikomori." *Neuropsychiatrie de l'Enfance et de l'Adolescence* 63 (5): 324–331.

———. 2015c. "Japanese Post-Modern Social Renouncers: An Exploratory Study of the Narratives of Hikikomori Subjects." *Subjectivity* 8: 283–304.

Tajan Nicolas, and Meiko Shiozawa. 2020. "Hikikomori wo saikōsuru – kaigai, tokuni furansu no jirei 「ひきこもり」を再考する—海外、特にフランスの事例" (Rethinking Hikikomori – Examples from France and Abroad), *Kyōiku to Igaku* 教育と医学. 3/4: 54–61.

Thrush, Laurence. 2008. *Tobira No-Mukō/Left-Handed*. http://tobiranomuko.com/index.html

Toivonen, Tuukka. 2008. "Introducing the Youth Independence Camp. How a New Social Policy Is Reconfiguring the Public-Private Boundaries of Social Provision in Japan." *Sociologos* 32: 42–57.

Ueyama, Kazuki 上山和樹. 2001. *"Hikikomori" datta boku kara* 「ひきこもり」だっ た僕から (From me, who was *hikikomori*). Tōkyō: Kōdansha.

Zielenziger, Michael. 2007. *Shutting out the Sun. How Japan Created Its Own Lost Generation*. New York: Vintage Books.

1 School nonattendance created the need for clinical psychologists

Introduction

When I read the special issue of *Japanese Psychological Research* on the "History of Psychology in Japan" (Satō et al. 2005), I was very surprised to find no mention of clinical psychology. I have been trained in French national universities (Bordeaux, Toulouse) where clinical psychology is a subdiscipline of psychology, inside psychology departments. I was expecting to find psychology departments (*shinrigakubu*) in Japanese national universities, but I had to come to a very simple and clear conclusion: psychology departments did not exist in the shape or form of which I was familiar.

In this chapter, I will explain some aspects of the history of Japanese psychology which remain widely unknown (note: for a full understanding of Japanese history of psychology before 1950, see McVeigh 2017). Then, I will underline that in Japan, psychology is never autonomous and often subordinated to educational science. Third, "Although the practice of clinical psychology seems to have a long history, clinical psychology is a new and confused academic area in Japan." (Satō 2007: 133). Fourth, it was the need to reduce school nonattendance (considered a problem to solve) that created the demand for clinical psychologists' services.

From scientific to clinical psychology

Birth of scientific psychology (1867–1927)

After a long period of closure, Japan's entry into modernity was marked by the Meiji era and a wide diffusion of Western knowledge. Between 1867 and 1888, the psychology that interested Japanese scholars and institutions was primarily a philosophy of education (Satō and Satō 2005: 53). It was a mental philosophy, as indicated by the title of one of the first foreign works translated – Joseph Haven's (1816–74) *Mental Philosophy Including Intellect Sensibilities and Will*, published in 1857. This book was translated in 1875 by Nishi Amane, a renowned intellectual of the time. He was one of the first to be sent abroad by the Edo Shogunate and was trained between 1862 and

1865 by Professor S. Vissering (1818–88) at the University of Leiden, the Netherlands. When he translated the work of Joseph Haven, Nishi Amane chose to simplify the title by keeping only two words, "Mental Philosophy," translated to *shinrigaku* 心理學 which stands as the current translation of "psychology" today.

In his 1874 *Hyakuichi shinron*, Nishi Amane had used *seirigaku* (性理学) to refer to psychology (Macé 2013: 186). In *Hyakuichi shinron, shinri* 心理 (mental) is distinguished from *butsuri* 物理 (physical) with "psychology" or *seirigaku* included in the category of *shinri* (grouping the intellectual sciences such as logic, politics, anthropology, etc.). When he translates the title of Joseph Haven's work as *shinrigaku* 心理學, he means a broader category than psychology – that is, mental philosophy – within which psychology (*seirigaku* 性理学) is included. However, the term *seirigaku* was quickly abandoned, and the exact reasons that led to the transition from *seirigaku* to *shinrigaku*, which corresponds to the current meaning of "psychology" 心理学 (*shinrigaku*), are not known. In 1875, the Ministry of Education sent some of its best students to the United States, to learn from the American system in order to build the Japanese system of Education. The first course of psychology was offered in 1873 at Tokyo University, and in 1877 was provided by the philosopher and sociologist Toyama Masakazu.

Motora Yūjirō can be considered the founder of psychology in Japan. In his career, a 5-year study trip to the United States played a crucial role. After arriving in Boston in 1883, he obtained a doctorate entitled "Exchange, Considered as the principle of social life" (Motora 1888) under the direction of Stanley Hall at Johns Hopkins, where he continued his training from 1885 to 1888. Upon his return to Japan, he first taught at Aoyama Gakuin University, then at the Imperial University of Tokyo between 1888 and 1890, where he was awarded the first chair of psychology (Satō and Satō 2005: 53–55). His interests were in psychophysics, philosophical theories of the mind, clinical psychology, and educational psychology. The text of his conference at the Fifth International Congress of Psychology in Rome in 1905 was published that same year in English: the conference was entitled "The Idea of the Ego in Oriental Philosophy," and the text, "An Essay on Eastern Philosophy." This was commented upon favorably in the journal *Revue de philosophie* by Ribot (1905: 642–645), and unfavorably in the *Revue neo-scolastique* by Théophile Gollier (1906: 346–348). Motora Yūjirō's lecture in Rome focused on his week-long experience in a Zen temple. He said that through the practices of Zen, one could reach a "pure" state of the ego, where no idea or sensory representation occurs. After being elected in 1902 as the first president of the Children's Studies Association, Motora conducted research with schoolchildren with learning difficulties and focused on the clinical and educational aspects of psychology (maintenance of concentration, attention, and learning to write). For him, children failing at school was not a situation of mental retardation, but one in which a method of concentration and a method for focusing their attention was lacking (Satō and Satō 2005: 56). He was the first

Japanese person to conduct research in the clinical psychology of children, published in 1911 in Germany a year before his death.

Motora's most notable student is Matsumoto Matatarō. After attending classes between 1890 and 1896, he moved to the United States to study experimental psychology with G. W. Scripture at Yale University. He became an assistant professor but was transferred by the Japanese government to Germany in 1897. He studied at Leipzig University with Wundt (but did not obtain a doctoral thesis) and visited some European laboratories. He returned to Japan and became professor of psychology at the Tōkyō Higher Normal School in 1900. Together, Motora Yūjirō and Matsumoto Matatarō opened the first laboratory of experimental psychology in 1903 at Tokyo Imperial University. A large wooden building, donated by the Department of Medical Pathology, was reformed into 12 rooms to allow for the conducting of experiments. In 1904, the first course in psychology began, which produced the first seven graduates the following year. Matsumoto Matatarō then went on to found the psychology department of Kyoto University, which he headed from 1906 to 1913, after which he left Kyōto to succeed Motora Yūjirō as the chair of psychology at Tokyo University. In 1927, the Japanese Psychological Association (JPA) was created with Matsumoto Matatarō as the first elected president.

If the beginnings of psychology can be embodied by Motora Yūjirō and Matsumoto Matatarō, another character is important to our understanding of psychology, Fukurai Tomokichi. The first student of Motora Yūjirō, Fukurai graduated in 1898 and quickly became interested in William James, translating several of his works. As a practitioner of hypnosis, he published Psychology of Hypnotism in 1906, and in 1908, he was appointed the Professor of Abnormal Psychology (*hentai shinrigaku* 変態心理学) at Tokyo University. *Hentai shinrigaku* is not the translation for psychopathology (*seishin byōrigaku*) and, therefore, describing him as the first Japanese to hold a psychopathology teaching position would not be accurate. The best translation for *hentai shinrigaku* is "abnormal psychology" because the discipline named at that time, *hentai shinrigaku,* developed from Abnormal Psychology, "Abnormal Psychology" being the title of a journal edited by Morton Prince (1854–1929). Japanese Abnormal Psychology includes the study of pathologies and spiritual phenomena, *hentai* being wider than *ijō* 異常 (*abnormal*). Fukurai Tomokichi was drawn to parapsychology and made experiments with two women, as early as 1910: one of them had, according to him, the ability to project the contents of her thoughts on a paper, or a photographic film (without using a camera). He named this phenomenon *nengraphy*. The problem is that the researchers, scholars, teachers, and intellectuals of the time who attended his experiments suspected a trick and their interest gradually declined. Even Motora Yūjirō urged him to stop his research in parapsychology. However, after the death of Motora Yūjirō in 1912, Fukurai (1913) persisted and published "Clairvoyance and Thought Writing," translated into English in 1931. Criticized by the lack of procedures for scientific verification,

Fukurai Tomokichi was marginalized in the intellectual community and forced to resign. After his departure, no one took over the chair of *hentai shinrigaku*, and Matsumoto Matatarō encouraged psychologists to return to the study of normal phenomena in order to regain credibility. The discipline named *hentai shinrigaku* was withdrawn from programs, and psychopathology, like clinical psychology, was "nipped in the bud" until the early 1950s. Here Fukurai's little history of developing parapsychology instead of clinical psychopathology meets wider historical processes: industrialization, militarism, and nationalism.

Psychology at University (1947–2000) and the invention of clinical psychology

The period following World War II was marked by scarcity and the American influence. Japanese intellectuals went to the United States with Fulbright scholarships in psychology, where they received training in the Jungian approach (Jung and Hisamatsu 1968), as well as client-centered therapy – Carl Rogers' "non-directivity." At the Institute for Education Leaders (IFEL), A.T. Jersild introduced Carl Rogers' texts, though his theories were already known in 1947 by Tomoda Fujio, who had learned from one of Carl Rogers' former students R.J. Fox, who had been head of the Student Advisory Service at Tokyo University of Letters and Science. In 1950, Fox obtained a position at the Christian University of Ibaraki and held the first workshop on non-directive therapy with Tomoda Fujio. At that time, it became the central place for training Japanese psychologists in Rogerian therapy. Carl Rogers, whose selected works were published in seven volumes in 1955 (Kitanaka 2003: 241), was invited to Japan in 1961 (Satō 2007: 139).

The period of reconstruction was followed by a baby boom, a standardization of education, and the creation of new schools and universities (Fumino 2005: 146). In this context, psychology had its first phase of expansion. Developmental psychology and educational psychology were made compulsory in the training of schoolteachers. Since the number of people who could provide this teaching was low, non-psychologists were enlisted to teach psychology as part of the curriculum in faculties of education (Fumino 2005: 148). After an initial period with educational psychology in the majority, the 1990s and 2000s saw its decline in favor of the emergence of clinical psychology. However, clinical psychology often still remained nestled in educational departments.

The rise of clinical psychology in Japan is inseparable from the formulation of "Japanese psychology," in both senses of the term: a Japanese mentality – or more exactly, discussions of "a Japanese heart," "the heart of the Japanese" (*Nihonjin no kokoro*), and various other *nihonjinron* (Befu 2001) – and a psychological discipline that is "authentically" Japanese. Clinical psychology has been able to develop in Japan only under the seal

Table 1.1 Three associations of psychology (JPA, JAEP, AJCP)

	Psychology (1927–)	*Educational psychology (1959–)*	*Clinical psychology (1982–)*
Japanese	日本心理学会 *Nihon shinri gakkai*	日本教育心理学会 *Nihon kyōiku shinri gakkai*	日本心理臨床学会 *Nihon shinri rinshō gakkai*
English	Japanese Psychological Association (JPA)	The Japanese Association of Educational Psychology (JAEP)	Association of Japanese Clinical Psychology (AJCP)
Members	7411 (2012)	6851 (2012)	25,545 (2013)
Journals	心理学研究 *Shinrigaku kenkyū* The International Journal of Psychology In Japanese (1926–) Japanese Psychological Research In English (1954–) 心理学ワールド *Shinrigaku wārudo* Psychology World In Japanese (1998–)	教育心理学研究 *Kyōiku shinrigaku kenkyū* The Japanese Journal of Educational Psychology In Japanese (1953–)	心理臨床学研究 *Shinri rinshō gaku kenkyū* Journal of Japanese Clinical Psychology In Japanese (1983–)
Certification	Psychologist (since 1990)	School Psychologist (since 1997)	Clinical Psychologist (since 1988)

of the Association of Japanese Clinical Psychology (AJCP). A Japanese Association of Clinical Psychology (*Nihon rinshō shinri gakkai*) had already been attempted in 1964 but failed five years later in 1969 in intractable debates over the establishment of a national certification system for psychologists (Kitanaka 2003: 241). The Japanese Association of Clinical Psychology (*Nihon rinshō shinri gakkai*) still exists and is much smaller than the Association of Japanese Clinical Psychology (*Nihon shinri rinshō gakkai*). Table 1.1 summarizes information on the three main psychological associations.

Before focusing on clinical psychology, let us mention as an example how the Japanese Psychological Association explains a certification system that was created in 1990 and its purpose: to increase the level of expertise and sense of identity of psychology specialists. Qualified individuals must (1) possess a bachelor's degree or above; (2) have lived in Japan for 2 or more years since they were 16 years old; and (3) earned academic credits designated by the JPA certification committee (JPA website consulted March 5, 2020). Other associations have developed selection criteria similar to these.

If we focus on psychology, and especially clinical psychology at the university level, by taking the example of Kyōto, Tōkyō, and Osaka universities, one notices that clinical psychology is systematically linked to education.

For example, at Kyoto University, clinical psychology is officially present in the faculty of education, which is composed of three divisions, including one of educational psychology: clinical psychology is alongside psychotherapy within the division of educational psychology, while "experimental" psychology is at the faculty of Letters. At Tokyo University, clinical psychology is also present in the faculty of Education, but it has a division of its own, among 10 others, including educational psychology. At Osaka University, we must look in the Graduate School of Human Sciences composed of nine "majors," among which are "psychology" and "clinical studies in education." In the psychology major, one finds fundamental psychology, social, applied, applied cognitive, environmental, and gerontology. It is in "clinical studies in education" that we find clinical psychology, alongside educational psychology, anthropology of education, and so on. Unlike most English-speaking and European countries, we do not find the common situation where clinical psychology exists as an autonomous field within psychology departments that are themselves independent of other disciplines. With this overview of psychological associations and the place of clinical psychology in Japanese national universities having been given, it is time to discuss the certification scheme for clinical psychologists.

Clinical psychologists and school counseling

As of 2017, Japanese universities issue only a master's degree; a national license for psychologists does not exist. The issuance of a Clinical Psychologist Certification is the mission of a private foundation: the Foundation of the Japanese Certification Board of Clinical Psychologists (FJCBCP). After obtaining a master's degree, the young graduate applies to the foundation and, if accepted, becomes a certified clinical psychologist (*rinshō shinri shi*). The certification is valid for a period of 5 years: a credit system allows the renewal of certification. Since the end of the 1980s to 2017, the increase in the influence of this foundation has been spectacular: the number of certified clinical psychologists was 1595 in 1988 and has increased continuously until the year 2000 (7912), reaching 13,253 certified psychologists in 2005. Between 2005 and 2012, the number of certified clinical psychologists almost doubled: in 2012 there were 26,329. The development of this foundation is parallel to that of the Association of Japanese Clinical Psychology (AJCP). It is not insignificant to note that the FJCBCP and the AJCP have been chaired several times by a small number of individuals, such as Kawai Hayao whom I will discuss soon. In 2013, the number of AJCP members (25,545) was close to that of clinical psychologists certified by the FJCBCP (26,329).

The Foundation of the Japanese Certification Board of Clinical Psychologists (FJCBCP) was established in 1988, when the Ministry of Education sent the first certified psychologists to junior high schools to respond to the growing problems of bullying, and school refusal. However, the Ministry of Education only began to recognize the profession of school counselor (*sukūru kaunserā*) later, during the education reform of 1995. Clinical psychology's official recognition is confirmed in 2004, when each junior high school is required to provide the services of a school counselor (Ingrams 2005). In the meantime, a multitude of certifications have emerged, and each association has developed its own certification. In 1990, the JPA started to certify "psychologists"; in 1995, the Japanese Association of School Counseling (JASC) started to certify "school counselors"; and in 1997, the Japanese Association of Educational Psychology certified "school psychologists." The list drawn up here is far from exhaustive, since there are more than 40 certifications in the field of counseling and psychology (Grabosky, Ishii, and Mase 2012: 223). These multiple certifications can actually confuse people seeking psychological care. On the other hand, among the clinical psychologists that I have met, all testify to a normative prescription: it is more or less mandatory to join the Association of Japanese Clinical Psychology (AJCP). They are implicitly required to do so. In a sense, on the question of the certification of clinical psychologists, the AJCP is presented as having won a competition in terms of popularity and number of members. This fight was won against other psychologists (those of the JPA and JAEP), and JASC certified school counselors, through the employment of clinical psychologists as school counselors. As of 2017, clinical psychologists are generally seen as best placed to fill this position. For instance, H prefecture, as we will see in the next chapter, requires that school counselor positions' applicants be certified clinical psychologists.

In 1995, school counselors were present in 154 schools (elementary, middle, and high schools) that participated in the Ministry of Education project, each accepting a school counselor: 134 were certified clinical psychologists and 20 were psychiatrists or university professors practicing in the field of education (Yagi 2008: 144). In 2006, school counselors were present in 10,158 schools, including 7692 colleges (three colleges out of four); 1697 colleges associated with a primary school; and 769 high schools. These services were employed for a total annual budget of 4217,000,000 yen. In view of the above, the growth of the profession of clinical psychologist, and that of clinical psychology as a discipline, can, therefore, be considered intrinsically linked to the establishment of the school counselor system, which has diffused considerably between 1995 and 2017. In order to enhance the coherence of my study, I will not mention the case of psychologists working in hospitals, who are potentially responsible for psychotherapeutic services. However, it seems necessary to say a word on the subject of psychotherapy, insofar as the question arises as to whether it constitutes a central part of school counselor services.

Japanese psychiatrists do not practice psychotherapy very much (Lock 1982, Kitanaka 2012); it has devolved to psychologists (Kitanaka 2003). Even still, psychotherapy is relatively uncommon, compared to Western countries where psychologists practice it a lot, and where it seems to constitute the most common identity of psychiatrists (Van Effenterre et al. 2012). In Japan, the practice of psychotherapy does not constitute the identity of psychiatrists, although it is part of their training (Fukushima and Hirayasu 2012). In terms of private practice, the Japanese counselor (*kaunserā*) may be considered the equivalent of the French "therapist," in the sense that the titles of "counselor" and "therapist" are not the subject of a restrictive national certification. In other words, there is great freedom in the use of the terms "counselor" in Japan, and "therapist" in France. As part of their private activity, Japanese counselors – in addition to the handling of face-to-face and group techniques – can also practice counseling online, by phone, or in cafés and restaurants, for a session cost that ranges from 10,000 to 20,000 yen (Grabosky, Ishii, and Mase 2012).

Now let us introduce a charismatic character, Kawai Hayao, and his theory. Kawai Hayao has played a leading role in the history of Japanese clinical psychology. His ideas have been widely disseminated in Japan, while remaining almost unknown to the broader international audience.

Japanese psychology according to Kawai Hayao

Kawai Hayao is revered by some and ignored by others. He was a professor at Kyoto University and a clinical psychologist who played a crucial role in the development of clinical psychology from the 1960s until the mid-2000s. Kawai Hayao's psychotherapeutic practice integrated Japanese Buddhism and Jungian psychology. As a scholar contributing to the history of psychological clinics in Japan, I felt I would be remiss not to mention Kawai and his influence. Here, I study a single book entitled *Yungu shinrigaku to bukkyō*, translated as "Jungian Psychology and Buddhism."

Kawai Hayao's Training

In the first part of his book, Kawai Hayao questions himself: "Jung? Buddhism? (*Yungu ka bukkyō ka*)." The questioning of his own identity is part of his research and is repeated in his writings. Kawai Hayao offers a number of explicit details about his personal life. He positions himself in the following terms: "as I am Easterner" (*watashi wa Tōyōjin desu ga*), and later, he writes "the state of my consciousness (*watashi no ishiki no arikata*), and my relationship to the unconscious differs from Europeans." The recognition of a Western consciousness – *seiyō no ishiki* (Kawai 1995: 39–40) – represents for him a cultural shock (*karuchā shokku*). Although he says he initially rejected Buddhism since the death of his younger brother when he was 4 years old, his stay in America allowed him to reconnect with his interest in Buddhism. He recalls several times during the period of World War II and his difference with peers, who blindly enrolled in the imperial army. He did not want to kill anyone: he was afraid of death and was convinced that Japan was going to lose. After several attacks by the US military, a soldier from the Japanese army came to explain to the group of students where he was, that in view of their long history, if the invaders could obtain some victories at first, the Americans would perish at the end. The American army trying to invade Japan was, according to the logic of this soldier, to lose the war. The young Kawai Hayao, who agreed with the first part of the argument, suddenly realized that it was Japan who had invaded first and concluded that his country was going to lose. Overwhelmed by this idea, he tried to drive it out of his mind until it became unbearable and he talked to his elder brother. The latter forbade him to tell anyone, not even his parents. After the defeat, he became aware of the irrationality of what he had been taught, and he was "ready to accept Western rationalism completely" (Kawai 1995: 31–32). If some turned to materialism and became communists, he turned to clinical psychology – little known at the time – and began lecturing at Kyoto University before he went to study in the United States (UCLA) in 1959. Trained in the Rorschach test with Dr. Bruno Klopfer, he met Jungian psychology, and after a year and a half of studies left the United States to study at the C. G. Jung Institute in Zurich. Studying Jungian dream analysis allowed him to reconnect with his own culture, through immersion in Japanese literature, tales, myths and legends, which he had rejected up until that point (Kawai 1995: 37).

During his training abroad, he underwent two periods of Jungian analysis: the first with a man (Dr. Spiegelman, Los Angeles), and the second with a woman (Ms. Lilian Frey, Zurich). As he was raised in a culture where the woman was subordinate to the man, he felt uncomfortable with "receiving the analysis of a woman" (*josei ni bunseki wo ukeru*): "I felt resistance to acknowledging a woman as superior to me, a man," he writes (Kawai 1995: 38). It was then that Ms. Lilian Frey appeared to him in a dream in the guise of the sun goddess Amaterasu. Because of this vision he changed his attitude toward her, as with other women in general. Here is a fragment he reports: "You were the Sun Goddess, weren't you?" "I am neither a goddess nor the sun. I am a human being. That Sun Goddess exists inside you" (Kawai 1995: 38). Kawai Hayao said he had difficulty accepting this, as he had negative feelings about Japanese mythology. Yet, his certification thesis at the C. G. Jung Institute in Zurich was about the myth of Amaterasu. Note also that in the Japanese text, he addresses his analyst by designating her by the term *sensei* (master, teacher), when he speaks to her. However, Ms. Lilian Frey did not speak Japanese. How did he address her in reality? Professor? Ms.? Doctor? In any case, the way in which he relates it reveals that he considered her to be a master, and that it was difficult for him to have a woman occupy such a position. Consequently, he deified her, denying her status as a woman, concrete, non-ideal. The story of Kawai Hayao makes it possible to highlight a point of resistance in his analytical process, which can be turned into a more general question: is it possible to envisage a therapeutic relationship in Japan, apart from a master–student relationship? Superior–inferior? Man–woman? This question is of primary importance in these three types of interpersonal relationships. "Master–student," because knowledge is engaged in a particular way in the analytic cure, what Jacques Lacan designated by the notion of the "subject supposed to know" (*sujet supposé savoir* in French). "Superior–inferior" because the hierarchical relationship compels us to think of a therapeutic relationship in terms of power relations and directive methods. And, "Man–woman" because gender inequalities are, even today, extremely strong in Japan as the Gender Equality Bureau yearly reports (GEB 2020).

To return to the Jungian analysis of Kawai Hayao, let us mention the fact that it lasted a few months, with two different analysts. His testimony is particularly rich, but it is impossible not to emphasize that his analytical training was interrupted at the beginning, especially on questions concerning money, knowledge, and the feminine. This was not without consequences in his clinical practice and future theorization, as we will see later. Here, I will focus on money, referred to as a fragment of the analysis of a dream. The analysis of dreams was first considered by him to be irrational. After having overcome this resistance, he tells a dream in which he sees a Hungarian coin playing the image of Taoist sage. The interpretation of the dream is as follows: Hungary is a bridge between East and West. This example, like the dream of the "analyst as Amaterasu," could surprise non-Jungian analysts, that is to say the vast majority of psychoanalysts. Indeed, whatever the theoretical orientation, one has difficulty considering these two examples as authentic dream analysis: it is rather a comment on dreams, made at the beginning of analysis and stopped prematurely.

An additional observation relates to this first anecdote. Kawai Hayao is recognized as one of the greatest exponents of Japanese identity discourse, *nihonjinron*, including the argument that the Western Self and the Japanese Self are intrinsically different. Kawai says that the Western Self is independent, relying on a cutting function to separate everything. In contrast, the Japanese ego holds its strength by containing without cutting. This opposition is based on his analytical experience, and on an exchange with his analyst regarding the reduction of the payment of the session. This account suggests his theory is based on his personal experience and, more specifically, refers to an event experienced in his analysis with Dr. Spiegelman. At the time, he had little money and wanted to reserve a share for his own entertainment. Embarrassed, he finally told this to his analyst, who agrees, after reflection, to reduce the cost of the session, saying to his patient: "I do not mind at all. Why do you mind?" But this only accentuated the patient's concern: "I felt that something important had been lost," he says (Kawai 1995: 41). He then decides to think about the proposal of his analyst, and to answer him the following week, in terms that caught my attention. He accepts the reduction of the session's fee, but he does not accept an idea of his analyst: the idea that the fact that "it is not a problem for the analyst" (I do not mind), should necessarily imply that the analysand does not have to worry, or does not worry (You do not mind). Seen through the lens of Lacanian theory, Dr. Spiegelman responded in the worst way possible, and it planted the seed of a problem that grew into his theories on cultural difference and personhood. Through such experiences he began to separate American logic from the Japanese attitude that supposes that one party makes no proposal without considering the implications for the other (Kawai 1995: 41).

I would now like to provide an interpretation of why these episodes played a crucial role in the life of Kawai Hayao. They also played a crucial role in the sociocultural and psychological life of Japan because Kawai Hayao was brought to influence the highest functions of the State as head of cultural affairs; he was also appointed to the highest positions in the university hierarchy, being a full professor at Kyoto University. My interpretation is, therefore, fraught with consequences and raises the following question: considering the positions of power occupied by Kawai Hayao, could it be that these two logical moments of his analytical course had a decisive role on the development of clinical psychology in Japan? And, therefore, the whole field of Japanese school counseling?

Kawai's male patients and the "constellation of negative Mother"

When he returned from Switzerland in 1965, Kawai Hayao wanted to start practicing psychotherapy, but as he wrote, "pay to talk" was unthinkable at that time. Clinical psychology was still seen as unscientific and he had to wait 10 years to present his work on tales, and 15 years on myths. His first patient was a 13-year-old boy in school – absenteeism. This teenager told him a dream: "I was walking in a field with a clover as big as me. Then there was a big swirl of flesh, I was caught inside, it was terrifying, and I woke up" (Kawai 1995: 45). For Kawai Hayao, this vortex that devours and regenerates symbolizes the archetype of the Mother. Without giving further details, he says that we find these spirals on the figures of the goddess of Mother Earth of ancient Japan. In his reasoning, the dream indicates the impotence of this boy in the face of the Mother's absorption force (Kawai 1995: 46).

The most amazing thing is in the paragraph that follows immediately. Kawai Hayao talks about returning to Japan after studying abroad. As usual, the extended family and friends had organized a small party and brought a sea bream. But an incident interrupted the celebrations. His mother caught a fish bone in her throat, and when she left the party to go to the hospital, he closed the taxi door on her arm. While denying an unconscious hostility toward his own mother, he associates this element of his personal history with the dream of his young patient, proposing the following idea: "When I heard the dream of this boy, I intuitively recognized that there was a constellation of Negative Mother all over Japan. All Japanese, myself included, are under the influence of this Mother. I think one of its manifestations is the spread of the phenomenon of school absenteeism." (Kawai 1995: 46–47) From a psychoanalytic point of view, this is an amazing conclusion. It can be hypothesized that he denies his own aggression toward his mother: he is angry with her for having caught a bone in her throat, and thus spoiling the party. Instead of recognizing his own feelings of hatred toward his mother, he assigns them to all Japanese mothers. What is more, from a single clinical experience: his first patient! In reality, the analysis of this boy's dream, like that of the event involving the therapist and his own mother, has barely begun. Obviously, their commented associations serve the argument of the author who then commits to the subject of absenteeism. It should be noted that he identifies a phenomenon of school absenteeism in the late 1960s and associates it with the "constellation of the negative mother." According to him, the "strength of the Mother archetype" (Kawai 1995: 47) is illustrated, for example, by the fact that the client becomes dependent on the therapist and projects the archetypal image of the Mother on the therapist.

Kawai Hayao often anticipates what his patients want to know. At the very beginning of the first part, he takes the example of a patient's question: "Why did my mother die when I was 3 years old?" Kawai Hayao says that the natural sciences response (e.g., she had tuberculosis but there was no treatment at the time), if rational, does not satisfy the patient: What this person wants to know is "why did my mother die when I was 3, leaving me alone?" His position is clear: he knows what his patients want to know. This is a decisive clue that allows one to place his practice outside the field of psychoanalysis. He is in the field of psychotherapy, and Jungian psychology. Moreover, if he knows what his patient wants to know, how can we not conclude that he knows what the Other (Lacanian *grand Autre*) wants? In any case, we can say that he knows what some of the little others (Lacanian *petits-autres*) who come to consult him want to know, and he knows that all the Japanese are influenced by the archetype of the Mother, without yet having met them one by one. This, too, supposes a cumbersome question: are the Japanese who are not under the influence of the archetype of the mother, Japanese? We see here that Kawai Hayao's theory is exclusive and prescriptive, such as in *nihonjinron*, Japanese identity discourses (Befu 2001). Kawai Hayao's theory aims to define and impose "what should be" Japanese identity, probably in disregard of the identity of Japanese people themselves.

Kawai's female patients and psychotherapeutic techniques

Another clinical example from his practice deserves our interest. It is titled, "I do not want to heal". Before mentioning the case of one of his patients, we must first point out that Kawai has introduced a new therapeutic process in Japan, adapting sandplay therapy (invented by Dora M. Kalff) in *hako niwa ryōhō*.

Sandplay therapy is a therapy (*ryōhō*) inspired by Jungianism where sand is mobilized in a defined space (a box: *hako*). The originality of its Japanization is the addition of the word "garden" (*niwa*) and, therefore, the relationship with the Japanese dry garden. This technique is used for both children and adults, for instance in the following example. When he was in trouble with a middle-aged woman whose symptoms did not give way, he had the idea to propose this therapeutic process. She is, therefore, actively arranging her sand garden for a whole session. He thinks, "It's good, now I can heal her." But when at the next meeting he invites her to continue her garden, she refuses. "Why?" he asks, surprised. "I do not want to be healed ... I do not come to be healed. – Then, why are you here?", he retorts. She replies: "I'm coming here just to come here." (*Koko ni kiteiru nowa, koko ni kuru tame ni kite iru dake desu*). Kawai (1995: 53) writes that, since then, he has understood that he cannot heal people, and while he has continued to receive her without wanting to heal her, her symptoms have disappeared.

We could rejoice at such a therapeutic success, but a problem persists: it is a clinical vignette, not a clinical case study. We know too little, we do not know her symptoms, and one question remains: did Kawai Hayao seize or miss the Freudian moment? Indeed, we see here the inaugural scene of psychoanalysis repeating, about a century after, that of the moment of refusal by a supposedly hysterical patient of the hypnosis of the master, the passage from suggestion and directivity to transference and free association. If this type of exchange were frequent, one could argue that it is not the Japanese who would be subjects foreign to transference, but rather the practitioners in charge with listening to them who, for personal and sociocultural reasons, would find it difficult to "step aside" (*pas de côté* in French), which is necessary to get involved in Freudian discovery. Taken from hierarchical relations that support them and from which they cannot be divested, openness to the Freudian moment and inclusion in the psychoanalytic discourse are a challenge that many current clinicians dodge. In Kawai Hayao's case, he approaches psychotherapy in a way in which he tries to make us believe that we should not distinguish the "healer" and "the one who is cured": when two people are there together, a "healing" happens as a side effect. Let it not be misunderstood: there is nothing Winnicottian when he claims to have been "trained" by his patients (Kawai 1995: 62). Above all, it is not enough to let someone talk in a non-directive way for lasting therapeutic effects to appear. Nor should one see in his practice a subversion of the therapist–patient hierarchy. Kawai Hayao was a master, and a hierarchy within the therapeutic relationship was present, especially as he integrates Buddhist philosophy with his practice, as we will see soon.

A final example from his practice illustrates how certain elements borrowed from Buddhist wisdom can be converted into interpretations. He receives a patient of old age who comes to complain about her daughter-in-law who, selected with care to marry her son, is proving to fail to serve her. Madam asks: what should I do? As Kawai listens, he remembers an old Buddhist story: *Ushini hikarete, Zenkōji mairi*. An old woman, greedy and a nonbeliever, is drying a fabric. The cow of the neighbor steals this cloth and the old lady runs after him, to find herself, without noticing it in the Zenkōji temple, where she prays for her afterlife, while her faith awakens.

After making sure that her client knew the story, he told her, "Your daughter-in-law is the Zenkōji's cow." Perplexed, the old woman was told: "By getting angry at your daughter-in-law, running after her, you end up coming to Zenkōji." (Kawai 1995: 78). This interpretation had no visible effect for several sessions, and she continued to complain about her daughter-in-law. She asked again if there was a good method but was opposed by a negative response from the therapist. She continued to come and was guided by her dreams, while deepening her interest in religion, preparing for great age and death. And Kawai Hayao concludes that while she came to complain about her daughter-in-law, she started looking for the Self, thanks to the story of Zenkōji he had used. This lady has returned several times, over a long period, and testifies of a progressive enlightenment. Once again, we must note the possible therapeutic effects, but the description of the psychologist does not allow us to know what triggered them: is it a step away from the patient caused by the therapist's "no"? Or a suggestion of the master who invites a religious conversion, a return to faith? In this regard, what would we say about a Western therapist giving biblical interpretations to his patient, citing a local version of anecdote X inspired by Gospel Y?

A vague relationship to Jungianism and Buddhism

Kawai Hayao thus has an open, "vague" relationship to Jungianism and Buddhism ("*Aimai na bukkyōto de aru.*" Kawai 1995: 62). He considers the advantage of Jungianism to be its flexibility, and Buddhism to be frankly open: "There is neither first nor last; neither beginning nor end. Buddhism shows the world as it is, invariable. No real change occurs." The type of psychotherapy he has led for 30 years is close to the *juji bon*, a sutra that illustrates the 10 steps to becoming a bodhisattva (Kawai 1995: 96–99). In his reflections, he alternates between Jungianism and Buddhism. He insists that Buddhism can heal the sufferings of the modern self (Kawai 1995: 57), but he also feels that Jungianism can also heal (Kawai 1995: 58). He says he has no problem in calling himself Jungian and Buddhist, but he is not a member of any Buddhist school because that would require him to choose, follow a doctrine, and practice rituals (Kawai 1995: 61). He suggests that the Jungians are Buddhists without a school, without ritual, and without doctrine, but who share the essence of Buddhism. Indeed, he argues these two approaches' essence is neither in their schools, nor rituals, nor in their doctrines ... but in the concept of heart/mind (*kokoro*).

Translating the title for Chapter Three of Kawai's work poses difficulties because of the use of the term *watashi*. The most accurate translation of this Japanese word is "what I am." Nevertheless, if we consider the use made by the author, it is possible to translate it as "I," which is also its usual translation when associated with *wa* or *ga*, for example. Chapter Three is, therefore, entitled "'*Watashi' towa nani ka,*" 'What is the 'I'?" It is translated into English in the original text as "What is 'I'?" This question is crucial for the author, unlike "Who am I?" (*Watashi wa dare ka*) whose answer would be, according to him, simpler. As he notes: "When you start thinking about 'I', the more you think about it, the more incomprehensible it becomes" ("*Shikashi, honto no tokoro wa, 'watashi' to iu no wa kangaereba kangaeru-hodo wakaranai sonzai desu.*" Kawai 1995: 121).

Kawai Hayao is interested in C. G. Jung and his developments in psycho-therapy. This goes through an affirmation: "I am Kannon." Kawai (1995: 119) testifies to the influence of *Jōdo shinshū* Buddhism in his practice when he takes up a story of Shinran Shōnin, the founder of this school, where Kannon appears to him in a dream. Kawai's (1995: 176) interpretation of Shinran Shōnin's dream leads him to claim that patients project Bodhisattva Kannon onto the therapist, who, consciously or not, tries to play this role. Also, he suggests there is equivalence between symptoms and *kōan,* para-doxical puzzles, and anecdotes used in the Rinzai school of Zen to evoke the limits of certain kinds of reasoning: "Concerning Zen, I have no experience of *sanzen* (interviews with a Zen master), and I have not read many books on the subject. But I had many opportunities to listen to acquaintances who had this experience. These were direct words, I had the answers to my questions without embarrassment, and I think I learned a lot. Listening to these stories, I felt that my work as a psychotherapist is, in a way, simi-lar to Zen." Let us remember that, while Buddhists in the Zen School can relate to those of *Jōdo Shinshū,* they are two distinct schools (the Zen School itself is divided into several schools). Both schools have been separated for centuries, and their practices, rituals, and doctrines differ. However, their common Buddhist background allows Kawai to invoke disparate elements such as the Kannon therapist (from the founder of the *Jōdo shinshū* school, Shinran Shōnin), and interpretation in the form of *kōan* (from the Zen school) for the purpose of socially withdrawn youths' treatment: "Instead of preaching to these apathetic young people the meaning of work and the value of social activity, we strive to find the *kōan* together." (Kawai 1995: 197–198). From this point of view, his approach is undoubtedly beneficial for patients who suffer from being labeled lazy and idle and summoned to work and contribute to society. This practice elaborated with reference to a Buddho–Jungian background has had, without a doubt, effects on the indi-viduals who met this therapist. Nevertheless, this is a practice manipulat-ing suggestion and calling on religious elements within it, via the protocol (e.g., the therapy envisaged from the *juji-bon* sutra); psychotherapy (similar to Zen); and interpretations (e.g., "your daughter-in-law is Zenkōji's cow").

When considering Kawai Hayao's contributions, we will see later that he helped to establish clinical psychology in Japan. In particular, despite all of the criticism that could be addressed toward him, one must acknowledge his contribution to the establishment of a vast system of school counselors: school counselors were only present in 154 establishments in 1995, whereas by 2006, there were 10,058. Kawai Hayao played a key role in starting meas-ures for students with special needs and their families, making the presence of a school counselor mandatory in each junior high school from 2004 onward (Ingrams 2005). In 2002, Prime Minister Koizumi Junichiro designated Kawai Hayao as head of cultural affairs, a rare position for a psychologist to attain. A charismatic figure, as much hated as he was adored, mentioning his work was inescapable in some circles and taboo in others. He supported the cultural reconstruction of Iraq desired by George W. Bush but also resonated with more liberal figures. He was considered the one and only confidant of the writer Murakami Haruki. The best selling author paid tribute to him in 2008: "When I talked using the word 'stories,' it was only Kawai-sensei who could correctly understand that meaning [...] Stories are very beneficial but very dangerous at the same time. Kawai-sensei really understood this. He was not a mere researcher. He had the excellence of a man who crosses a battlefield because he actually examined patients" (Koyama 2008). My research could not avoid the importance of this character who has marked the history of Japanese clinical psychology. It remains to be seen in more detail the exact role played by Kawai Hayao in setting up the clinical psychologists' certification system, and their hiring through the school counselor system. How was the decision to create the school counseling system made, while Kawai Hayao was in the Ministry of Education "in charge of cultural affairs"? If the latter has played a role, it remains to describe all the dynamics of the actors who allowed the spread of the school counselor system, at the national level and in each prefecture. It remains to be seen, by an in-depth study, who were the actors who led to the birth of Japanese clinical psychology by attributing to Kawai Hayao his rightful place, without idealizing him and without silencing his name, as is often the case.

Before providing the details of my interviews with clinical practitioners in the next chapter, it is necessary to describe what a Japanese junior high school is, and how teachers work there. In conducting my research, I would try to find out if the school counselor was performing duties that were formerly assigned to teachers, and whether he or she was assuming new functions specific to his specialization in clinical psychology. I would also examine the emergence of school absenteeism as a matter of concern, as students in this situation are the ones that the school counselor had to deal with.

Educational and psychological guidance

The bond with school and teachers

In Japan, the municipalities have a local education committee (*kyōiku iinkai*) and an administrative apparatus headed by a director of education (*kyōikuchō*). The *kyōikuchō* supervises local or prefectural administrative services of education. This administrator appointed by the *kyōiku iinkai* is under the control of the elected officials of the local or prefectural assembly.

The school head (*kōchō*) exercises his authority by delegation of the *kyōiku iinkai*. The prefecture issues guidelines and recommendations that influence local choices. The statutory working week of teachers is 40 hours at the national level but, in reality, teachers work between 52 hours and 60 hours per week: 20 hours are devoted to teaching, and more than half their time is devoted to meetings and various commissions (Satō 2007: 22, Lévi-Alvarès 2007: 157). Teachers have a bachelor's degree (4 years in Japan) and are recruited by exams set up in each prefecture: they hold their position only in this prefecture, which is a significant difference compared to many countries. They are transferred, within the same prefecture, every 6–7 years, and every 3–4 years for their colleagues who have become heads of institutions. This development dates from the early 2000s, because previously, teachers remained in the same district all their lives.

The mission of the middle schools as defined by Japanese legal texts is teaching, the formation of the person, the learning of collective life, and the acquisition of moral sensibility (Lévi-Alvarès 2007: 168). This mission is conducted through various activities: moral education (*dōtoku katsudō*), special activities (*tokubetsu katsudō*), group-management class (*gakkyū katsudō*), activities of the student association (*seitokai katsudō*), club activities (*kurabu katsudō*), and organization of the different collective manifestations of the school (*gakkō gyōji*). Globally, one often hears that the teaching profession does not correspond to the expectations of young recruits. However, one of the significant differences with many Western countries is that speaking at meetings is discouraged for newcomers, as it does not correspond to the expectations of the teaching profession. Implicitly, young recruits are expected to start speaking when they have more experience and knowledge of the institution. It can last several years, but at the age of 35, it seems that one can begin to make one's voice heard (Lévi-Alvarès 2007: 175). One of the reasons given to explain this is a principle of seniority – the older one is, the higher the status – where peer recognition depends on active and prolonged immersion in the school environment. For example, school management (*gakkō keiei*) books clearly define the teacher's career: at age 20, he works exclusively with students as a teacher and facilitator; at age 30, he thinks of the insertion of his activity in the educational project of the establishment; at age 40, he assumes administrative responsibilities; and at age 50, he can choose a career as principal or deputy (Lévi-Alvarès 2007: 175). Hierarchy is everywhere. In the school field, it is between the different staff members, between the teacher and the pupil, between the pupils, and between the schools. There is always an inferior and a superior: there is always an older colleague, or a friend of a higher class (*senpai/kōhai*), and establishments are classified according to an index, the *hensachi*. Hierarchy is a benchmark that allows individuals to situate themselves, to orient and limit their possibilities, and to focus their choices.

Another powerful, central idea I regularly encounter is that school is an institution that manages almost the entire life of young people, from primary school to their professional life – whether it is post-high-school or post-university. Teachers are charged with missions that their counterparts in many other countries never practice. The most striking examples are the organization of club activities or sports events during summer holidays, home visits, and patrols during school holidays. The responsibility of the teacher extends far beyond the school's spatial boundaries: teachers patrol at regular intervals during the summer holidays to observe "hot spots"; they identify bicycles in front of a karaoke, where alcohol can potentially be drunk (Letendre 1995: 178). These "holidays" are, therefore, not a period of rest detached from school obligations; only the nature of their work changes. When Shimizu Hirokichi observed how classes at a junior high school in Ōsaka operated in the late 1980s and early 1990s, he was confronted with teachers who made more than a hundred home visits a year. The teachers' strategy for students who had difficulties was as follows: "The further away a student is from the required level, the more problems there are, the more relentlessly he or she will be guided" (Shimizu 2007: 126). Depending on one's point of view, the school can be considered good or bullying, monitoring, or harassing. For example, the theme of home visits in the 1990s was the subject of debate: violation of privacy for some, a way to better understand children for others, and even a way of keeping Japanese culture alive (Tsuneyoshi 2007: 146–148).

The work of Gerald K. Letendre is interesting here to help us better understand the school of the early 1990s and to identify current changes, especially on the subject of school absenteeism. He recounts a case of school absenteeism reported by a teacher at a meeting in the establishment where he practiced in 1992 (Letendre 1995: 171–172). When visiting the student's home, she was able to talk to the mother and the child on the doorstep. The latter, at the mention of the school, systematically avoids discussion. We learn that the father died of cancer, and the mother thinks that he is afraid of dying himself: go see a counselor? She does not know any, so the teacher gives her an address. After 40 minutes on the front porch with the dog, the conversation changes to a book of animals that the mother has offered to her son, but he is interested, she says, only in dogs. She wonders about using the dog to try to install routines in her son's life, such as getting him out, etc. The teacher approves because it would give him a sense of compassion (*aijō*). Although there was a school counselor at this school, it was the teacher who continued to make visits to the home of this child, bringing books dedicated to dogs. In addition, she tried to introduce him to other children in the neighborhood who would have the same interest in dogs, and asked class members to make visits to their comrade's home.

The discipline in Japanese schools is another dimension that I must mention. There are strict regulations defining routines and good habits: storage, cleaning, care of uniforms, marking of names (shoes), physical appearance (hair), and accessories (bracelets, necklaces, piercings). The nurse records the students' complaints and then forwards them to the teacher and guidance service. In Gerald K. Letendre's survey, teachers regularly examine hair, nails (the fact that they are gnawed or discolored is considered a sign of mental or emotional problems), and coordinate nutritional programs for parents. The students have a meeting with the teachers, morning and evening. Cleaning and inspection of uniforms is done once a month. These routines focus on detecting and preventing student problems. Among the important issues in these activities for teachers in the early 1990s were the following: Were jacket buttons open? Had the student cleaned vigorously? In addition, sleepovers on a weekday were frowned upon. Similar concern was directed toward other behaviors such as girls wearing bracelets. For minor incidents, the student received harsh admonitions from the head teacher, and the head of the guidance service. For example, after the end of classes, a person who had disturbed the class must kneel before the teacher, while he lectures him about his behavior (this situation is unimaginable in schools today, as will be seen in the next chapter). Also, attempts were made to facilitate parent–teacher–student communication with the holding of a notebook (*seikatsu dayori/nōto*), where the student notes his daily activities (study time and time watching television). The teacher would regularly consult the student's notebook (Letendre 1995: 176–178).

While a number of these elements are no longer current, this description of Japanese schools in the early 1990s suggests the strict nature of the school, and unmanageable expectations imposed on teachers, students, and parents. Searching for runaways, being on patrols, and home visits took considerable time. Teachers were not trained in the treatment of absenteeism, school violence, or the various psychopathologies that were just beginning to be recognized, such as anorexia, bulimia, Obsessive-Compulsive Disorder (OCD), developmental disorders, and autism. How was the school of the 1990s different from today's school? What changes have occurred since the 1990s? More specifically, how are students treated when their difficulties are psychological? These are questions I will address in the next paragraphs.

School bashing

A first element to answering these questions is the school counselor system that was gradually introduced starting in 1995. Three factors contributed to the introduction of this system, identifiable as early as the 1980s: first, the increase in violence and truancy; next, the advent of neoliberal projects in the field of education; and finally, the gradual recognition of clinical psychologists as agents of "students' health of the heart (*kokoro*)." The scientific literature on educational issues seems to demonstrate the following fact: difficulties that emerged in school before 1980 could be solved and/ or were not well publicized. But from 1980 on, insoluble problems with young people and their families began to attract more and more attention. It was at this point that Japan's policies were progressively included in a neoliberal project.

Three events illustrate my point. First, in 1984, The ad hoc Commission on Education (*Rinkyōshin*), decreed by Prime Minister Nakasone Yasuhiro, allows a deregulation in the field of education with the slogan "the end of modernity": privatization, liberalization, individualization, and degreasing (*surimuka*) of the public sector (Satō 2007: 31). Second, in 1995, an employers' organization that affects education issues, *keizai dōyūkai*, produces a report entitled "Twenty-First Century School Design," in which it advocates for public education limited to three areas: language competence (Japanese language), logical reasoning (mathematics), and Japanese identity (moral and national history). All other disciplines (sport, music, fife sciences, arts, economy, the humanities, social sciences) would then be delegated to cram schools (*juku*). Third, in 2000, the private consultative commission "Japan for the 21st century" considers "the 3 days' week." In this context, it would be the myriad of *juku* available in the archipelago that would take over in the context of activities chosen by the parents and the child (Satō 2007: 36–37).

In this context, a discourse denigrating public schools and their teachers had developed, namely, school bashing (*sukūru bashingu*). This negative discourse on public education grew stronger and corresponded with the increasing implementation of neoliberal policies. Moreover, rhetoric around violence and school absenteeism started to develop. To treat what has since appeared as real difficulties, two options have been favored. On the one hand, a private support network outside compulsory school has spread. This shadow education consists of private tutoring companies, the *juku*, which can be of different types: some upgrade the "dropouts" and the children in difficulty by offering them targeted support for certain topics, allowing them to catch up. Others are aimed at good students, those who, with their parents, want to increase their performance in order to enter the best schools.

On the other hand, according to Satō Manabu, the teachers of the public school designated as responsible for the evils of Japanese society have responded thusly:

> …by the multiplication of the bureaucratic devices of surveillance of the children, in the hopes of limiting the manifestations of the crisis. When a problem arises at school, the group of teachers in charge of discipline becomes dominant, and there is a general tendency to strengthen club activities and engage students after classes and weekends. All this in order to limit the risks of delinquency and deviant behavior. This approach generates work overload, and the hostility of students and parents faced with authoritarianism and school bureaucracy.
>
> *(Satō 2007: 28)*

In 1998, of the 550 students in the junior high school in which Satō Manabu investigated, 36 were in extended school absenteeism, or 6% of students, which were about two to three students per class. This is three times higher than the national average, which in 1998 was more than 100,000 cases of prolonged school absenteeism (more than 30 days), of which 80% were in junior high school (Satō 2007: 24). This development was confirmed to me by a statement of a retired teacher, who has today invested in assisting people with *hikikomori* (Mr. Sano): "When I started teaching, there was only one dropout in the school. When I retired, there was one in each class."

One of the findings, noticeable around the year 2000, seems quite clear: the management of problems such as absenteeism, violence, petty crime (even if the pupils in question are followed by the police ...), bullying, and material damage (broken tiles and deteriorating toilets), represents a considerable workload for teachers. Naturally, the interest in examining the evidence of school counselors is, at this point in the study, manifest. Because it is they who, very gradually since 1995, have been responsible for relieving teachers of a significant workload: that of students in difficulty. The titles of some articles in *The Annual Report of Educational Psychology in Japan* around the year 2000 (Oono 1998, Fujioka 1999, Hashimoto and Shiomi 2001) illustrate the transfer of missions that were happening between teachers and school counselors: "A Definition of School Counseling Services by Teachers in Japan" in 1998; "Current Issues in Clinical Practice in Schools: Toward the Construction of School Counseling Activities specific to Japan System" in 1999; and in 2001, "Roles, and Functions of School Psychologists in Schools." Nevertheless, collaboration between school counselors and teachers still remains particularly delicate today.

Well-being at school

Teachers have always been a resource for counseling, guidance, and some type of psychological support. With regard to psychological support, their action is, however, not comparable with that of clinical psychologists who, through their training and specific knowledge, can approach the interviews in a clinical way and hope for therapeutic effects from their interventions. One of the questions I ask practitioners in the next chapter is: Do Japanese school counselors carry out psychological assessments or observations in class? What kind of clinical interviews do they practice? Psychotherapy? In and/or out of school? Before I attend to my own findings, however, several data from the scientific literature is requisite. Indeed, it seems that the function of Japanese school counselors has gradually been oriented toward the health and well-being of students. Their interviews with teachers and parents should aim to maintain a pleasant climate within the school (Yagi 2008). According to Yagi, each class has a principal teacher with a triple mission: counseling, academic orientation, and personal development of students. Three other categories of teachers complete this system. Some assist their colleagues on issues of discipline and education. Others assist colleagues working in classrooms where some students have personal or family problems. Others, finally, have an assistant function for each year, by level, with their colleagues, and work in classes where some students have academic difficulties in specific subjects. Each of these teachers is supposed to work in a network with the school counselor. To the homeroom teacher and to these three categories of teachers is added the nurse (who also works in a network with the school counselors); social workers (whose positions were created in 2008, and with whom school counselors must cooperate); and finally, the educational advisors (*shidō shuji*). Basically, if we add health and social services out of school, we could think that the Japanese system is similar to other countries' systems. However, I will try to show how these appearances are deceptive. Japanese schools are a powerful institution coupled with a complex organization that is much denser and more complex than what the non-Japanese public may know.

In their article on teachers' collaboration with the school counselor, Kuwabara and collaborators state that Japanese teachers have "a strong sense of responsibility" toward students. These authors take up the idea that problems that originate in school must be treated in school or in the field of *kyōiku iinkai* (Kuwabara et al. 2008: 267). Beyond a very understandable recognition of the authority of the local education committee, these authors argue that the activities of school counselors must move from a "medical" model (intended for special "problem" children) to a "nurturing" model that would benefit all children (Kuwabara et al. 2008: 268). These perspectives lead us to think a positive and a negative side of the school: the permanence of the relationship to school is both a way of preserving traditions, fostering exchanges, and maintaining a living social bond, but this can also be experienced as an oppressive form of surveillance and control, which no one can escape. On the other hand, why should the school be "nurturing?" Why should we de-medicalize support for special needs of students in order to promote the well-being of all students? If I am raising these questions, it is because the school counselor is thought to be one of the actors favoring generalized well-being. The overlapping of counseling, support, and guidance provided by several professionals within the school is not the result of a bad outcome, but the product of a deliberate policy that serves specific goals. It is not uninteresting to note that scholars who support this "nurturing" model (Kuwabara et al. 2008) write in a journal founded by Kawai Hayao and are located in his school of thought. In their article, he is quoted to legitimize the views that the Japanese Self is different from the Western Self, the *leitmotiv* of the discourses on Japanese identity (*nihonjinron*). The relative popularity of these ideas helps to define the role of school counselors, especially since Kawai Hayao played an important political role, both for the recognition (certification of clinical psychologists), and employment (creation of the school counselor system) of emerging clinical psychologists in the late 1990s, and in the course of the 2000s.

Kuwabara and collaborators see the school as having always been a place of counseling. Other authors regret the confusion between counseling and psychology, because counseling is taught in psychology at the university (Grabosky, Ishii, and Mase 2012: 222). There are also those who deplore the current state of the Japanese system for psychology and counseling (Yagi 2008: 151). I think that a certain logic governs the fact that clinical psychologists occupy the position of school counselor. In this logic, psychologists must participate as a school counselor for the well-being of students, with other staff of the school. If there can be an overlap of missions between teachers and psychologists, it is to better work together for individual and collective well-being. This perspective is illustrated by Kuwabara et al. (2008: 275) when they say that in Japan, teachers and school counselors are in one and the same room, and "collaborate as individuals with a fundamental sense of unity." This emphasis on unity is prescriptive, with ideological overtones that resonate with "the hegemony of homogeneity" that Befu Harumi refers to when talking about *nihonjinron*. These discourses define what is "authentically" Japanese, and in turn what is good to do in the context of schools. Instead of turning to a critique of *nihonjinron* (Dale 1986, Befu 2001), I will try to understand how the school counselor system works, for which one of the most famous leading voices of *nihonjinron*, Kawai Hayao, played an important role.

In Japan, the emergence of clinical psychology involves the affirmation of a Japanese psychology, in the sense of a Japanese mentality but also of an academic discipline that would be the science – not of the psyche – but the *kokoro* (heart and mind). The implications of this distinction should not be underestimated: what we know in the West as "psychology" is not the Japanese variant of a "science of the heart" (*kokoro no kagaku*), which develops within a "world psychology." The insistence of Japanese psychologists to manipulate a common language term, *kokoro* – meaning an irreducible "heart/mind" instead of a "psyche" – could go as far as this: everything that has developed so far in Western psychology is partly true, but partly false, because Westerners have ignored the heart (*kokoro*). For psychology to become popular in Japan, it had to be formulated in such a way as to fit into the historical, sociological, and anthropological coordinates of the archipelago. It was necessary to preserve a reference to Western science, while affirming an "Eastern" peculiarity and a Japanese uniqueness.

This gradual development during the last quarter of the 20th century and the beginning of the 21st century saw a proliferation of clinical psychology as a discipline, and a considerable increase in the number of clinical psychologists. Yet the school counseling system made to reduce violence and school absenteeism still needs to be improved. Faced with this observation, Kuwabara and collaborators propose the exit of the medical model toward a nurturing model, and the promotion of the well-being of all the students. Would it be at the expense of care for those who are struggling the most? Does thinking about the school as a nurturer make it possible to distinguish students who suffer from psychopathologies and to offer them appropriate treatment? Does the promotion of the well-being of all foster a sense of being surveilled by teachers and parents, or does it contribute to a better mental health for students?

Withdrawal from school

School refusal (tōkō kyohi)

One of the first social science surveys of school refusal came from Canadian anthropologist Lock (1986). Lock (1986: 99) examines *tōkō kyohi* as "a form of resistance to social pressures and expectations," whose treatment has devolved to health professionals. Note that in Japan, doctors can pre-scribe and sell drugs themselves, so they can agree on arrangements with pharmaceutical companies. In these cases, the doctors make a profit; this is favored by the fact that, according to Lock (1986: 101), the implicit influence of Confucian ideology "encourages a reductionist approach to illness [...] and a willingness to resort freely to medication to try to alleviate (but not necessarily cure) a range of problems on the part of not only physicians but also of patients." The Japanese health system of the early 1980s operates by means of a system of points attributed to pathologies that give rights to a certain type of reimbursement. Some particularly harmful effects are also identified: doctors spend a lot of their time on "paperwork" and they spend little time talking with their patients. Let us now consider two cases of school refusal described by Lock.

The first case (Lock 1986: 101–102) is that of a 15-year-old boy who first developed stomach pain and was diagnosed as a child with school refusal syndrome. During the pediatrician's unsuccessful investigations, the symptoms increased. After the teacher had repeatedly humiliated him (as the student was entering from the hallway during class, for instance), he became violent at home: for example, beating his mother, one of his sis-ters, and throwing objects on the walls. After a month of withdrawal at home, the consultation of a school counselor led to his hospitalization for 14 months. The treatment (psychotherapy and medication) focused on the re-acquisition of the good habits of life (routines), and he was able to rein-tegrate into the school system. The parents, on the other hand, reduced their expectations in terms of academic results. While attending a monthly parent group, the father admitted that he was colder and more distant with his son than with his daughters.

The second case (Lock 1986: 102–103) is of a 12-year-old boy who comes with his mother to the guidance center, on the advice of teachers. The par-ents describe him as selfish (*wagamama*), lazy (*ōchaku*), with a nervous temper (*shinkeishitsu*), and one who finds the junior high school exercises difficult. The father locates the origin of the problem as springing from an episode of bullying in primary school. It is noted that he once went to jun-ior high school wearing a kendo uniform (he changed between home and school so that his parents did not see it), and a series of events related to a scar were mentioned.

After this brief account of clinical vignettes of school refusal, let us look at the interviews with doctors (Lock 1986: 104–105). Their moralizing tendency is sometimes surprising, especially when a psychiatrist says to a child: "You used to say that you were afraid of your father. How about now?" "Sometimes I'm afraid," he answers. The psychiatrist retorts, "That's because you don't do what he says!" (Lock 1986: 106). Another doctor, Dr. Nagai, denounces the egoism of mothers who treat their child like a domestic animal, while enjoining him to enter the University of Tokyo. For him, the goal of treatment is to encourage the mother to change her behavior. Dr. Sakama runs several clinics specializing in school refusal, where the main treatment is ... a diet. Indeed, a bad diet (he is, for example, formally opposed to sugar and white rice) is considered the cause of school refusal and mental illness. If this doctor agrees that bullying and a bad parent-child relationship may precipitate school refusal, the underlying problem would be nervous exhaustion (*shinkei ga tsukare sugiru*), caused by a poor diet, a lack of exercise, and excessive attention to school.

A former teacher (the only nondoctor but holding a position of responsibility toward these young people on the local education committee), Mr. Maeda, asserts that parents and children are selfish: absent fathers, mothers over-involved in the education of children, who spend their time watching television or manga, instead of playing in groups. Having grown up in a village where he felt that everyone and everything was watching him (villagers, mountains, nature, ancestors), he deplored the fact that everyone was talking about freedom; he wished for a restoration of strict authority. He acknowledged that some children who do not attend school have a mental illness but for the most part would only need regular family counseling. Finally, Dr. Tajima, as a psychiatrist, considers that school refusal is a symptom, but that the cause of the problem lies in the fact that the mother has no purpose in life (*ikigai ga nai*). As a result, she cannot let her child become independent. It also points to a society that has become too competitive, where the child who does not perform well in school is criticized by his parents, teachers, and peers, and who thus loses confidence in himself. He wants the education system to recognize that not all students are the same, and that school refusal is too publicized.

Dr. Tajima is partly right because in the early 1980s, school refusal was not an epidemic. Although the media encouraged this image by frequently reporting cases of school refusal, in 1982, they represented only 0.36% of college students (Lock 1986: 103). It gradually became a social issue around the year 2000, signaling the end of the use of the term of *tōkōkyohi* and especially, the popularity of its more neutral equivalent – school absenteeism (*futōkō*) – which has effectively become an "epidemic" measurable by national statistics. For Yoneyama Shoko, school refusal is very close to school phobia (as described by Berg and his collaborators in 1969), but he wishes to provide a more precise description: school refusal as a subcategory of school absenteeism, but distinct from school dropout and separation anxiety. Since the mid-1970s, the increase in cases of school refusals identified by the Ministry of Education is spectacular: there were less than 10,000 schoolchildren in this situation in 1975, but more than 70,000 in 1997, 1.9% of college students (Yoneyama 2000: 80). And, in 2005, there were even more, 2.73% of college students, a figure to put in perspective with that of 1982 cited previously: 0.36%. In 1990, the Ministry of Education developed a speech that stated "school refusal can affect everyone," rhetoric that can be observed a few years later in the context of depression (this "cold of the heart" *kokoro no kaze*), via a recourse to the notion of *kokoro* (Kitanaka 2012).

Yoneyama Shoko emphasizes the role of school refusal (*tōkō kyohi*) in the crisis of the education system and describes four types of discourse on school refusal: psychiatric, behavioral, citizen, and sociocultural. In psychiatric discourse, school refusal is a mental illness. It is a sign of the individual's maladaptation to society and is necessary, according to Saitō Tamaki's master, Inamura Hiroshi, to rebuild their foundation as a human being (cited by Yoneyama 2000: 83). In one of the famous associations supporting these young people (Tōkyō Shure), only 24% of them had consulted a psychiatric clinic (Yoneyama 2000: 83), even though 41% had suicidal thoughts (Yoneyama 2000: 84). In behavioral discourse, school refusal is a form of laziness, selfishness, and idleness: the solutions proposed are discipline and punishment, going as far as corporal punishment. Citizens' speech was largely opposed to these ways of considering the situation of children. One of his slogans was "school refusal is not an illness": it is resistance to school, and the opportunity to change the education system. In the sociocultural discourse, school refusal is the result of physical and psychological overwork, a "social disease" which is also linked to an imbalance of the autonomic nervous system. Yoneyama Shoko's strong hypothesis is that school refusal corresponds, for students, to an empowerment process, a way of seeking their own subjectivity (Yoneyama 2000: 77). It reveals four stages in students: "I cannot go" (lassitude); "I would like to but I cannot do it" (physical symptoms); "I do not go there" (critical consciousness); and finally "I will not go" (rejection, empowerment) (Yoneyama 2000: 87). By illustrating his conception of the refusal to go to school as a form of empowerment, he provides several testimonials that I will mention next.

A 14-year-old boy said he was a model student, but the impossibility of being himself, in any place, made him progressively exhausted. Following an episode of bullying, he stopped attending school (Yoneyama 2000: 88). A 14-year-old girl reports that she stopped attending school, without knowing why, and without being bullied; some days she did not want to see anyone. As everyone around her tried to find a solution, her health deteriorated, and terrible headaches appeared (Yoneyama 2000: 88). A 15-year-old student writes about his experience, using the metaphor of reloading energy:

the room is conceived as a place where one relies on energy lost in social activities (Yoneyama 2000: 89). Another student writes haunting thoughts – "being trash," "everyone has to go to school no matter what" – which he only released after a year of school refusal (Yoneyama 2000: 89). A 13-year-old schoolgirl writes that if she originally thought "it was wrong not to go to school" and that she was not "a good human being" because everyone was going there, today recognizes that it was not an incapacity but a choice because the school did not suit her (Yoneyama 2000: 90). Another boy describes the reasons for his academic refusal: "I thought I was going to lose myself, that I was controlled by the school" (Yoneyama 2000: 90). Another student sees school as a waste of time; another considers that he feels better than before and has forged his character as well; and another does not want to travel the common rails, but would rather create new ones (Yoneyama 2000: 91).

Finally, when Yoneyama brings together the scattered elements of the speeches of these adolescents to make school refusal a form of empowerment – a process by which they (re) find their subjectivity – we could reformulate it as follows: the situation described in terms of school refusal can be a way for these adolescents to experience a subject formation they cannot achieve within the Japanese school system.

School nonattendance (futōkō)

A survey published in *Social Science Japan* (Shimizu 2011) shows through a study of terminological changes in ministerial documents that the Ministry of Education (MOE) has ceased to define school refusal as a psychiatric disorder in their census. Between 1980 and 1987, one category was named "refusal because of a mental disorder, considered an early stage of mental illness" (Shimizu 2011: 175). Starting in 1988, however, this category disappeared because it was too infrequently rated. In the summer of 1997, the MOE decided to no longer use the term "school refusal" (Yoneyama 2000: 93), and in 1998, the term "school refusal" disappeared from ministerial documents for the benefit of the term "school nonattendance," which is more neutral. Until 2006, the factors of absenteeism were divided into five categories (Shimizu 2011: 178–179): (1) school (bullying, other problems with friends, problems with teachers, unsatisfactory academic performance, maladjustment to club activities, problems with school rules, maladjustment when entering school, change in school or class); (2) circumstances related to the home (rapid changes in home conditions, problems with parents, conflicts within the home); (3) individual problems (absence due to illness, other individual problems); (4) other; and (5) unknown.

The term "school nonattendance" (*futōkō*) now occupies an important place among caregivers, teachers, parents, but also in the media and official texts. According to the MOE, the factors of withdrawal are identified through five categories, two of which remain particularly imprecise: "Other" and "Unknown." For 2011, the MOE estimates that 112,437 students were absent from school for more than 30 days. The majority of them were college students (91,079).

From a psychiatric standpoint, Saitō Tamaki defined four subtypes of *futōkō*: excessive adaptation (which would cause frailty), passive (reaction to academic pressure or friendship), impulsive (immaturity), and complex (has the characteristics of several types). This psychiatrist also defined four phases of absenteeism: preparatory (somatic symptoms, internal conflicts, and anxiety); beginning of refusal (beginning of absenteeism and disagreements with the family); *hikikomori* period (with avoidance of father); and, finally, reunion with society (cited by Furuhashi et al. 2013).

Before concluding, a survey published in *Culture, Medicine, and Psychiatry* (Borovoy 2008) deserves to be reported here. The American anthropologist Amy Borovoy stresses that the refusal to marginalize "different" children is manifested by regular schooling with significant support for parents and family. This is valid for children with psychiatric disorders, because "doctors, aware of the sensitivity of families, avoid diagnosing a major psychopathology to the extent that is possible." (Borovoy 2008: 556). When a school counselor has to tell a parent that it is necessary for their child to see a psychiatrist, or receive special education, it is a high-tension moment, and parents struggle to give their authorization. Take, for example, the case of a child who got lost in the mountains during a school trip. The school counselor informs the anthropologist Amy Borovoy that this child had a developmental disorder, noticed by him and the teachers, a disorder that manifests itself by a significant motor incoordination and a delay in verbal abilities. The school uses the mother for the outings, and the child is assigned an educator who promotes his participation in the class. Added to this is an extra course twice a week, and a *juku*. One year after the event, Amy Borovoy participated in an appointment between the school counselor and the mother: the child had still not been diagnosed, and he was not considered different from others by his parents. According to the counselor, children raised in a healthy environment will naturally grow up healthy (*kodomo wa kankyō ga yokereba sukusuku sodatsu*), which corroborates the discourse that "a child is always better when the parents take care of him" and reinforces the discourse of some parents: "If parents cannot help the child, how can a specialist do it?" (Borovoy 2008: 561–562).

Amy Borovoy's research shows that, for a large number of children, psychiatric pathologies or psychological difficulties (cognitive or affective) are not treated, and attendance by the school counselor or nurse is inappropriate, or insufficient, in view of the difficulties they encounter. In another example reported by the anthropologist, the mother of a child with Asperger's syndrome had to follow the class secretly on a school trip, and sleep in a nearby hotel, in case the teachers needed her help. This situation illustrates the idea that mothers have to take care of family members in difficulty and be the main resource on socialization issues, in a context that resists medicalizing or psychologizing children's problems: "The presence of middle-class women at home in relatively large numbers compared to other industrialized nations, and the notion of the home as a sphere of social support, has created the very conditions for the phenomenon of *hikikomori*, making it possible for poorly functioning youths to retreat in the home and continue to be fed and cared for." (Borovoy 2008: 566).

Clinical psychology has developed simultaneously with the emergence of school refusal and school absenteeism as a social problem, and today it is the clinical psychologists who have to treat children who are absent from school. In the next chapter, I report on my interviews with three clinical psychologists and a child psychiatrist, examining the difficulties they face in the fight against school nonattendance.

References

Befu, Harumi. 2001. *Hegemony of Homogeneity: An Anthropological Analysis of Nihonjinron*. Melbourne: Trans Pacific Press.

Borovoy, Amy. 2008. "Japan's Hidden Youths: Mainstreaming the Emotionally Distressed in Japan." *Culture, Medicine and Psychiatry* 32: 52–56.

Dale, Peter N. 1986. *The Myth of Japanese Uniqueness*. Nissan Institute, London: Routledge.

Van Effenterre, Aude, Marion Azoulay, Xavier Briffault, and Françoise Champion. 2012. "Psychiatres... et psychothérapeutes ? Conception et pratiques des internes en psychiatrie." *L'Information Psychiatrique* 88 (4): 305–313.

Fujioka, Takashi. 1999. "Current Issues in Clinical Practice in Schools. Toward the Construction of School Counseling Activities Specific to Japan." *The Annual Report of Educational Psychology in Japan* 38: 142–154.

Fukurai Tomokichi 福来友吉. 1913. *Tōshi to nensha* 透視と念写. Tōkyō: Hōbunkan.
———. 1931. *Clairvoyance and Thoughtography* (augmented translation of Tōshi to nensha). USA: Kessinger publishing.

Fukushima, Hiroshi, and Yoshio Hirayasu. 2012. "Postgraduate Training in Japan: The Road to Subspecialty." In *The 108th Annual Meeting of the Japanese Society of Psychiatry and Neurology*, 397.

Fumino, Yoh. 2005. "Establishment of New Universities and the Growth of Psychology in Postwar Japan." *Japanese Psychological Research* 47 (2). Special Issue: The History of Psychology in Japan: 144–150.

Furuhashi, Tadaaki et al. 2013. "Etat des lieux, points communs et différences entre des jeunes adultes retirants sociaux en France et au Japon (Hikikomori)." *L'Evolution Psychiatrique* 78 (2): 249–266.

Gender Equality Bureau. 2020. *Women and Men in Japan 2020*. Tōkyō: Cabinet office, Government of Japan. Available at: http://www.gender.go.jp/english_contents/pr_act/pub/pamphlet/women-and-men20/index.html

Gollier, Théophile. 1906. "An Essay on Eastern Philosophy, by Motora (Professor of Psychology, Imperial University, Tokyo)." *Revue Néo-Scolastique* 13 (51): 346–348.

Grabosky, Tomoko Kudo, Harue Ishii, and Shizuno Mase. 2012. "The Development of the Counseling Profession in Japan, Past Present and Future." *Journal of Counseling and Development* 90: 221–226.

Hashimoto, Hidemi, and Kunio Shiomi. 2001. "Roles and Functions of School Psychologists in Schools." *The Annual Report of Educational Psychology in Japan* 40: 177–189.

Ingrams, Elizabeth. 2005. "Depression. Long-Taboo 'Mood Disorder' Is Now Being Seen as the Common and Crippling Disease It Is." *The Japan Times*. http://www.japantimes.co.jp/life/2005/07/10/to-be-sorted/depression/#.UkjbMyQfbeY.

Jung, Carl Gustav, and Shin'ichi Hisamatsu. 1968. "On the Unconscious, the Self and the Therapy: A Dialogue." *Psychologia: An International Journal of Psychology in the Orient* 11: 25–32.

Kawai, Hayao 河合隼雄. 1995. *Yungu shinrigaku to bukkyō* ユング心理学と仏教 (Jungian Psychology and Buddhism). Tōkyō: Iwanami Shoten.

———. 1996. *Buddhism and the Art of Psychotherapy* (translation of *Yungu shinrigaku to bukkyō*). Texas: Texas A&M University Press.

Kitanaka, Junko. 2003. "Jungians and the Rise of Psychotherapy in Japan: A Brief Historical Note." *Transcultural Psychiatry* 40: 239–247.

———. 2012. *Depression in Japan, Psychiatric Cures for a Society in Distress.* Princeton, NJ: Princeton University Press.

Koyama, Tetsuro. 2008. "Storyteller Murakami Plumbs Depths of the Soul." *The Japan Times*, April 16, 2008. http://www.japantimes.co.jp/news/2008/04/16/national/storyteller-murakami-plumbs-depths-of-the-soul/#.UjbS6rwfbeY.

Kuwabara, Tomoko, Haruka Sudo, Chihiro Hatanaka, Masaki Nishijima, Kenichi Morita, Chihiro Hasegawa, and Yasuhiro Oyama. 2008. "A Study on the New Paradigm in Collaboration Between Teachers and School Counselors." *Psychologia: An International Journal of Psychology in the Orient* 51: 267–279.

Letendre, Gerald K. 1995. "Disruption and Reconnection: Counseling Young Adolescents in Japanese Schools." *Educational Policy* 9 (2): 169–184.

Lévi-Alvarès, Claude. 2007. "L'adhésivité d'un monde professionnel." In *Enseignants et écoles au Japon – Acteurs, système et contexte*, edited by Claude Lévi-Alvarès and Manabu Satō, 157–190. Paris: Maisonneuve et Larose.

Lock, Margaret. 1982. "Popular Conceptions of Mental Health in Japan." In *Cultural Conceptions of Mental Health and Therapy*, edited by Anthony J. Marsella and Geoffrey White, 215–233. Dordrecht: D. Reidel Publishing.

———. 1986. "Plea for Acceptance: School Refusal Syndrome in Japan." *Social Science & Medicine* 23: 99–112.

Macé, Mieko. 2013. *Médecins et médecine dans l'histoire du Japon.* Paris: Les Belles Lettres (Collection Japon).

McVeigh, Brian J. 2017. *The History of Japanese Psychology. Global Perspectives.* London: Bloomsbury (SOAS Studies in Modern and Contemporary Japan).

Motora, Yūjiro 元良勇次郎. 1888. *"Exchange, Considered as the Principle of Social Life".* PhD Diss., Johns Hopkins University.

———. 1905. *An Essay on Oriental Philosophy.* Leipzig: Voigtlander.

Oono, Seiichi. 1998. "A Definition of School Counseling Services by Teachers in Japan." *The Annual Report of Educational Psychology in Japan* 37: 153–159.

Ribot, Théodule. 1905. "Motora – An Essay on Eastern Philosophy, Leipzig, Voigtlander." *Revue Philosophique* 60: 642–645.

Satō, Manabu. 2007. "Les enseignants japonais dans une période charnière." In *Enseignants et écoles au Japon – Acteurs, système et contexte*, edited by Claude Lévi-Alvarès and Manabu Satō, 21–44. Paris: Maisonneuve et Larose.

Satō, Tatsuya et al. 2005. *Japanese Psychological Research* 47 (2). Special Issue: The History of Psychology in Japan.

Satō, Tatsuya. 2007. "Rises and Falls of Clinical Psychology in Japan: A Perspective on the Status of Japanese Clinical Psychology." *Ritsumeikan ningen kagaku ken-kyū* 13: 133–144.

Satō, Tatsuya, and Takao Satō. 2005. "The Early 20th Century: Shaping the Discipline of Psychology in Japan." *Japanese Psychological Research* 47 (2). Special Issue: The History of Psychology in Japan: 52–62.

Shimizu, Hirokichi. 2007. "Le 'roman de formation' dans les collèges - Éducation et sélection dans l'orientation scolaire." In *Enseignants et écoles au Japon – Acteurs, système et contexte*, edited by Claude Lévi-Alvarès and Manabu Satō, 115–136. Paris: Maisonneuve et Larose.

Shimizu, Katsunobu. 2011. "Defining and Interpreting Absence from School: The Debate in Ministerial Discourses in Japan." *Social Science Japan Journal* 14 (2): 165–187.

Tsuneyoshi, Ryōko. 2007. "L'esprit de groupe et l'école japonaise." In *Enseignants et écoles au Japon – Acteurs, système et contexte*, edited by Claude Lévi-Alvarès and Manabu Satō, 137–155. Paris: Maisonneuve et Larose.

Yagi, Daryl Takizo. 2008. "Current Developments in School Counseling in Japan." *Asian Journal of Counseling* 15 (2): 141–155.

Yoneyama, Shoko. 2000. "Student Discourse on Tōkō Kyohi (School Phobia/Refusal) in Japan, Burnout or Empowerment?" *British Journal of Sociology of Education* 21 (1): 77–94.

2 The resistance to students' psychological care

Introduction

In-depth qualitative research interviews with four Japanese mental health practitioners working in H. city were performed during a fieldwork period lasting 3 years. The names of the individuals interviewed, who gave authorization to be audio-recorded and quoted (Tajan 2015), have been anonymized in order to respect their privacy. In this exploratory investigation, I used an open questionnaire in Japanese in which I asked subjects to describe the following: first, the period between graduation and present work; second, a typical day; third, clinical practice and the patients met; fourth, school discipline and norms; fifth, the role of the clinician in the institution (school, guidance center, university); and sixth, their career's best and worst experiences. I will be sharing highlights from these interviews in order to provide scope for discussing contemporary psychological clinics and student counseling practices, and to improve the support to school absentees in Japan.

Clinical psychologist and school counselor

I would like to share responses from my first series of questions covering the period between graduation and present work that were directed to Ms. Otsuka, a certified clinical psychologist and member of the Association of Japanese Clinical Psychology (AJCP). (She was interviewed, mainly in English, on the 10th of April 2013 for 2 hours and 30 minutes, of which 1 hour and 45 minutes was audio-recorded.) Her situation is unique in which she obtained her master's degree from a university that is not accredited by the Foundation of the Japanese Certification Board of Clinical Psychologists (FJCBCP). In cases such as this, an applicant who wants to become a certified clinical psychologist (*rinshō shinri shi*) must first have 2 years of experience in Japan. In some prefectures, certification is a prerequisite for working as a school counselor; this was, in fact, a peculiarity of H. prefecture; however, their mode of operations cannot be extrapolated to all the Japanese prefectures. Since the certification of clinical psychologists is provided by a private foundation, it is not compulsory for public institutions (i.e., hospitals and schools) to require certification from private foundations.

Ms. Otsuka began her career as a non-certified psychologist in a hospital and later in an institution for individuals with disabilities. After this period of work, she then became a certified clinical psychologist and school counselor in H. prefecture. Once certified, she had to register with the AJCP. (As I have noted in the previous chapter, the vast majority of Japanese clinical psychologists are members of this association.) The local board of education (*kyōiku iinkai*) dispatches the counselors to one of the prefecture's schools after completing a questionnaire in which the applicant expresses his wishes (working in primary school, junior high, or high school); indicates whether he owns a car; and how far he can move within the prefecture. At the end of the first year, the school in which the counselor is assigned indicates, through its director, whether he wants to change or keep the counselor. If the director does not say anything, the counselor stays there for 3 years, like the teachers (5–6 years maximum). Unlike teachers, school counselors' nontenure contract is renewable every year. Each school counselor is assigned to one junior high school and to one or two primary schools (not all elementary schools currently have school counselors). At the end of the interview, I tell my interviewee that part-time employees, or those who do part-time jobs (*arubaito*), do not contribute to their retirement pension, and I ask: what is the situation for school counselors? "It is identical," she responds. "They do not contribute to their retirement." According to her, it is a vulnerable and unsecured position.

Clinical practice at school

The second series of questions focused on what a typical day looks like for a school counselor. Ms. Otsuka works 1 day/week as a school counselor in a junior high school and the other days in a hospital. In her role as school counselor, a typical day involves 7 hours of work from 12 to 7 pm. She meets the teachers between 12 and 1 pm, and between 6 and 7 pm. From 1 to 6 pm, she offers counseling to students and their parents (usually mothers) but is not performing psychotherapy in the school setting, only counseling activities that help the patients to cope with their problematic situations. Most school counselors have 30-minutes sessions, she adds. Also, it might happen that the director asks the counselor to take care of the teachers' mental health as well, but as this is not included in the contract, it is up to the counselor's discretion. Psychological testing, often considered a big risk for damaging the relationship between the school and the parents, is never done inside a school setting—only in guidance centers or medical institutions.

I also investigated if school counselors could help the exhausted teachers described in the educational literature – 100 home visits per year (Shimizu 2007: 126), 52–60 hours of work per week (Satō 2007: 22) – but it appears that it is still the teacher, rather than the school counselor, who does home-visits (*katei hōmon*):

MS. OTSUKA: Not necessarily only for school refusal, some children have serious family problems, where the parents are not there, or the parents are severely sick, or they themselves never go home. In these cases, teachers visit the student's home, sometimes with the police, for example, and they visit a lot. In some cases, they do it every day, like at 9 or 10 pm in the evening they still may be visiting the homes of their students.

N.T.: I've also read about patrols during summer vacation, with teachers patrolling the city around several spots such as karaoke bars to see if the students are behaving well. Is this still going on?

MS. OTSUKA: Yes, sure (...) they do that.

Some school counselors do it, but it is not in the contract, which is part-time, that is, they are not supposed to work on weekends and holidays, and what is more they have no insurance to do it. Some do it, but never officially. As for group therapies, she herself has not engaged in this practice, and they seem uncommon. During the past 5 years, interviews with both parents and their child together in the same room never happened, and there was only one interview with both parents. Even though fathers can be met with early in the morning or in the evening, they just do not come: mothers come 99% of the time, and often because their child is not attending school anymore. I ask if she investigates both the childhood of the parents and the child during consultations:

MS. OTSUKA: I personally do. A lot, that's what I do during the first few sessions (...) ask them about the history of the child, the student himself, how was it when he was born, how has it been, and at the same time after a few sessions I start asking about the parents themselves, but some parents don't want to talk about it, so I don't push them, of course, and I never really collected data of what I've done or what I've heard, but I have a very strong impression about children who have problems with school refusal: their parents likely had the same problem when they were in junior-high school or around the same age, or they had horrible experiences at school; this happens a lot, so I always try to ask them how they perceive the school.

However, she gets criticized by her colleagues because she asks the parents about their own experiences as children. They tell her school counseling is not the place to go deeper with the person who is not the person who has the problem: it is not the place to ask personal questions to the parent. Ms. Otsuka does not agree because she thinks that, since parents raise the child, their stories as children have a significant impact on their own child. In other words, she must justify to her colleagues that the story of the child, and the story of the parent as a child, can be part of the treatment. (This is not the case in France, where most psychologists would agree with Ms. Otsuka on this point, even without being psychoanalysts.) Nevertheless, one can ask the question of whether identification is a psychological or psychoanalytic concept. If one refers to the Japanese situation, it seems to be a psychoanalytic concept. Let us not underestimate this. Identification is a mechanism in which psychic life is transmitted through the generations. Would the type of psychology underway in the archipelago not suppose that identification is a mechanism in which psychic life is transmitted through the generations? How would it be possible? How is the psychic life transmitted through the generations, if not by identification? Another question: does psychology, as conceived in the Japanese archipelago, imply a theory of the psychic apparatus, a theory such as psychic elaboration, or a construction of psychic life? As I introduced in the previous chapter, the promotion of a notion such as "heart/mind" (*kokoro*), instead of a "psyche", has become popular. A different generational logic seems to prevail. Theories and psychological practice are built by making psychology a "science of the heart" (*kokoro no kagaku*) that dodges the concept of identification, while trying to guarantee a conception of identity.

Discipline

Japanese school discipline in primary schools has already been described (Cave 2007); it seemed useful to check the accuracy of specific aspects described in junior-high schools during the 1990s and the 2000s, however, which was accomplished in the fourth part of my interview. For example, cleaning the classroom and the school facilities (*sōji no jikan*) is typically done after lunch and takes 15 to 20 minutes, but because there is a turnover between groups and classes, a student would not clean the classroom, the toilets, or the stairs on a daily basis: "When the teachers don't control (...) the students, they play in the toilets and it's never clean," Mrs. Otsuka says. Of course, Japanese junior-high school students wear uniforms, and take off their shoes when entering the school building: they put on slippers (*uwabaki*) upon which they previously had to write their names (otherwise they would not recognize them: they are all the same). The rules related to hair are simple: when it touches the shoulders, it has to be cut. Hair should be black (natural color), and if someone colors their hair, for instance, the delinquents called *yankii*, then teachers spray their hair black before they enter the school area; these students rarely come to school and are not supported by school counselors: "They want to act, not to talk," Ms. Otsuka remarks. Nails should be cut and not painted, which is difficult to check during winter, when students arrive by bicycle with gloves on their hands. Even at high school, no makeup, no bracelets, no earrings, no piercings, and no necklaces are allowed: "Anything that's not necessary for studying: 'no'. You're not allowed to be an individual (...) you have to be a part of the group, so they don't like anything that shouts out your individuality. That is seen as a threat to the group, where you're supposed to look the same and behave the same." (Ms. Otsuka).

I ask her about self-harming practices which, according to her, spread as in a "mass hysteria". In general, when such issues arise, she discusses it with the teenager identified as the main source and invites him to speak instead of acting out. She then tries to contain what is happening in the classroom, because cutting the wrists, or forearms (*risuto katto*), spreads very quickly to other students. Students with eating disorders, such as ano-rexia and bulimia, are not supported in junior high schools: these cases are already hospitalized, or they stay at home, and it is the homeroom teacher who makes home visits. According to her, scarification and self-injury can be handled inside the school by the school counselor, unlike teenagers with eating disorders who are generally very severe cases and require a lot of medical support. They are most often out of school.

Still in the field of school life and discipline, I mentioned the issue of corporal punishment (*taibatsu*). Teachers today are particularly nervous in this regard, especially since the media have repeatedly echoed teachers being fired for this reason. Recently, in her school "a young teacher threw something – what he had in his hand – to a student and unfortunately reached him, and it became a huge scandal [...] In Japan, teachers are not used to sitting with students, talking with them, explaining things to them; but it's more discipline – telling them what's right and wrong. It's changing a lot lately, it's a real challenge [...] teachers are very nerv-ous about scolding and especially punishing their students ... they do not know what to do ... and what happens is that they try to become their stu-dents' buddies [...] often the young teachers – but not only them – develop a relationship of friends with their students, because it's simpler, and they call their teacher *chan* [...] it is not unusual for a student to call his teacher X-*chan*." I then point out to my interlocutor that "scolding, in itself, does not fall under corporal punishment (*taibatsu*): it depends on the words we use," to which she replies: "Yes, but if you have a loud voice, students tell their parents that their teacher is really aggressive, and you have prob-lems. So I think teachers are in an extremely difficult situation: they really do not know what to do." (Ms. Otsuka).

Other changes regarding discipline have occurred. The example given by Letendre (1995) – a student kneeling on the floor while being scolded by the teacher after class – seems impossible in today's Japan: "I think a lot of teachers are really afraid, they'll never do that, they don't want to risk anything, and that will be considered inappropriate if it ever comes out, under the light: if you ask your student to sit on the floor on their knees, it's not good." (Ms. Otsuka).

In other words, we are witnessing a considerable and problematic shift of teachers' authority from an excess of discipline to a lack of it. As she says very well, "they don't know what to do" and it is both the media and the parents who have a role in changing the exercise of authority by teachers. Therefore, if there is a positive side of policies that favor the participation of students' parents as users of educational services or the empowerment of parents and students themselves (e.g., there would be fewer cases of corporal punishment), there is also a negative side, because teachers do not know anymore how to exercise their authority: if they raise their voice, they will be subjected to considerable pressure and are likely to create a scandal, especially if parents take for granted students' account. What is happening in Japan today is a dramatic transformation in the way teachers exercise authority.

"The teacher is here to accuse me of not sending my child to the school"

I was also interested to know more about the type of population with which the psychologist works, and the psychologist's place in the school. She is contacted by parents, teachers, and the student, directly or through the nurse or the home room teacher:

> I wrote an essay every month in the school newspaper – some schools impose what they want you to write—I was talking about some psychological things: some students told me they read it, and that's why they came, and parents too, that's how they learned that I was there, and they came to see me. It's not really "with the system" that we will see the school counselor, it's more in relation to a personal idea that they decide to come to see you ... It's pretty close to go see someone freely in your private time, the system does not impose it on you, it is rather: "I want to speak to someone and I go to see the school counselor."
>
> *(Ms. Otsuka)*

For her, psychosis and neurosis are medical diagnoses, not psychological, and she works more from the student's complaint. The most common reason for consultation is a complaint about bullying (*ijime*). She takes the example of a student who, behind a complaint about bullying, was witnessing her parents' divorce: according to her, this teenager felt bad and projected her distress, which was confirmed by the discussion with the teacher who had never noticed that she was especially mistreated by others. These feelings of threat and this projection are the psychological aspects diagnosed.

Ms. Otsuka never encountered sexual harassment cases involving students, but she notes that the cases of pregnant girls pose serious problems: it is systematically girls who meet older men outside of school. Here, my interlocutor does not speak of high school prostitution (*enjo kōsai*). We are in junior high school, and what she describes does not necessarily imply this type of commodification, but rather the situation of girls who meet older boys. Boys of the same age are very immature, which girls complain about, and they do not mix with girls because gender division is strongly marked in the school context.

The major reasons for consulting are complaints about bullying (*ijime*) which is consistent with official data at the national level. In fact, as for 2012, the MOE estimates that 75,000 primary and junior high school students suffered from *ijime*. Also, teachers are divided in two groups that are highly gendered. The first group is mainly composed of men in charge of students' guidance and discipline (*seito shidō gakari*) as opposed to the group composed mainly of women who provide comprehensive guidance to the students (*kyōiku sōdan gakari*). One of the major difficulties is that "teachers express themselves towards the students, but do not let the students express themselves, do not provide a space for the students' words: always instructions, advice to do, or not to do this or that, because of this or that." (Ms. Otsuka).

I asked her to tell of two episodes from her clinical practice (one positive and one negative) that could also be interesting from the point of view of relationships with teachers and the institution. The first case involved a girl with depressive symptoms, suicidal ideation, self-harming behavior and family problems. She was counseled and "towards the end when she was graduating, the situation was getting more and more chaotic, and it was hard for her to come to see me constantly, so I tended to lose contact," she says. Ms. Otsuka informed the teachers that she needed a lot of attention, especially in high school; she wanted the teachers to contact the high school because she had made one serious suicidal attempt. However, this girl came back to the junior-high school 1 or 2 months after entering high school and asked for counseling: Ms. Otsuka wasn't there, but when it was reported to her, she understood that the teachers hadn't contacted the high school. After insisting again with the teachers, the student could then access counseling in her high school. It was one of Ms. Otsuka's hardest experiences.

Additionally, she mentions that it is not recommended to refer students and parents to one's private practice.

> It's not forbidden, but they always tell you to refer whoever you're seeing to a public one because it doesn't involve money, and when things happen, again it's a risk that the Ministry of Education might be accused, or held responsible for whatever happens (…) There's no law for that. I think it is partly because we're not legal yet (…) We don't have a national license.
>
> *(Ms. Otsuka)*

I would like to conclude the interview with Ms. Otsuka with a successful experience. She counseled the mother of a student who was described as depressed and who had been skipping school for a few weeks. During the consultations with the mother, it appeared that the family was falling apart (divorce and financial problems), and the mother had intense feelings of persecution. Whenever the teacher came over for home visits, he was not allowed to enter the house or meet the student. The mother felt persecuted, thinking "it's my fault that the child is not doing well, and the teacher is here to accuse me of not sending my child to the school". But Ms. Otsuka found a solution in order to communicate with the child. Nobody was allowed to enter the house and meet the student, but the school handouts were allowed. So Ms. Otsuka told the teacher to write a few words in the handouts like "how are you? You're not catching any cold?": it was a way to connect with the child, not by saying "you must go to school," but by offering a human space to speak at a time when her home life was full of problems. After 3 weeks, she went back to junior-high school, not *during* classes but after, and she started recovering.

Clinical psychologist and coordinator at guidance center X

Mr. Sakurai is a certified clinical psychologist and the manager of guidance center X (created in 2003 and intended for students enrolled in public schools in the city and their parents). The interview took place on April 24, 2013 from 2 to 3 pm and was recorded (55 minutes with the agreement of Mr. Sakurai). Ms. Otsuka played the role of intermediary between me and Mr. Sakurai, agreeing with him at the time of the appointment and remaining present during the interview. It seems important to clarify this, because in many of my interviews, the questioning of a person has often involved a third interlocutor, without the latter being reduced to an intermediary or a translator. The subtlety of social relations lies behind all these interviews, where one is introduced to others according to particular circumstances and according to predefined social codes: Predefined social codes, because one speaks to people like Mr. Sakurai or Dr. Matsuda with a certain "reverence," on the one hand related to their status, and on the other hand within the framework of a testimony of gratitude linked to the precious time they gave me; special circumstances, because I met Ms. Otsuka, Dr. Matsuda, and Prof. Kubo via symposia that I co-organized at Kyōto University. Without this effort – to volunteer to organize a conference – I could never have met them. In Dr. Matsuda's case, which I will describe later, it even took the form of an exchange, because after listening to my lecture, he improvised a lecture, which was part of the interview process with him. I will return to this topic later.

The purpose of center X (created in 2003) is to cultivate the health of children (*mokuteki wa sono kodomotachi no kenzen ikusei*) through students' and parents' guidance and counseling. It is composed of two teams: the clinical psychologists' team (n: 40), called *kyōiku sōdan* (educational guidance), and the teachers' team (n: 30), called *seito shidō* (student discipline). The peculiarity of this center is to coordinate these two teams, whose school culture and representations of education differ. Mr. Sakurai is supervising these two teams in a vast open space associated with a third team, a network of employees (n: 30) scattered across the city, proposing various activities (tutoring, sports, etc.). In total, a hundred employees are working for the guidance center, but most of the clinical psychologists are part-timers.

They mainly offer counseling to the students, their families, and also to the teachers working in the public schools. The number of sessions per year is around 15,000, and the number of individuals (children and parents) being counseled is between 800 and 1000. Children and adolescents rarely come by themselves, but many parents come alone. The center welcomes students between the ages of 6 and 18, and only those registered in public schools, as those enrolled in the private education system may have support provided by their school. If this is not the case, they must move to a private mental clinic (*mentaru kurinikku*) or a private mental health practitioner (such as counselor: *kaunserā*). The center does not systematically accommodate those who do not go to high school, because high school is not compulsory. In terms of funding, the center is 100% supported by the city, unlike school counselors who are partly funded by the Ministry of Education, and partly by the resources of the cities. This type of guidance center is, therefore, always dependent on the wishes of the mayor, his team, and their constituents. Situations can be addressed by teachers in schools in the city, but parents can also spontaneously contact the center after browsing their website or having received a prospectus. Mr. Sakurai feels that these cases are the most numerous. Staff activities are, therefore, primarily aimed at parents and young people, mainly in the form of counseling, but they also focus on the link with the school in terms of support (*shien*), discipline, and guidance: guidance center's staff works with schools' staff, in the city, and gives them advice on absentees, offenders, and families in distress. In counseling, most professionals practice individual therapy (*kojin ryōhō*) and some *hako niwa ryōhō* (Japanese sandplay therapy or miniature garden therapy). There is one self-help group—called "parents' training"—for parents raising a child with developmental disabilities (*hattatsu shōgai*).

School nonattendance (*futōkō*) represents 50% of the cases, quite a few come because of bullying (*ijime*), and the number of students with developmental disorders (*hattatsu shōgai*) is increasing. Mr. Sakurai says, "here there is no guidance on psychosis/mental illness ... as there are no doctors." This statement is, at first glance, somewhat surprising unless one puts oneself in a different sociocultural context where mental health and psychological counseling are well separated. There is, among the clinical psychologists, no hypothesis put in terms of structure (according to Lacanian psychoanalytic doctrine; psychosis, neurosis, and perversion are three normal subjective structures of being) and there is no psychiatrist in the center, except for during team supervision. The term "psychosis" is always seen as a medical diagnosis, and a situation that is beyond the purview of clinical psychologists.

Most of the time, those with developmental disorders are referred to the guidance center J. (*jidō sōdanjo*) to consult with child psychiatrists, and where it is possible to perform psychological testing (*shinri kensa*). In this city, there are, therefore, several guidance centers: the literal "guidance center" (*sōdan sentā*) created recently which includes Mr. Sakurai and the "child and adolescent guidance center" (*jidō sōdanjo*), a much older institution, which includes the child and adolescent psychiatrist that I will examine later. The first center receives children and adolescents: these two centers are, in fact, "child and adolescent guidance centers," but the first is psychoeducational, while the second—the *jidō sōdanjo*—is medico-psycho-educational. In the first case, there is no medical doctor (there are only psychologists and teachers), whereas in the second, there are 11 medical doctors. My two interlocutors agree that in the context of counseling, there is not really a culture of evaluation, in the sense of an interest and practice of psychological tests: it is not considered important. Assessments are made by medical institutions rather than these counseling services. I shared how the French context differs with my interlocutor, to which they responded as follows. According to Mr. Sakurai, when you tell the parents psychological testing will be necessary, they resist (*teikō*) and fear that their children could be mentally ill. If a psychological test is proposed, the parents immediately say: "Does my child have an illness?" Also, it is difficult in everyday clinical practice to gain the trust of the parents and to obtain sufficient information from them about their history, and to find a good balance with what they want to say and what they do not. Major problems appear when it comes to dealing with developmental disorders, neglect (*gyakutai*), and single-parent households. Mr. Sakurai adds that Japanese institutions propose counseling for situations where there is violence between the parents, or violence from the parents towards the child. However, when it comes to violence between the children, or from the children to the parents, no specific counseling exists at the moment.

A child and adolescent psychiatrist at guidance center J

I met Dr. Matsuda for the first time at a conference I had given on the prevention of school dropout in France. At this conference, I mentioned the absence of child psychiatrists in the guidance center X, and during the discussion, Dr. Matsuda intervened to affirm that there was a second guidance center in this city, where 11 child and adolescent psychiatrists were present. After the conference, we invited Dr. Matsuda to have dinner with the speakers, and good relationships were created between Dr. Matsuda, Mr. Nobutomo Kenji, and myself. Subsequently, we agreed on an interview and a visit to his center.

To prepare for the interview, I first translated the available data I gleaned from their website concerning the child and adolescent guidance center (*jidō sōdanjo*), which is part of a child and adolescent welfare center (*jidō fukushi sentā*) and included in social welfare institutions (*shakai fukushi hōjin*). The website consists of two parts: the "register for consultations" (*sōdan no mōshikomi*) and the "content of consultations" part (*sōdan naiyō*). Under the "register for consultations" section they note, first of all, that it is possible to report a case of abuse to these services and to receive consultation to this effect, 24 hours a day, 7 days a week, and 365 days a year. Second, it is possible to consult by phone, email, or in person. They repeatedly note that, whatever the medium, confidentiality is respected (*puraibashī wa kataku mamorimasu*). Third, the center conducts scientific assessments conducted by qualified professionals: the need for testing is emphasized, and as evaluation, consultation, and treatment progresses, problems are solved, one after another. Finally, the center offers various effective methods for the child, in collaboration with the parents.

Within the website's "content of consultations" section, two consultation centers are listed. The first is the guidance center J (*jidō sōdanjo*), which lays out these four guiding principles. First, consultations offered are related to the education of the child and the family atmosphere (*kodomo wo sodateru katei kankyō ni kansuru sōdan*); here the focus is on the difficulties of "education/breeding" (*kosodate*) of the child. Second, consultations offered make it possible to raise one's children well (*kodomo wo yori sukoyaka ni sodateru tame no sōdan*); here, it is the children who encounter difficulties at school who are concerned: children who do not go to school (*gakkō he ikenai kodomo*), children who suffer from bullying (*ijime*), or who have problems of discipline (*shitsuke*). Third, other types of consultations are offered for persons who wish to become a foster family (*sato oya*). Fourth, some consultations are proposed in cases of abuse (*gyakutai*) and to report a situation of abuse: "As soon as you realize that a child suffered abuse, contact us as soon as possible" (*Gyakutai sareteiru to omowareru kodomo wo mitsuketara sugu tsūkoku wo*).

The second center of consultation noted on the website is the developmental guidance center (*hattatsu sōdanjo*), which is still part of the guidance center J but addresses three specific population types: (1) Those who have a developmental delay (*hattatsu no okure*), an anxiety related to their hearing and words (*kikoe ya kotoba no fuan*), and those who are concerned with the development of their body and their heart/mind (*kokoro ya karada no hattatsu*); (2) people over the age of 18 who have a intellectual disability (*chiteki shōgai*) and; (3) people with autism and developmental disorders (*jiheishō nado no hattatsu shōgai no aru kata*). Included in developmental disorders (*hattatsu shōgai*) are autistic spectrum disorders (*jiheishō supekutoramu*), attention deficit hyperactivity disorder (*chūi ketsujo tadōsei shōgai*), and learning disabilities (*gakushū shōgai*). It is proposed to relieve the family of people with developmental disabilities through guidance (*sōdan*), assistance (*shien*), development support (*hattatsu shien*), employment support (*shūrō shien*), and dissemination of better information about these problems (*fukyū keihatsu kenshū*). Also, a few words are included affirming that people with developmental disabilities are irreplaceable individuals (*kakegae no nai kojin*).

The assistance that guidance center J offers is in the form of interviews (*mendan*) on the spot, or by telephone. The center has also set up parents' meetings (*kazoku gakushūkai* or *kazoku mītingu*), whose objective is to improve the understanding of the disorder among them. The parents' meetings are held at the childcare site. Social clubs (*sōsharu kurabu*) or workshops are organized, and small group activities take place there. All activities take place from Monday to Friday, from 9 am to 12 pm, and from 2 to 5 pm. Employment support (*shūrō shien*) targets adults with developmental disabilities and their parents, who are involved in job search activities set up at the center. The public awareness training project on issues related to developmental disabilities holds lectures, workshops, regular training seminars for caregivers (*shiensha*) and receives trainees. The center employs people who are qualified to treat autism spectrum disorders. As part of the guidance program for parents and legal guardians of the child (*chokusetsu shidō puroguramu* and *hogosha jissen gakushūkai*), seven meetings are planned: the team gives lectures for them and provides the basic knowledge needed to support the targeted people. The personal experiences of parents and legal guardians are considered. Some meetings (out of 11 in total) are specifically planned for parents and guardians of children with Asperger syndrome (*Kōkinō jiheishō, asuperugā shōkōgun hogosha gakushūkai*). During these meetings, they try to cultivate a better understanding of the syndrome: the people concerned can be present, and everyone can talk about their personal experience.

Interview at center J

The visit and the recorded interview took place on August 15, 2013, between 2 and 6 pm, in the presence of Nobutomo Kenji who, when I had difficulties with comprehension, was the interpreter. The half-day was structured in three stages: an introductory interview in an ophthalmological consultation room on the third floor (20 minutes); a visit of the establishment (1 hour); and a long interview (2 hours and 35 minutes). I would like to underline that the fact that a doctor devoting 4 hours of his time to a foreign doctoral student is rare and highly unusual.

In order to prepare for the interview, I had previously sent a set of questions and reserved a second set for the interview itself. Dr. Matsuda had answered the first series of questions sent by email in the form of a very well-crafted PowerPoint©. Let us mention here some historical elements before proceeding to the interview. The current *jidō sōdanjo* was first created under the name of *jidōin* (児童院) in English "House of Children". It was part of the child welfare and maternal child protection services which were in charge immediately after the war to protect mothers and orphans. Today, it is part of the child welfare (*jidō fukushi*) system. Dr. Matsuda's detailed explanation (about 4 hours) met my expectations without me having to formally ask all the questions I had. In a sense—and unlike the other interviews—it was Dr. Matsuda who "directed" the interview. However, I consented to this situation for the following reasons. In the Japanese social context, medical authority is well established: Dr. Matsuda spent a whole half day, and the agreement of this privilege deterred me from any attempt to conduct a semi-directive interview in good and due form, since our interlocutor had decided otherwise. Further, seeing that I had met Dr. Matsuda following my own lecture, and in a way, by providing a PowerPoint© and commenting extensively on it, he himself wished to return the favor in this scholarly format. This appointment was, therefore, the second time of the exchange.

Dr. Matsuda controlled the meeting from beginning to end, and instead of letting me conduct a research interview, he produced a private, semi-directive conference with respect to his two interlocutors. When we sat down and started talking, Dr. Matsuda paused, saying "good, now the interview." I had a brief moment where I was going to start asking my first question but was interrupted by a long discussion commenting on his PowerPoint© presentation. I am not complaining about this situation, but rather mentioning it as a way of indicating how a Japanese medical doctor can control the situation from beginning to end and leave very little room for input from the "patient." Luckily, Dr. Matsuda let me ask several questions, allowed by the length of the meeting and the fact that I was there, not as a patient, but as a researcher. However, the range of time he has met with us (between 2 and 3 hours), is comparable to the duration of the first session of the patients he meets. In the first 20-minute interview, Dr. Matsuda explained that the main building is spread over three floors. On the third floor is a clinic (*kurinikku* or *shinryōsho*) where consultations are held with doctors (pediatrician, psychiatrist, ophthalmologist, orthopedist), and where eight nurses (*kango shi*) work, three of whom are under the direct authority of child psychiatrists. On the second floor is the rehabilitation center. On the 1st floor the main child and adolescent guidance center (*jidō sōdanjo*), where social workers (*kēsu wākā*) and psychologists are located. The third floor really looks like a hospital; its appearance and atmosphere are very different from the first floor where social workers and psychologists are located, and where the developmental guidance center is (*hattatsu sōdanjo*). In other words, the doctors and nurses are separately located on the third floor, and the others on the second and first floors.

In an adjacent building, there is a boarding school where young people can stay for 6 months to a year. Another building serves as an elementary school. Several other buildings are scattered in other parts of the city and some remain "secret" that are associated with the center. Child and adolescent psychiatrists are eleven, and six people practice psychological assessments for children and adolescents. Other psychologists handle issues of abuse and emotional disorders (*emoshonaru na mondai*) and practice psychotherapies.

The increase in the cases of developmental disorders (*hattatsu shōgai*)—particularly noticeable from 2005, according to Dr. Matsuda—caused an institutional reorganization that saw the creation of the center of developmental guidance (*hattatsu sōdanjo* abbreviated *hatso*), in a *jidō sōdanjo* specializing in the treatment of developmental disorders (*hattatsu shōgai wo senmon ni shien suru*). Indeed, this guidance center is the only one in the prefecture to treat children and adolescents with developmental disabilities. Dr. Matsuda drew our attention to a graph showing the number of psychiatrists per capita, and by prefecture. The guidelines of the Ministry of Health, Labor, and Welfare indicate that this number must remain at least 1 psychiatrist for every 80,000 inhabitants: the prefecture where I investigated is in a good position with a psychiatrist for every 35,000 inhabitants, unlike the Hokkaido prefecture, for example, which is close to one psychiatrist per 80,000 inhabitants. Another graphic also held our attention. It showed the considerable increase in the number of consultations for truancy: the increase was particularly spectacular over the 3 years of junior high school. We noted the low attendance of high school students, which was also observed in the guidance center X.

Children, families, and disability

In this prefecture, hospital beds are available for junior-high-aged students in four or five hospitals or clinics, although students are typically only referred to one of them. The practice of home visits is common, and physicians can participate, but its frequency depends on the services. The demographic distribution and its particular characteristics within the city must be noted. He tells us that, south of the city station, people can make more use of social assistance and entrust their difficulties. It is precisely in certain southern neighborhoods that I attended the activities of an NPO supporting *hikikomori*. These neighborhoods are associated with stigmatized groups in Japan: children of Korean migrants (*zainichi*), discriminated communities (*burakumin*), and poor people. The NPO receives few requests from the city center where traditionally middle and upper class families live. Applications for social assistance and mental health differ by neighborhood. According to Dr. Matsuda, the middle and upper classes do not give away their family secrets (*ie no himitsu*). When there is a child with developmental disabilities, for example, those family members who can, will take care of them rather than rely on public services: the difficulties and secrets remain within the family. According to Dr. Matsuda, the fact, for example, that the grandparents accept the grandson as he is, is a positive point. But the negative point is that nobody talks about it, that it remains hidden. When discussing these issues, Dr. Matsuda raised the idea that poor nuclear families in some southern neighborhoods of the city can "open their secret" to social assistance, unlike the wealthier families in the city center. Dr. Matsuda said that this was valid for this city but that each prefecture has its own culture.

As family issues began to emerge in Dr. Matsuda's speech, I asked him about the theoretical possibility of trauma transmission from the generation of grandparents to the grandchildren, via the parents. To do this, I used an example of the trauma caused by the suicide of a grandparent which can be transmitted, by the parent, to the grandchildren, via the mechanism of identification. I explained that in France, there is a theory of the transmission of psychic life between generations (Ciccone 1999, Halfon, Ansermet, and Pierrehumbert 2000, Guyotat 2005). If trauma occurs in the grandparents' generation, it is possible that it is transmitted, in some cases, to the generation of grandchildren. In this sense, Pierre Legendre proposed the expression "symbolic permutation of places over generations," and a more psychopathological dimension was built in the case of "the relic child" (Legendre 1996). As part of the reflections on family secrets undertaken by Nicolas Abraham and Maria Torök, the psychopathological dimension is represented, in part, by the notion of a "crypt," defined as the "burial of a shameful and unspeakable experience." I did not explain these ideas to my interlocutor, but I did tell him that in this context, for example, the psychosis of a grandchild may be related to the suicide of a grandparent, as part of a theory of psychic causality through the development of the concept of identification (or lack thereof). However, it seems that there are no such theories in Japan. This cultural difference was already mentioned, at least in one of its aspects, in Lock's (1986: 105) work: "Unlike their Western counterparts, in Japanese psychotherapies, exploration of family dynamics in terms of the affective responses of family members towards one or the other is very rarely undertaken." Nevertheless, Dr. Matsuda added one clarification for the Japanese context. According to Dr. Matsuda, in Japan, transmission is seen at the social and biological level, but not psychologically. For example, he said that there is a phenomenon called *kakusei iden*, which has not been systematically theorized, but nonetheless touches upon how symptoms (e.g., low intelligence, physical symptoms, *shinkeishitsu*) skip a generation. As a concrete example he explained how a trait of a grandparent, like scratching his hand, can be found in a grandchild without going through the parent. Dr. Matsuda explained the phenomenon to us without any theory implying a psychological cause of the symptom. In other words, a physical symptom skips a generation, but the type of causation invoked is not included in an explanatory and systematic theory. This insistence on the biological and the social, to the detriment of the psychological, has been highlighted in Kitanaka's (2012) ethnographic survey. Beyond this insistence on the biological and the social, I have already emphasized the presence of a third element that is neither completely biological, nor social, nor psychological: it is "the heart" (*kokoro*), irreducible to "psyche."

Child and adolescent psychiatry

Dr. Matsuda detailed his career as a means to discuss the issue of training in child and adolescent psychiatry. After joining the department of medicine at X University, he wanted to become a researcher but gave up when the national university became institutionalized and bureaucratized in the direction of privatization. What our interlocutor refers to as the abbreviated term *doppoka* is a set of measures established between 2001 and 2006—during the government of Prime Minister Koizumi Junichiro—under the name *dokuritsu hōjinka*. Dr. Matsuda found this "very boring," and therefore abandoned research. He was trained in internal medicine (*naika*); anatomy and developmental biology; and pediatrics (*shōnika*); but finally pivoted his career by becoming a child and adolescent psychiatrist. He repeatedly mentions his training under his teacher who instructed him in child and adolescent psychiatry.

Indeed, there is no university path in medicine to become a child and adolescent psychiatrist. Those who are child and adolescent psychiatrists are doctors—and some are already psychiatrists—who have done additional individual training with a specialist and recognized medical doctor. In many universities there are none, and at X University there is only one. The doctor does a training course with him, as part of an individual master-student relationship. Although child and adolescent psychiatrists are doctors, their consultation activities are not completely reimbursed by medical insurance, which makes their clinical practice in a private office difficult for financial reasons. In the guidance center J, child and adolescent psychiatrists are paid by the city. Brief consultations giving rise to the prescription of psychotropic medication are reimbursed, but not psychotherapy sessions of half an hour or an hour. This is one of the concrete reasons for the small number of child and adolescent psychiatrists in Japan, another reason being the weakness of academic societies (*gakkai*). Note that the Ministry of Health, Labor and Welfare authorizes very few psychotropic drugs for children (e.g., Prozac® is not allowed), but refuses simultaneously to refund consultations if, for example, Concerta® (for ADHD), Olap® (for autism), or other Selective serotonin reuptake inhibitors (SSRIs) are not prescribed.

Regarding the relations with the other guidance center, it should be noted that the child psychiatrists of guidance center J supervise psychologists and teachers of guidance center X. If the latter provides for consultations and a school for the *futōkō* children, it sends to guidance center J the cases "resistant to care": the referral is operated in consultation with child and adolescent psychiatrists. The act of referring a patient from one center to another can be marked by making an appointment with a child and adolescent psychiatrist, or a request for psychological assessment. This involves the recognition of professionals and parents that the child or adolescent has a psychiatric condition, or serious mental and cognitive difficulties. The 10 other child psychiatrists in the center usually take about 2 hours for the first appointment, but in his case, it can last up to 4 hours. "Like Winnicott?" I naively asked Dr. Matsuda. "Not really," he replied. He said he sees about 10 people a day from 9 am to 5 pm. The duration of the psychotherapies is 1 hour—as for most of his colleagues at the center—in what he stands out from his master in child and adolescent psychiatry who received more than 80 patients a day, each 5 minutes. He uses many different theories and techniques within his therapeutic practice. He asserts that this center is very special, and that one can absolutely not generalize to all centers and child and adolescent psychiatrists in Japan: "In this guidance center, there is a specific child and adolescent psychiatry culture," he told us.

As we have seen with Dr. Matsuda, the situation of Japanese child and adolescent psychiatry is complex. He himself is a doctor, but not a psychiatrist, and even without being a certified child and adolescent psychiatrist, he works as a child and adolescent psychiatrist. He is not alone in this case. At the national level, not all Japanese child and adolescent psychiatrists are certified doctors (*ninteii*) of the Japan Society for Child and Adolescent Psychiatry (JSCAP). The list of certified doctors in this association, therefore, offers the minimum measurable number of Japanese child and adolescent psychiatrists (206). The actual figure of doctors or psychiatrists working with children and adolescents, as child and adolescent psychiatrists, is, therefore, higher, without it being possible to obtain—for the moment—their exact census. On the other hand, we know that child and adolescent psychiatrists who are not certified by the Japanese Society for Child and Adolescent Psychiatry (JSCAP) are certified by other associations. They are mainly distributed into four associations: The Japanese Society of Psychiatry and Neurology (JSPN), The Japanese Society of Pediatric Psychiatry and Neurology (JSPPN), The Japanese Society of Psychosomatic Pediatrics (JSPP), and The Japan Pediatric Society (JPS). As of April 1, 2013, the 206 Japanese doctors who are certified doctors by the Japanese Society of Child and Adolescent Psychiatry (JSCAP) are unequally distributed in the territory. Forty-eight of these certified child and adolescent psychiatrists work in forty-six universities. The name of the place of practice of child and adolescent psychiatrists certified by the JSCAP mentions the term *kokoro* (heart) in 20 cases. Of these, he is employed with the term *shinryō* (clinic) in eight cases; the term *kurinikku* (heart clinic) in three cases; and it is associated with "care" in two cases. Four university departments where these child and adolescent psychiatrists work include the term *kokoro* in the name of their service. According to Dr. Matsuda, there are actually 206 JSCAP-certified doctors today, but in 2008, there were only 150, and in 1992 we know that they were at least 103. Dr. Matsuda was himself a part of this academic society, but left it recently because of overly expensive annual dues. He complains that there is no third-party institution that certifies specialists (*senmon.i*). As of April, 2020, there are 388 Japanese doctors who are certified by the Japanese Society of Child and Adolescent Psychiatry (JSCAP).

Guidance centers nationwide

In Table 2.1, we observe that child and adolescent guidance centers (*jidō sōdanjo*) are the privileged place for the treatment and management of intellectual disability, with impressive increases in certain kinds of consultation

Table 2.1 Number of "first consultations/initial intakes" (*kensū*) in guidance centers (*jidō sōdanjo*) nationwide between 1954 and 2008 (Kawasaki et al. 2013: 64)

Consultations	1954	1961	1972	1989	1990	2002	2003	2008
Motor disorders	2755	14,456	16,956	16,697	16,123	11,581	7,705	6849
Sight, language, hearing disorders	1236	3426	14,072	23,495	–	–	–	–
Language development disorders, etc.	–	–	–	–	28,237	19,642	19,694	14,865
Intellectual disorder	4861	23,016	41,327	87,624	88,780	149,627	111,085	131,778
Autism	–	–	1542	3693	4051	11,927	10,178	14,864
School nonattendance	–	3329	3858	8378	13,933	10,234	10,948	7557
Discipline and education (*shitsuke*)	–	10,902	28,299	20,666	18,705	12,118	11,330	7719

between 1989 and 2008. In less than 20 years, the number of consultations for people with autism more than quadrupled (3693:14,864). In order to facilitate a clear reading of this table, let us specify that the number of consultations listed here concerns the first consultations (*kensū*). In other words, for the year 2008, 14,864 cases of autism were registered in Guidance centers *jidō sōdanjo*. This figure is significantly lower than the number of children and adolescents with autism in Japan, because they can be supported by other structures (hospitals, clinics, NGOs, NPO).

Regarding the number of initial consultations for children in school absenteeism, we note that after a sharp increase in 1990 (13,933), it stabilized around 10,000. Then, it decreased significantly in 2008 (7557), returning to a figure comparable to that of 1989 (8378). We can explain this figure by the multiplication of initiatives around absenteeism: not only the expansion of the network of school counselors but also the creation of services such as guidance center X. Today, guidance centers *jidō sōdanjo* are not the privileged place of care for children and adolescents in school absenteeism: it hosts a subcategory of them that have posed multiple problems to professionals upstream: domestic violence, psychiatric pathology of a parent, absence of parents, precarious social situations, and delinquency.

We also observe the appearance of categories of consultations. As early as 1961, consultations on the grounds of absenteeism (*futōkō*) and on grounds of discipline (*shitsuke*) took place. In 1972, consultations began to be identified for reasons related to autism, and in 1990, consultations were held on the grounds of "language development disorder, etc." Conversely, certain categories disappeared such as disorders of sight, language and hearing (1990), as well as various forms of rehabilitation.

Counseling at University with Prof. Kubo

I had met Prof. Kubo many times from April 2011 onward, but the first long informal conversation I had with him took place during a specific event in July 2013 when I worked as a Japanese-English translator for a foreign researcher visiting Japan during a conference. After the symposium, some participants met for dinner, during which I was able to schedule an interview with Prof. Kubo. We met on October 29, 2013, from 10 am to 3 pm where I conducted an interview in Japanese without an interpreter present. The recorded research interview lasted 2 hours and 12 minutes in total, but the meeting, including lunch, was spread over 5 hours of conversation. At 10 o'clock in the morning, I was on a campus with 100-year-old trees and a new university library powered by solar panels visible from the outside. The university was under renovation, and Prof. Kubo could not receive me in her office. On the way, she informed me that the university was created after World War II, in facilities that were used by the imperial army until their defeat. Today, this university has a junior high and a high school and enjoys a solid reputation in the field of education studies.

Counseling and psychotherapy

The interview with Prof. Kubo started with a naïve question: "What is the difference between counseling and psychotherapy?" Prof. Kubo evoked the past and present regulations of psychotherapy implemented by the Ministry of Health, Labor and Welfare. Then, she showed a pamphlet describing the university's guidance services (*sōdan shitsu*, lit. "consultation room"). This pamphlet illustrated the difference between psychotherapy and counseling: although the words psychotherapy (*seishin ryōhō*) or therapy (*ryōhō*) were never mentioned, *sōdan* (meaning "consultation," "guidance," or "counseling") was systematically written. In people's minds, psychotherapy designates "what is reimbursed by medical insurance (*iryō hoken*)," Prof. Kubo says. *Kaunseringu* (counseling) and *sōdan* are not reimbursed, as clearly explained in the pamphlet. In this sense, a consultation room is rooted in the Japanese tradition where clinical aspects of a student's psychology are founded on the basis of educational assumptions: here, located in the faculty of education (*kyōiku gakubu*) of a university of education (*kyōiku daigaku*). This heritage can also be seen through the name of the consultation space: *shinri kyōiku sōdan shitsu*. *Kyōiku sōdan* means "educational guidance," *shinri kyōiku* means "psycho-education," and "*shinri kyōiku sōdan shitsu*" could be translated as "psycho-educational consultation room" or "psycho-educational guidance space."

I expressed my surprise and told her how I felt psychotherapy was poorly represented at the 108th Symposium for the Japanese Society of Psychiatry and Neurology (JSPN). I asked Prof. Kubo: "Do Japanese psychiatrists have an interest in psychotherapy? Is psychotherapy the job of psychologists or psychiatrists? Her answer was based on Ministry of Health and Labour documents available on the Internet:

> "Is this the job of psychiatrists? Oh ... well, it's therapy, isn't it? "Therapy". But ... if you think that what the clinical psychologists do is psychotherapy, then that's not always the case ... clinical psychologists can do counseling outside of the medical insurance, and psychotherapy is reimbursed by it [...] concerning psychotherapies in Japan, to answer simply: It's both!" Prof. Kubo says.

I then specified that psychotherapy lasts 20–30 minutes (generally and at least) and that it is unlikely that Japanese psychiatrists, as a whole, can devote so much time to their patients. Obviously, I have encountered exceptions such as Dr. Matsuda, psychiatrists from Nagoya University, and some other independent psychiatrists–psychoanalysts, but they do not represent the majority of Japanese psychiatrists, especially those of the JSPN. I insisted that psychiatrists have little time and supposed that psychotherapies are more practiced by clinical psychologists. Prof. Kubo seemed to understand my reasoning and showed signs of approval: indicating that the practice of psychiatrists is similar to other forms of medical consultation (*shinsatsu*) rather than being a therapy in itself. She distinguished big hospitals, where a large number of patients come every day for consultations, and smaller clinics, where practicing physicians (*kaigyōi*) are in charge of psychotherapies. It depends on the clinic, and the "way of thinking and doing" of the doctor in charge of the clinic, according to Prof. Kubo.

After my years of fieldwork and clinical practice in Japan, I came to the conclusion that only a minority of Japanese psychiatrists are practicing or are interested in psychotherapy. Although I almost exclusively met with this nonrepresentative minority, this conclusion concurs with the previous research (Lock 1982, 1986, Kitanaka 2003, 2012), and Prof. Kubo confirms this fact.

Family therapy and parallel consultation

I was surprised at almost never having met Japanese practitioners consulting parents and children together in the same room. They offer counseling to the parent; the child alone; sometimes the parents together; more rarely the mother and the child; and very exceptionally father, mother, and child together. My first impressions were "This is not really family therapy" and I asked, "What do you think of this method, this way of doing interviews (*mensetsu hōhō*)? Prof. Kubo laughed, no doubt, because of the abrupt nature of my reasoning, and slight embarrassment. As a specialist in family therapy, Prof. Kubo's answer is highly relevant. She asked to read my question and reacted in the following way: "We don't have any other choice!", meaning that it was difficult to gather the three members of the family together, and even dangerous (*kiken*) without sufficient training in family therapy. The setting of the parallel consultation (*heikō mensetsu*) is quite common: usually, mother and child come at the same time to be counseled separately by two psychologists. If the child comes alone, he pays 1500 yen; if the mother comes alone, she pays 1500 yen; but if they come together, at the same time, they pay 2000 yen in total, and they are each received by a different psychologist, in a different room. This parallel consultation practice consists of receiving mother and child at the same time, by two different people, who can then communicate about the situation in the meeting. She adds that the parallel consultation is practiced in other guidance centers, such as guidance center X, which I was not aware of until now. She adds, "interviews with parents are frequent, but there are also cases where mother and father are received at the same time separately." Because we are in a university that trains psychologists, Prof. Kubo supervises the two psychologists together after each counseling session.

Then she asked me what I meant by "true family therapy." I answered that the setting must involve mother, father, and child together in the same room. According to her, in this sense, even though the parallel consultation is not "true" family therapy, if the child and the mother are not in the same room, we can still talk about family therapy. In other words, it is not necessary to gather all the members of the family to use the term family therapy: "family therapy" is conceived as "a way of thinking" (*kangaekata*) where the family plays an essential role in the therapy. Today, she is no longer doing family therapy in the sense of therapy where the whole family is received, a family interview (*kazoku mensetsu*), although she had practiced it regularly during her studies. The parallel consultation—which is practiced in her university and which, as she reminds us, is very widespread in Japan—is used with a particular intention:

> There are things that the mother doesn't want her child to know, and there are things that the child doesn't want his/her mother to know. So in Japan, we think that it could be okay to treat them separately, in different rooms, in order for them to say what they deeply feel to the counselor.
>
> *(Prof. Kubo)*

Finally, Prof. Kubo adds that the most difficult thing about meeting patients is when adults simply give up and abandon a student. For example, teachers have to care about a lot of difficult situations concerning students and parents, and when a student becomes delinquent, the burden is so heavy that the teachers hope he or she will drop out of school as soon as possible. In this sense, the most difficult psychotherapies are those when a high-school student drops out. Because high school is not a part of compulsory education (*gimu kyōiku*), the awareness of the necessity of continuing to go to school is particularly low among the teachers, the parents, and the students. Students think "maybe I could work part-time?", and because their parents and teachers often do not support them, they drop out. According to Prof. Kubo, the lack of recognition that "high school dropouts are a problem" is itself a serious problem.

Conclusions

What we have learned

This investigation describes how psychological counseling spread, mostly due to the issue and treatment of school nonattendance, especially at the junior-high school level. It is the responsibility of the school counselor (e.g., Ms. Otsuka), and, in guidance center X., truants and their parents represent 50% of the cases. The pervasive influence of education is striking: *kyōiku sōdan* (educational guidance) and *seito shidō* (student discipline) are two important traditional markers of Japanese school culture. They extend their influence to guidance centers. In other terms, they contribute to structuring counseling practices outside the school setting by nurturing them with educational assumptions, one of the main problems being the insistence on "compulsory education." As we have seen in the four interviews, the strong support in junior-high school suddenly and brutally stops in high school, provoking an abandonment of the dropouts.

Supplementary aspects should be discussed, such as the parents' refusal of psychological testing due to fears that the child could be diagnosed with a mental disorder (Borovoy 2008). It should be underlined that the Japanese educational system is now experiencing a considerable and problematic shift of teachers' authority from an excess of discipline to a lack of discipline. This phenomenon could be put in perspective with the problems related to an aging society (e.g., the number of children is decreasing) and the competition among schools to attract students (a subject worthy of further investigation).

These interviews help to clarify the complexity of Japanese psychologists' and counselors' certifications and its underlying issues. In brief, the AJCP maintains, on one hand, its control of the clinical psychologists' certification through the FJCBCP. On the other hand, nearly 50 academic societies form the Japanese Union of Psychological Associations (JUPA), advocating for a national psychologist license (*shinri shi no kokka shikaku*). It should be noted that the AJCP and FJCBCP are members of the JUPA but have no interest in the JUPA succeeding in establishing the national licensing system because it would mean the end of the FJCBCP's business. As of 2016, the JUPA did not succeed, partly because of the heterogeneity of the affiliated associations, and partly because of the popularity of the AJCP, which, through the FJCBCP, developed a well-established system of certification. Consequently, it is not possible to know the total number of psychologists with a clinical practice in Japan. Because some of them have two or more certifications, it is not possible to establish an accurate number by collecting the JUPA's data. The most reliable number is the number of certified clinical psychologists (26,329), which is the minimum number of psychologists with a clinical practice in Japan. The most reliable number of medical doctors working as child and adolescent psychiatrists is also a lowest estimation, namely 206 child and adolescent psychiatrists certified by the JSCAP.

From the point of view of child, adolescent and youth studies, an important question should be discussed: What does it mean to be a child in Japan? As we have shown, the consequences of a powerful educational system invading every sphere of individuals' lives might reach to the extent of reducing the child to a student. What are the consequences in terms of the adolescents' development, maturation, and identity? What does it mean to be an adolescent in Japan when your identity is defined only as a student? Also, some individuals dropping out during high school might never make the transition from "student" to "worker," and they could spend years as "shut-ins" in a situation that some would call "never-ending adolescence" (Saitō 1998, 2013). I suggest that the overwhelming role that education plays in Japanese society might prevent an increasing number of students from being effective adolescents and delay the experience of adolescence until adulthood. It may also contribute to a problematic emerging adulthood (Arnett, Žukauskienė, and Sugimura 2014) as I will explain in the last chapters.

Proposals

I would like to make proposals that could stimulate new countermeasures in Japanese politics regarding youth and adolescence. The school counselor system should be strengthened. This is primarily because it is too weak at the junior-high school level, and second because the status given to school counselors remains dramatically different from one junior-high school to another. In fact, school counselors are available in almost every junior-high school, but the ways in which they cooperate with the teachers' teams are very different, depending upon the school. This prevents the establishment of a clear school counselor image for students and their parents. Since the employment contract is renewed every year, the lack of job security remains a major problem in the Japanese school counselor system. In some cases, it might result in a feeling of insecurity among the students, their parents, and the teachers themselves (Will the counseling continue next year with the same psychologist?), as well as the reinforcement of hierarchical and authoritarian positions among tenured employees and others. In this sense, the school counselor's status should be strengthened.

The number of high school dropouts could be contained by assuring the continuity of counseling between junior-high school and high school. Counseling services should be implemented in high schools in order to prevent students from dropping out. The best solution may be to reinforce the school counselor system, which is too weak at the high school level. It is not well-developed because high school is not compulsory, but we have to keep in mind that it is during high school that student dropouts can start becoming shut-ins (*hikikomori*), or developing major psychopathologies. An expansion of school counselor systems from primary school to high school requires sufficient specialized training of professionals. In this respect, clinical psychologists and counselors working in high schools should be sufficiently trained in adolescent psychopathology and family therapy. Emphasizing their presence among high schools is necessary because teachers are not trained in psychopathology, psychotherapy, or psychoanalysis, and also because psychological counseling implies a meeting with someone whose status is different from that of a teacher. Also, it should be underlined that Japanese teachers' overwork (e.g., a hundred of home-visits per year, city-patrols, and 52–60 hours of work per week) could damage their mental health and classes' quality.

These proposals for the reinforcement of psychological counseling of adolescents are ways to better prevent school nonattendance, dropouts, and social withdrawal. As a whole, this study takes into account deep changes in Japanese society and discusses the impact of education on adolescence and emerging adulthood. Eventually, it becomes the responsibility of psychologists and counselors to invent a practice that fits Japan's contemporary social setting and cultural heritage. In further investigations, the pervasive rhetoric that emphasizes the role of *kokoro* (heart and mind) in health and education should be an item for deeper analysis.

What's new

In 2015, I wrote that a controversial topic lay in the following question: Should it be required that every school counselor be a certified clinical psychologist?

Obviously, certification does not always mean high competency, but a strong certification could clarify the professional identity, mission, and role of the counselor. Regarding the issue of "certification," we have described a complex situation. If the certification of clinical psychologists (*rinshō shinri shi*) is satisfying, the monopoly of the FJCBCP and the influence of the AJCP could be considered a problem. Nevertheless, a unique certification established through the JUPA seems impossible because of the heterogeneity of its affiliated associations. On this point, Japanese psychologists' and counselors' academic communities should find solutions to allow for a certification of psychologists and counselors with a clinical approach that could make things clear for parents, students, and teachers (Tajan 2015).

The decision for a national license was made in 2017, and Japan produced its first licensed psychologists (*kōnin shinri shi*) in September 2018. What are their qualifications? First, there is a transitional measure stipulating that applicants must have at least 5 years of psychological support experience. Second, beginning in 2019, the standard qualification procedure requires applicants to have studied necessary courses in undergraduate and graduate schools (i.e., possess a master's degree), or studied necessary courses in undergraduate school and worked in specified institutions for at least 2 years. Consequently, it is not mandatory to have a master's degree or a certification from a private organization to become a licensed psychologist.

As of the beginning of this year, many of the applicants hold a master's degree and a certification from a private organization. Applicants include clinical psychologists (*rinshō shinri shi*), school psychologists (*gakkō shinri shi*), and family psychologists (*kazoku shinri shi*), among others. There are more than 40 certifications related to psychology and counseling (Grabosky, Ishii, and Mase 2012), and, among them, the growing importance of the certification of clinical psychologists, provided by a private foundation, raised serious issues and concerns. The very fact that these certifications are granted by private organizations, and that some of them are made compulsory to be recruited into universities, welfare services, and hospitals, urges control initiatives by the State. Public institutions prefer to rely on public licenses. Are certifications going to disappear with the rise of licensed psychologists? It is possible that the majority of clinical psychologists will take the exam and become licensed psychologists. However, it is not clear if the number of licensed psychologists will be controlled or limited. On the other hand, it seems likely that licensed psychologists will maintain their memberships in at least one association to reinforce their professional identities and sense of belonging in a community.

It is likely that the number of clinical psychologists will drop dramatically in the years to come. Up until 2017, the title of clinical psychologist, normatively constraining, filled a role that will now be filled by licensed psychologists. Should clinical psychologists become licensed psychologists? Would it make sense to hold this certification and the license simultaneously? It seems obvious that a great number of current clinical psychologists will abandon their certification and become licensed psychologists, while a relatively small number might remain clinical psychologists or hold both a certification and a license. Due to financial and training constraints, it will be too expensive and unnecessary for most people to hold both a certification and a license. The exception will be for those who feel a strong sense of belonging to that community or who are implicitly pressured by their peers, employers, or mentors.

Satō (2007) wrote that clinical psychology was "a new and confused academic area in Japan." While we are certainly witnessing a decrease in the influence of clinical psychologists, what about the clinical knowledge of licensed psychologists? What about the pluralism of the Japanese counseling culture? While the rise of licensed psychologists is undoubtedly a sign of increasing control of counseling professions by the State, it is still uncertain if this profound transformation of the field will bring more professionalism, creativity, recognition by consumers, and therapeutic efficiency. Most of all, what about the dropouts? What about children who do not go to school? They have long been invisible, and their voices unheard. But they caught the public eye (Horiguchi 2012) when shut-in adults *hikikomori* became widely discussed in the Japanese media.

References

Arnett, Jeffrey, Rita Žukauskienė, and Kazumi Sugimura. 2014. "The New Life Stage of Emerging Adulthood at Ages 18–29 Years: Implications for Mental Health." *Lancet Psychiatry* 2014 (1): 569–576.

Borovoy, Amy. 2008. "Japan's Hidden Youths: Mainstreaming the Emotionally Distressed in Japan." *Culture, Medicine and Psychiatry* 32: 52–56.

Cave, Peter. 2007. *Primary School in Japan. Self, Individuality and Learning in Elementary Education.* London: Routledge, Japan Anthropology Workshop Series.

Ciccone, Albert. 1999. *La transmission psychique inconsciente.* Paris: Dunod.

Grabosky, Tomoko Kudo, Harue Ishii, and Shizuno Mase. 2012. "The Development of the Counseling Profession in Japan, Past Present and Future." *Journal of Counseling and Development* 90: 221–226.

Guyotat, Jean. 2005. "Traumatisme et lien de filiation." *Dialogue* 168: 15–24.

Halfon, Olivier, François Ansermet, and Blaise Pierrehumbert. 2000. *Filiations psychiques.* Paris: Presses Universitaires de France.

Horiguchi, Sachiko 堀口佐知子. 2012. "Hikikomori: How Private Isolation Caught the Public Eye." In *A Sociology of Japanese Youth, From Returnees to Neet.* Edited by Roger Goodman, Yuki Imoto, and Tuukka Toivonen. Oxon: Routledge.

Kawasaki, Fumihiko 川﨑二三彦, Tsunefumi Fujii 藤井常文, Tetsuo Takenaka 竹中哲夫, Kōichi Ishida 石田公一, Takayuki Suzuki 鈴木崇之, Tamio Koide 小出太美夫, and Rintarō Aizawa 相澤林太郎. 2013. *Heisei 22·23 nendo kenkyū hōkokusho - Jidō sōdanjo no arikata nikansuru kenkyū—jidō sōdanjo nikansuru rekishi nenpyō—* 平成22·23年度研究報告書 - 児童相談所のあり方に関する研究—児童相談所に関する歴史年表—(Research and History of Guidance Centers – Studies of years 2010-2011). http://www.crc-japan.net/contents/guidance/pdf_data/H22-23jisou.pdf.

Kitanaka, Junko. 2003. "Jungians and the Rise of Psychotherapy in Japan: A Brief Historical Note." *Transcultural Psychiatry* 40: 239–247.

———. 2012. *Depression in Japan, Psychiatric Cures for a Society in Distress.* Princeton, NJ: Princeton University Press.

Legendre, Pierre. 1996. *Filiation, leçon 4, suite 2 : Fondement généalogique de la psychanalyse.* Paris: Fayard.

Letendre, Gerald K. 1995. "Disruption and Reconnection: Counseling Young Adolescents in Japanese Schools." *Educational Policy* 9 (2): 169–184.

Lock, Margaret. 1982. "Popular Conceptions of Mental Health in Japan." In *Cultural Conceptions of Mental Health and Therapy*, edited by A. J. Marsella and G. M. White, 215–233. Dordrecht: D. Reidel Publishing.

———. 1986. "Plea for Acceptance: School Refusal Syndrome in Japan." *Social Science & Medicine* 23: 99–112.

———. 1995. *Encounters with Aging. Mythologies of Menopause in Japan and North America.* Berkeley, CA: University of California Press.

Saitō, Tamaki 斎藤環. 1998. *Shakaiteki hikikomori — owaranai shishunki* 社会的ひきこもり—終わらない思春期 (Social Hikikomori – Adolescence without End). Tōkyō: PHP Shinsho.

———. 2013. *Hikikomori: Adolescence without End.* Translated by Jeffrey Angles. Minneapolis: Minnesota University Press.

Satō, Manabu. 2007. "Les enseignants japonais dans une période charnière." In *Enseignants et écoles au Japon – Acteurs, système et contexte*, edited by Claude Lévi-Alvarès and Manabu Satō, 21–44. Paris: Maisonneuve et Larose.

Satō, Tatsuya. 2007. "Rises and Falls of Clinical Psychology in Japan: A Perspective on the Status of Japanese Clinical Psychology." *Ritsumeikan ningen kagaku kenkyū* 13: 133–144.

Shimizu, Hirokichi. 2007. "Le 'roman de formation' dans les collèges – Éducation et sélection dans l'orientation scolaire." In *Enseignants et écoles au Japon – Acteurs, système et contexte*, edited by Claude Lévi-Alvarès and Manabu Satō, 115–136. Paris: Maisonneuve et Larose.

Tajan, Nicolas. 2015. "Adolescents' School Non-Attendance and the Spread of Psychological Counselling in Japan." *Asia Pacific Journal of Counselling and Psychotherapy* 6 (1/2): 58–69.

Žukauskienė, Rita, et al. 2016. *Emerging Adulthood in a European Context*. London and New York: Routledge (Psychology Press).

3 Is social withdrawal a mental disorder?

A brief historical overview: Japanese psychiatry and social withdrawal

Stagnation of vital energy and nervous temperament

Although Japanese psychiatry was born at the beginning of the Meiji era, a number of mental illnesses were already present in the archipelago. This is particularly the case for the melancholy known in premodern times as *utsushō*. We are interested here because social withdrawal is one of its major symptoms: "Originally imported from China and incorporated into Japanese medical knowledge by the 16th century, *utsushō* was a category that indicated pathological stagnation leading to a wide range of symptoms including lack of energy, dejection, and social withdrawal." (Kitanaka 2012: 21). The melancholy of the time was characterized by a stagnant vital energy (*ki*) resulting in several symptoms including social withdrawal. In the premodern period, it is more generally a conception of mental illness in terms of the circulation of vital energy that predominates.

In modern conceptions, the role played by vital energy loses its importance in favor of a conception where the nerves (*shinkei*) are apprehended as the cause of mental illness. *Shinkei* has been present in the vocabulary of Japanese doctors since the publication of the Japanese translation of the treatise of anatomy of Johann Adam Kulmus in 1774 signifying the point when "nerves" as understood in Western medicine were translated into Japanese: "The most remarkable in the terminology adopted is the creation of new terms to designate parts of the body that Chinese medicine did not name." (Macé 2013: 103). In other words, the term *shinkei* was created in Japan by a small group of intellectuals, doctors, and translators in 1773, but its wide dissemination did not take place until the beginning of the 20th century via the appearance of discourse on "nervousness." With the popularization of this discourse the medicalization of ordinary suffering also began.

Concepts close to "neurasthenia" appear in works of the father of Japanese ethnology (*minzoku gaku*), Yanagita Kunio, in terms of nervous exhaustion (*shinkei suijaku*), and Morita Shōma in terms of "nervous temperament" (*shinkeishitsu*). Social withdrawal is one of the possible symptoms among neurasthenic or nervous-tempered individuals (appropriating the term *shinkeishitsu* or being labeled by others) that simultaneously tend to introspect in the context of a solitary life.

The famous writer Natsume Sōseki saw in the neurasthenia of him and his contemporaries, the manifestation of a sudden arrival in a modernity that they had not chosen. In 1903, one of his students – Fujimura Misao – jumped from the legendary waterfalls of Nikko. A sign of freedom for some, this event was welcomed by some of the doctors of the time as a means of weeding out the weak in society. In a speech published in the 1906 Journal of Neurology, Ōkuma Shigenobu – whose brother had a mental illness – said that "Those who jump off of a waterfall or throw themselves in front of a train are weak-minded. They do not have a strong enough mental constitution, and develop mental illness, dying in the end. How useless they are! Such weak-minded people would only cause harm even if they remained alive. [applause]" (cited by Kitanaka 2012: 59). As suggested in Ōkuma's statement, Fujimura's suicide also inaugurated the denigration and cruel treatment of suicides and the mentally ill, particularly by those who would treat them. For instance, the forensic scientist Katayama Kuniyoshi stated that suicides "dispersing poison in society [and that the nation must] strengthen its body and mind so as it can eliminate such pathological molecules" (cited by Kitanaka 2012: 58). Statements such as these were not uncommon at the time, suggesting the violence of medical judgment with regard to suicides, mental patients and people with *shinkeishitsu*.

Shinkeishitsu, while falling within the framework of the vocabulary of nervousness, escapes medical definition, insofar as non-physicians and patients appropriate a term, using the term to refer to a type of personality or temperament. In a sense, *shinkeishitsu* can be considered the ancestor of the term *hikikomori*, especially in terms of the discomfort that it causes in medical doctors and psychiatrists who can hardly treat it. *Shinkeishitsu* is consistently associated with the name of its most fervent promoter, Morita Shōma, inventor of "Morita Therapy" (Morita 1928). He conceived the key to treatment was encouraging the patient to realize that what he is suffering from is not a real illness but simply his way of being: 60% of patients would be cured in less than 40 days, proving that neurasthenia was not an incurable hereditary predisposition. According to Kōra Takehisa, patients suffering from *shinkeishitsu* could return to their normal state thanks to the psychological changes induced by the Morita therapy. If this therapy is relatively well-known internationally, it is anecdotal today in the Japanese psychiatric care landscape. The interest of citing it here stems from the resonance between the negative discourse of *shinkeishitsu* and recent discourse that look down upon men who do not correspond to the dominant masculine norms, which will be discussed later.

Psychiatrists and socially withdrawn youths

In some ways, we can speak of Japanese psychiatrists' ambivalence toward the *hikikomori*, or perhaps more accurately, their embarrassment. Since some of the *hikikomori* individuals suffer from psychiatric pathologies, and others do not, the *hikikomori* phenomenon is considered a prerogative of the Ministry of Education and the Ministry of Health, Labor and Welfare, concerning the measures for young people: prevention, assistance, occupational integration, and mental health. If, as we will see later, the NPOs play an important role, it is the psychiatrists who, insofar as they incarnate a recognized authority, are entrusted with a responsibility of which they do not know what to do, for it is uncertain as to whether these people are sick in the ways commonly conceived in psychiatry or psychology.

Japanese psychiatry developed under German influence between 1870 and 1930 and was characterized by biological and hereditary conceptions of mental illness, associated with a social Darwinism policy favoring the private and exponential detention of deviants. As a tool of oppression, exclusion, and stigmatization, the psychiatric tradition conceived mental illness as an infectious, shameful disease that must simultaneously remain secret (Kitanaka 2012: 42–43). The post-war period was marked by the American occupation, and characterized by a situation that remains quite unknown: "There was a brief period in Japanese psychiatry, in the aftermath of World War II, when the predominance of neurobiology was fundamentally shaken by the onslaught of psychoanalytic American psychiatry." (Kitanaka 2012: 48). At that time, the American model of "mental health" spread through new academic departments of psychoanalytic orientation, as well as by the American-led National Institute of Mental Health. In many ways, psychoanalysis imported to Japan in the aftermath of the Second World War was seen as the "psychiatry and mental health" component of the American occupation (1945–1952). Yet, it was also resisted because of this perception. In Japan, the books on neurosis (*noirōze*) became bestsellers and the media echoed worries about the increase in psychotropic prescriptions. Although there was much disagreement among Japanese psychiatrists with regard to American psychiatry, the great majority nevertheless agreed to define the object of psychiatry as "the biological mechanisms of psychosis," excluding any psychology of neuroses. It was the latter, in the form of American psychoanalysis at the time, which was gradually and overwhelmingly rejected by the psychiatrists of the archipelago. Japan, under the Occupation, therefore, on the one hand accepted the influence of American biological psychiatry, and on the other hand, resisted the influence of American psychoanalytic psychiatry.

More specifically, Japanese psychiatrists rejected an ego-psychology associated with drug prescription and psychotherapy, to achieve a theoretical renewal of neurobiology in psychiatry, boosted by expansion of private clinics and psychiatric hospitals, nationwide. The number of beds in psychiatry increased gradually from 173,000 in 1965, to 278,000 in 1975, and finally 334,000 in 1985 (Kitanaka 2012: 50). Instead of a deinstitutionalization, the common trend in Europe and North America, we have witnessed in Japan a boom in the institutionalization of the mentally ill. Takemi Tarō – the director of the Japanese Medical Association – ridiculed psychiatrists by calling them "stock farmers" (Kitanaka 2012: 50). Why might he say such a thing? The high growth period saw the multiplication of private psychiatric hospitals and clinics, resulting in many psychiatrists making large profits, and even positioning themselves as business leaders at times. Although I do not choose to undertake it here, let me emphasize that a history of Japanese psychiatry, particularly concerning its conflicted development in the second half of the 20th century, remains to be written. (Note: For an understanding of Japanese history of psychiatry, see Nakamura 2013: 35–69.)

Current Japan is in an atypical situation from a mental health perspective. Japanese psychiatry focuses on the continuous and important institutionalization of the mentally ill but remains perplexed by those who express their distress in the form of neuroses, or conditions such as social withdrawal (*hikikomori*). It is felt that the responsibility for their treatment lies with psychiatrists, but as we saw earlier, Japanese psychiatry always focused on heavy pathologies, excluding neuroses. It is quite likely that a non-negligible part of the *hikikomori* people are in situations where the prescription of psychotropic medications – a therapeutic mode largely proposed by psychiatrists – is insufficient, and where hospitalization is abusive. Psychiatrists, in addition to the fact that they rarely have time to devote themselves to these questions, find themselves triply embarrassed: First, they know that they can only treat a portion of these young people; second, NPO caregivers are not sufficiently trained in psychopathology, clinical psychology, and psychotherapy; finally, care is usually expensive, and some users refuse to view their situation as an illness. At least two subgroups of the *hikikomori* population actually in distress are not receiving appropriate care: those who refuse to be considered ill, and those who have modest incomes without community support.

Since the early 1980s in Japan, psychiatry has become part of the mental health field. At the same time, social withdrawal grew to become one of the major concerns of the youth policies of a nation the demography of which has been declining for three decades. I will now try to show how *hikikomori* became a topic of the psychiatric community.

First work of a psychiatrist on *hikikomori*

An author and his work

After completing his medical education at Tsukuba University in 1990, Saitō Tamaki first practiced as a psychiatrist at Sōfukai Sasaki Hospital in Funabashi City, east of Tōkyō, and now practices in a psychiatric clinic hosting *hikikomori* people. In April 2013, he became a professor of psychiatry at Tsukuba University. He is the author of numerous books on *hikikomori* (Saitō 1998, 2002, 2003, 2010a, 2012a, 2013), the "otaku subculture" (Saitō 2006, 2010b, Saitō and Azuma 2011), and popularizes Lacanian psychoanalysis (Saitō 2012b). He is a regular guest on television or print media and more recently advocates for open dialogue.

Shakaiteki Hikikomori – Owaranai Shinshunki (Social Hikikomori – Endless Adolescence) is the first book on *hikikomori* as a social phenomenon and mental health problem. It is broken down into two sections. The first section is entitled "What's going on?" The author questions himself about *hikikomori* (Chapter 1) and describes the symptoms and treatment of *hikikomori* (Chapter 2). Then, he describes the troubles that can accompany this situation (Chapter 3) and wonders if *hikikomori* is a disease (Chapter 4), to conclude by speaking about a "*hikikomori* system" (Chapter 5). In the second part, entitled "How to deal with *hikikomori*," he unfolds successively different themes, such as the need to go beyond our tendency to sermonize or lecture (Chapter 1). Then, he gives important information for the families (Chapter 2), describes the evolution of the treatment (Chapter 3), and daily life (Chapter 4), the sadness that underlies domestic violence (Chapter 5), the return to society (Chapter 6), and concludes by speaking of *hikikomori* as a "social pathology" (Chapter 7).

In the introduction to his book, Saitō states that he personally had to treat, for 10 years, 200 cases of *shakaiteki hikikomori*, and that his use of this name does not designate a disease (*byōmei*), but a symptom (*shōjō*) (Saitō 1998: 6). This psychiatrist thus presents three ways of considering the situation: It could be related to mental disorders (*seishin shōgai*), a reflection of the problems of the society, or related to family pathology (*kazoku byōri*) (Saitō 1998: 7).

The first lines of his first chapter (Saitō 1998. 16) are intended to impress the reader: He mentions the case of a schoolboy who was beaten to death by his father with a baseball bat. Here, a comment is needed. In Jeffrey Angles translation, the first sentence of the first chapter is as follows: "In November 1996 a tragic incident took place: a middle school student took a bat and beat to death his father, who was an office worker in Tōkyō." (Saitō 2013: 17) However, the Japanese version states: "*Heisei 8 nen 11 gatsu ni, Tōkyō no kaishain ga chūgakusei no musuko wo batto de nagurikorosu to iu, itamashii jiken ga arimashita,*" which means, "In November 1996 a tragic incident took place: an office worker in Tōkyō took a bat and beat to death his son, who was a middle school student." In other words, a schoolboy was beaten to death by his father, and not the opposite as in Jeffrey Angles' translation. Saitō points out that this boy was violent with his family members and had stopped going to school. A few weeks after the mother left home in November 1996, this schoolboy, one of the characteristics of which was his situation of social withdrawal, was killed by his father.

Typification and originality of Saitō Tamaki

The author presents four clinical vignettes. They are inspired by real cases treated by him, as well as others he has not treated, but as he himself acknowledges (Saitō 1998: 22), are fictitious cases. These cases are not pure fantasies, but are built by psychiatrists to illustrate certain typical aspects of a particular condition (Kato et al. 2012, Teo 2010). In other words, it is a research and dissemination methodology. Much like in quantitative methods, where no individual falls exactly on all averages, no case is purely typical. Consequently, the real cases are voluntarily typified by psychiatrists in order to construct an ideal-type of *hikikomori* that can enable them to conduct research. Needless to say, this ideal-type does not correspond to any real case. The argument that the motivation is to maintain the anonymity of the people is invalid, since other psychiatrists work from real cases without disclosing the identity of patients. However, I am not here to criticize this method, it is one way among others of thinking about a phenomenon and of obtaining results.

Saitō Tamaki's typification continues: *hikikomori* people are middle class or upper class, have a hard-working father who participates very little in child-rearing, and an overprotective mother (Saitō 1998: 22). Many Japanese could recognize themselves in this family portrayal. The young *hikikomori* reverses his day–night cycle, avoids his parents, and barricades himself in his room. In some cases, there is violence and suicide attempts. In general, they are rather worried. It was recognized that there were too few places of care in 1998 and that the socially withdrawn person found they could never escape the situation in which they found themselves.

When this author evokes the problems of diagnosis, he delivers a personal conception that opposes that of "other psychiatrists." According to him, the latter systematically diagnose the symptoms that accompany withdrawal instead of considering the withdrawal itself: A person in a state of withdrawal will be said to be suffering from obsessional neurosis (*kyohaku shinkeishō*) when they exhibit obsessional symptoms (*kyohaku shōjō*) or else will carry the diagnosis of "interpersonal fear disorder" (*taijin kyōfushō*) when they display corresponding symptoms (*taijin kyōfu shōjō*). This would be the conception of "other psychiatrists" that Saitō Tamaki opposes: for him, *hikikomori* has become a unique clinical situation. In order to understand how unusual this psychiatrist's conception is, let us be more precise. By writing "symptoms that accompany the withdrawal," he "decenters" the classic conception of psychiatric pathologies, because withdrawal is systematically considered as a symptom: Indeed, in the classifications, it is always withdrawal that constitutes one of the symptoms of a pathology, and never the pathology of withdrawal that would be accompanied by symptoms x or y. In other words, Saitō places withdrawal "in the center" and symptoms "around," while psychiatric classifications place a pathology P "in the center" and symptoms x or y (including social withdrawal) "around." And he takes the example of a case from his practice to illustrate this. It is a *hikikomori* patient who presents olfactory hallucinations; however, during treatment, this patient goes out of social withdrawal and develops a paranoid delusion, and finally obsessive-compulsive symptoms. Saitō Tamaki concludes that if we diagnose a case only from the symptoms, then the diagnosis changes with the symptoms (in this case, 3 times).

This psychiatrist is presented in Japan and the English literature as "Lacanian" but, for those who know Lacanian psychoanalysis, he delivers his own peculiar interpretation. Moreover, we can notice that through this example, he introduces, without ever saying it explicitly, an opposition between a classic psychiatric diagnosis, based on categories of classifications such as the DSM® or the ICD, and a diagnosis of structure as thought by the Lacanians. However, instead of talking about structure (*kōzō*), subject (*shutai*), and structure of the subject (*shutai no kōzō*), Saitō Tamaki speaks of "*hikikomori.*" This psychiatrist develops rather a hybrid conception, where one perceives, in addition to the antipsychiatric tendencies and the psychoanalytical orientations, a reference to the heart/mind (*kokoro*) typical of Japanese identity discourses: "social withdrawal is a problem which finds its origin in the heart," and it should not be thought in terms of cerebral pathology or psychosis. For him, *hikikomori* occurs when the adolescent fails to become an adult: This withdrawal situation reflects a lack of maturation and is experienced in a confrontational way by those concerned and who, in general, refuse care and any external intervention (Saitō 1998: 30–31).

First investigations about hikikomori (1983–1988)

The second chapter deals with symptoms and the development of social withdrawal. The author mentions the study he conducted between January 1983 and December 1988. The survey's inclusion criteria (Saitō 1998: 32) are different from those that were subsequently developed to define *hikikomori*. Here the survey focuses on young people who have neither schizophrenia (*sukizofurenia*), manic-depressive psychosis (*sōutsubyō*), nor endogenous psychosis (*kishitsu seishinbyō*). The withdrawal period is limited to 3 months before the first consultation; they had at least 6 months of treatment until June 1989, and came at least 5 times (this criterion is added because parents often come alone). These criteria made it possible to enroll 80 patients in the study. The age of the first consultation was between 12 and 34 years (mean age 19.6 years) and at the time of the survey, the age of the participants was between 13 and 37 years (average age 21.8 years).

The results are as follows (Saitō 1998: 33) the withdrawal period is on average 3 years and 3 months. Men are more numerous. The age of onset is 15.5 years, and 68.8% are related to absenteeism (*futōkō*). Subsequently, he mentions the fact that 90% of them (86% for a period of at least 3 months) experienced an episode of absenteeism (Saitō 1998: 39). It cannot be said that all students absent from school will experience *hikikomori*. However, among *hikikomori* people, the majority experienced a period of school absenteeism. Finally, families are middle-class and very few are divorced or live separately for professional reasons.

These results describe quite well part of the *hikikomori* population, but only a part. As Saitō Tamaki himself wrote, a number of patients were not enrolled in the study – all who came less than 5 times. Let us say that there are a lot of situations where the parents are coming to counseling sessions, and unless we make a home visit, we cannot meet the *hikikomori* person. The population met by Saitō Tamaki is already a subcategory within the *hikikomori* population. Also, there is a lack of information about the methodology that has allowed the collection of data, perhaps because the book targets a nonspecialized readership. Indeed, researchers can hardly use the fact that some of these patients ranging from 12 to 37 years of age have symptoms of interpersonal fear, others have obsessive symptoms, others are uncomfortable on the bus because they are looked at, others have dysmorphophobic symptoms that they treat without success through cosmetic surgery, others still sleep in their mother's bed or cannot sleep in another room, others are violent, others are persecuted, others are depressed, others have suicidal thoughts, and others have eating disorders. The same applies to his analogy that school absenteeism is to *hikikomori* as cold is to tuberculosis (Saitō 1998: 37–38). However, he uses an interesting notion that will be mentioned in the explanation of depression (Kitanaka 2012), menopause (Lock 1995), school refusal (Yoneyama 2000: 86), and *hikikomori* (Ueyama 2010). Indeed, Saitō Tamaki himself uses an explanation mobilizing the notion of equilibrium of the autonomic nervous system (*jiritsu shinkei no baransu*) when he evokes the reversal of the nycthemeral cycle of socially withdrawn individuals: An imbalance of the autonomic nervous system would be linked to lifestyle habits such as living at night, doing nothing and watching television, and therefore their difficulties in relaxing (Saitō 1998: 47). He also uses this notion when referring to his *hikikomori* patients who have eating disorders (Saitō 1998: 56).

In Chapter 3, Saitō insists again that "*hikikomori* is not the name of a disease," and works to distinguish it from schizophrenia. Indeed, *hikikomori* and schizophrenia both have the symptom of social withdrawal in common. Without going into the details mentioned by this psychiatrist to argue how these two conditions differ, let us mention two essential points. According to him, schizophrenia is endogenous, responds immediately and favorably to drug treatment, and is difficult for the analyst to put himself in the place of the patient who, for example, deploys strange behaviors such as bursts of laughter when he is alone, or suffers from strong delusions. According to him, *hikikomori* people differ in an essential but rather simple way: One can put oneself in their place. In other words, *hikikomori* people do not present the kind of difficulty in empathizing with which one has with the strangeness of people with illnesses such as schizophrenia. When *hikikomori* people have delusions or hallucinations, this psychiatrist distinguishes them from schizophrenics because they are, in the case of *hikikomori* people, caused by the situation of social withdrawal itself (Saitō 1998: 66). Finally, he recounts a technique learned from Dr. Kasugai Takehiko to distinguish social withdrawal the causality of which is psychogenic with the one with endogenous causality (e.g., schizophrenia). This technique, the effectiveness of which has been largely demonstrated according to Saitō Tamaki's own clinical experience, is to send a letter to the family who then transmits it to the patient: If the patient takes it in his hands and reads it or shows an interest, then the withdrawal is psychogenic and the diagnosis of schizophrenia can be rejected (Saitō 1998: 68). In the remainder of this third chapter, he demonstrates why *hikikomori* must also be distinguished from avoidant personality disorder (*kaihisei jinkaku shōgai*), or borderline personality disorder (*kyōkaisei jinkaku shōgai*), borderline (*kyōkairei*), delusional adolescence syndrome (*shishunki mōsōshō*), depression, schizoid personality disorder (*bunretsu byōshitsu shōgai*) or schizothymia (*seishin byōshitsu*), and cyclothymia (*junkansei kibun shōgai*).

An investigation of psychiatrists' representation (1992)

The fourth chapter is devoted to another way of answering the question of whether *hikikomori* is an illness or not. Saitō conducted a survey to see the representation of social withdrawal by psychiatrists in Japan, between April and May 1992. Of 303 people contacted, 99 were professors of psychiatry, 103 child and adolescent psychiatrists (members of the Japanese Society of Child and Adolescent Psychiatry), and 101 psychiatrists practicing in clinics or hospitals. Too few responses (102 questionnaires were returned), and their disproportion according to the three groups interviewed did not allow a rigorous study, but Saitō believes that some results were worth sharing. In this survey, psychiatrists were asked to consider patients in a situation of continuous social withdrawal for more than a year, whose situation would be of a psychogenetic nature, would have developed before 30 years, and would not have other symptoms (or some secondary symptoms: interpersonal fear, obsessive symptoms, domestic violence, mild feelings of persecution, etc.). The results were as follows:

Fifty-seven percent of psychiatrists had met this type of patient but did not think that their number had increased; 29% thought that their number had increased.

Fifty-seven percent believed that existing classifications can provide a diagnosis but are not accurate enough, while 22% would like a new diagnostic category.

Thirty-six percent of psychiatrists diagnosed an avoidant personality disorder; 2% said they diagnosed the symptoms that accompany the condition; and 23% diagnosed a withdrawal neurosis.

Fifty percent believed that treatment (*chiryō*) was necessary; and 48% believed that the need for treatment should be assessed on a case-by-case basis.

Eighty-seven percent believed that the treatment method (*chiryōhō*) should be psychotherapy (*seishin ryohō*); 67% drug therapy (*yakubutsu ryōhō*); and 37% considered treatment as part of hospitalization.

By "psychotherapy" 54.2% opted for family therapy (*kazoku ryōhō*), and 51.3% opted for a person-centered therapy (*raidansha chūshin ryōhō*) on an outpatient unit (Saitō 1998: 85–86). Note that the term *kazoku ryōhō*, if translated as "family therapy," can be misleading because family therapy was difficult to administer in Japan in 1992, and it still is today. It is very difficult to offer counseling to a father, mother, and child together; it is a little more common to gather mother and child; and it is very common to consult with the mother alone. It is therefore better to understand (here in this survey) *kazoku ryōhō* as a consultation first aimed at the parents, but ultimately it is the mothers who come, and in some cases the father or the patient, as we have seen in the previous chapter. Sixty percent of psychiatrists expected a change even if parents came alone. Regarding the activities that could help these patients to return to society, 56% of psychiatrists suggested a day care center, 34% a part time job (*arubaito*), and 22% a workplace adapted to the mentally disabled (*seishin shōgaisha no tame no sagyōjo*).

"Hikikomori system"

In Chapter 5, the author deepens his thinking about the "*hikikomori* system." He first tries to differentiate *hikikomori* from apathy (*mukiryōku*) or student's apathy syndrome (*gakusei mukiryōkushō*), while bringing his inquiry closer to that of addiction via the notion of vicious cycles (*akujunkan*). These vicious cycles would be present in the three systems that make up the *hikikomori* system of the individual, the family, and society. In addition, it accentuates the problems associated with relationships with others (*taijin kankei*), the lack of communication (*komyunikēshon no ketsujo*) of people in a *hikikomori* situation, and the disconnection (*kairi*) from the family system and social system (Saitō 1998: 106–108). Saitō Tamaki implicitly evokes here what I will describe later in terms of "double-*hikikomori*": The person concerned folds on itself, and the family, in turn, hiding the situation of the child, isolates him from the rest of society. This isolation of the family is accentuated by the fact that the child does not create an alliance with another family group. The developments on the "*hikikomori* system" are also extended in the second part of Chapter 5 where he discusses domestic violence. He considers that most of the *hikikomori* subjects he met who had shown domestic violence against their parents eventually admit that they were "terrible" (*dame na ningen*) with them: *hikikomori* subjects are daily torn between self-blame and reproach to others. In particular, he reports the example of a young man who stopped all violent acts against his mother as soon as his sister's fiancé came to live at home. He also mentions the possibility of calling the police but urges parents not to use private security companies. Another solution, in some cases, is to exclude the family.

He describes in great detail the story of a family where the young man became more and more violent until his mother fainted under his blows. Panicked, this young man was eager to tell his father to call for help. This crisis situation was then monitored by the psychiatrist who communicated regularly with the parents to show them how to react. Following this incident, the psychiatrist encouraged them not to mention the place of hospitalization and not to return home. In the evening, the father, from the hotel where he was going to spend the night, called his son who was staying at home: His son was worried that his mother would be dead or disabled and have to go to prison. The father replied that it was not so bad, but that she had to stay in the hospital and take exams. The psychiatrist told the mother that she should not communicate too much over the phone (a maximum of 5 minutes a day), and it was decided that she would go live with one of her sons for an undetermined period of time. The father returned home, and lived alone with his son. During a telephone call from the mother, the *hikikomori* son apologized very much at the beginning and then, seeing that the mother did not come back, thought that she was going to abandon him and reproached her for loving only the little brother. It was only after 2 months of absence from the mother that the patient really calmed down. The extra step was for the mother to come and pick up something she needed at home. The *hikikomori* patient replied that he would never let her come home. But on D-day, he was not at home. They did not see each other for 3 months. Very gradually, the mother came back to the home to spend a few nights, and later fully reintegrated after 5 months: The violence completely disappeared, and the *hikikomori* subject began to come out more and more.

How to rescue hikikomori individuals

The second part of the book is quite surprising: It could be described as the first self-help manual written by a Japanese "Lacanian" psychiatrist. This is claimed by the author who wants to tell parents how to deal with their child. Especially designed for the general public and parents, this second part was the draft of what the author would concretize 4 years later in a book called "Hikikomori Rescue Manual" (Saitō 2002). Despite its simplistic tone, a number of useful elements can be found. It is noted that the author manages to introduce the idea that the child wants to say something via his symptom (Saitō 1998: 122), and tries to raise awareness of the problem of mother–child interdependence, which is a recurring characteristic of *hikikomori* situations. Also, he invites us not to consider the young as lazy, but rather to restore a broken relationship of parent–child trust, and gives examples of sentences that disturbed parents: "If I'm miserable now, it's because of you.

You are my parents, you raised me so, so you are responsible"; "You forced me to go to school when I did not want it"; "If you had enrolled me in a *juku*, I could have joined a university and I would not be in that state"; "You never saw me being bullied at school. You do not know how hard it was"; "We lived in a pitiful neighborhood, but you never wanted to move"; "I would like to remake college. I would like to go back in time and redo everything."

It can even go as far as requiring the parent to give financial compensation and apologies (Saitō 1998: 142), which falls into a family rationale where one "seeks the criminal" (*kazoku no naka no "han.nin sagashi" no riron*). Saitō Tamaki makes this clear through the phrase "look for the criminal," a logic of reproach within the family where a *hikikomori* person resides. I was also able to identify these tendencies in the course of my own investigation among those I interviewed: Mr. Ueyama, Ms. Hayashi, and Mr. Onishi attest to a presence of feelings of guilt or assignment of responsibility to the other, or rejection of responsibility by the parents. In this logic, the parental couple can also be torn apart: The father rejects his responsibility and blames the failure of the mother who is supposed to educate the child, and she in turn reproaches him for his lack of interest and involvement at home. Saitō Tamaki points here at the situation of fathers who take refuge in their work to flee the difficulties in the home, and finally, he denounces toxic situations where maternal sacrifice only reinforces their feeling that the child cannot live without them. He insists and speaks to her: It is not good to stay around the clock with your child. Even if she does not like to leave the house, she has to force herself, because this will allow the child to consider her as an individual who has an existence separate from him (Saitō 1998: 146–149).

Chapter 4 of the second part goes even further in the advice given to parents. The clinical experience of this psychiatrist leads to a recognition of the deterioration of family relationships, as individuals must relearn to speak to each other as human beings. Learning to say simple words of everyday life: greetings when leaving the home for example, and not using degrading personal pronouns with an aggressive tone (in Japanese, it will be *kimi* and *omae*); respecting each other's private life by knocking before entering the room and waiting for the child's answer; deciding on pocket money and continuing to give it even if he starts working part-time. Finally, he recommends private clinics created by the new generation of child and adolescent psychiatrists, rather than university hospitals (Saitō 1998: 185, Saitō 2013: 156), while recognizing the effectiveness of some mental health centers (Saitō 1998: 190, 2013: 160–161). He describes the conditions of successful care (Saitō 1998: 192–193, Saitō 2013: 161–163) that inspired many nonprofit organizations created in the 2000s. As early as 1998, Saitō predicted that the increase in the number of *hikikomori* individuals in their forties would be inevitable, given the small number of facilities that can support them when they are younger. In 2013, the aging of *hikikomori* is a concern for many parents with a child in this situation, as will be indicated by one of them (Mr. Yamamoto). Saitō Tamaki rightly asserts that when a person is *hikikomori* for more than a decade, as a psychiatrist, he cannot close his eyes and say that everything is fine: The likeliness of a psychiatric pathology must be raised, so that any possible disability might be recognized and appropriate subsidies given (Saitō 1998: 199, Saitō 2013: 167).

Saitō Tamaki's conclusions

In the last chapter, he is led to position *hikikomori* as a pathology produced by society (*shakai byōri*). He recalls the discourse on the apathetic youth of the late 1970s, but for him, this phenomenon was nothing but the sign of a conflict of values between generations (Saitō 1998: 203, Saitō 2013: 171). He writes that "social withdrawal is a pathology of adolescence. This suggests that the problem of withdrawal is closely related to our current education system." If this point of view is understood and widely held, that is not the case with the point of view that the education system compels students to deny castration (*"Kyosei wo hinin saseru" kyōiku shisutemu*). By the term "castration," Saitō Tamaki refers to the psychoanalytic concept of the same name: He explains that castration means the renunciation of the all-powerful infant. According to him, non-castrated people (in the symbolic sense) cannot participate in society. This is a universal statement based on the idea that the suffering of repeated losses while growing up is that of castration. In addition, Saitō argues that the Japanese education system maintains the illusory belief that its students can do anything, and at the moment when they should accept castration, they are forced by the education system to deny it. Saitō also draws attention to the gender differences in the field of education and mental health, through the consideration that 80% of *hikikomori* are men (Saitō 1998: 208). Finally, he concludes his last chapter by affirming that young shut-ins are the victims of an educational system that forces them to deny castration and keeps them in an endless adolescence. According to him, *hikikomori* is the pathology that best represents our time.

In a foreword to the American edition, 14 years after the publication of his book, Saitō reviews the 2010 guidelines on *hikikomori* produced by the Ministry of Health, Labour and Welfare [Ministry of Health Labour and Welfare (MHLW) 2010]. A study was conducted with 5000 people aged 15–39 years, which provided an estimate of 696,000 youths who had been in a state of withdrawal at home for more than 6 months (Saitō 2013: 1). Saitō Tamaki takes into account these figures and is willing to admit that the *hikikomori* would be around 700,000. At the same time, he dissociates himself from governmental works in which he himself participated (Saitō 2013: 7). According to him, there were problems with the reporting behavior in the study because *hikikomori* is considered a shameful situation in Japanese society (Saitō 2013: 3). This allows him to maintain, 14 years after the publication of his eponymous book, that the *hikikomori* population is more likely to be between one million and 1,500,000, which would be considered an overestimation by some. Saitō Tamaki's statement that respondents hide that their child is *hikikomori* because this situation is a source of shame, could belong to a Japanese identity discourse essentializing Japan as a shame society. *Hikikomori* is a situation that can be lived in shame, and considered as shameful, but it needs to be considered on a case by case basis and described in detail. In other words, the idea that "we do not talk about *hikikomori* because it is shameful" is a hypothesis, and one could just as well make another hypothesis: There are respondents that falsely claim to have lived in *hikikomori* circumstances. Indeed, if we question them further, we could perhaps find that the people concerned continued, for example, to have contacts with friends and go out for their hobbies, which would make them less so *hikikomori* than NEET (Not in Education, Employment, or Training).

Despite the influence and insights of Saitō Tamaki, one cannot escape questioning his methods. In his 1998 book, as in the preface to his English translation, he advances his own results without really explaining how he got them. When citing authors, he does not systematically mention his references or sources. When he does, one realizes that he uses shortcuts that misrepresent other scholars' findings. He says, for example, that 250,000 young people under 25, in Britain, are homeless (Saitō 2013: 6), but the article he cites is more nuanced. This article mentions young people sleeping in modest hotels, living under sublets, or sleeping with friends. In this very brief article of 2004, it is written that the figures were obtained by charity associations and cross-referenced with the data of the local English authorities, which estimated 250,000 homeless people under 25 years. Similarly, he quotes the figure of 300,000 *hikikomori* in South Korea, and includes those who are "addicted" to online games. But he does not cite any epidemiological study, nor any bibliographical reference to support this figure, and does not try to explain the connection between *hikikomori* and Internet addiction among young South Koreans.

Is *hikikomori* a Japanese culture bound syndrome?

Social withdrawal has long been seen as a symptom of mental disorders such as depression, schizophrenia, or social anxiety disorders. It is only recently that in Japan an epidemic of *hikikomori* led researchers to consider social withdrawal as a mental disorder in itself (Saitō 1998), and more specifically as a Japanese "culture-bound syndrome" which could be introduced into the DSM-5 (Teo and Gaw 2010). It is now recognized that *hikikomori* in Japan is the phenomenon of social withdrawal that affects some hundreds of thousands of individuals, in which the individual shuts his/herself in their room, generally at their family's home, for several months or years without physical social relationships. Although the number of articles on this topic is increasing, a thorough review of the literature is lacking. The purpose of this section is to provide a review of psychiatrists' studies on social withdrawal. To do this, I reviewed the literature and selected 53 studies – books, guidelines, and articles from 1978 to 2014 – investigating idioms of distress and social withdrawal within and outside of Japan. I collected articles available on Japanese and international databases such as CiNii, JAIRO, JSTAGE, Web of Science, PubMed, and Scopus. The inclusion criteria include the overall quality of the article and its methodology. Findings are broken down into four sections.

Idioms of social withdrawal in Japan

Social withdrawal as a social problem emerged in the second half of the 1970s. Among the terms directly related to *"hikikomori,"* we find "retreat neurosis" (*taikyaku shinkeishō*) (Kasahara 1978) and "student apathy" (*apashi shindorōmu*) (Kasahara 1984). Student apathy is the phenomenon that affects masculine individuals who retreat from academic tasks while pursuing other activities. Apathetic students avoid competition and are afraid to fail, despite good abilities, and sometimes present obsessive-compulsive disorder with identity conflict (Uchida 2010). Whereas retreat neurosis and student apathy were described by psychiatrists during the end of the 1970s and the beginning of the 1980s, the term *"hikikomori"* appeared during the mid-1980s. In 1991, the Ministry of Health Labour and Welfare (MHLW) launched a pilot project to support youth suffering from social withdrawal (*hikikomori/futōkō jidō fukushi taisaku moderu jigyō*). In 1997, Shiokura Yutaka published reports in *Asahi Shinbun*. In 1998, Saitō Tamaki published *Shakaiteki Hikikomori: Owaranai Shishunki*, a book that is considered a major milestone in the history of *hikikomori* studies, as explained earlier. Here, Saitō Tamaki's research estimates put the *hikikomori* population at over one million individuals, a statement that was impossible to prove, but something that nonetheless contributed to the widespread attention given to the subject.

For 2010, estimates placed the *hikikomori* population at 696,000 [Ministry of Health Labour and Welfare (MHLW) 2010]. The first guideline structuring the phenomenon of *hikikomori* was established 7 years earlier [Ministry of Health Labour and Welfare (MHLW) 2001, 2003] and describes withdrawn individuals as not participating in society, staying at home for 6 months or more, and distinguishing them from individuals with mental disorders such as schizophrenia (Kaneko 2006). Later, American psychiatrists Teo and Gaw (2010), proposed the following criteria: a lifestyle centered at home; no interest or willingness to attend school or work; symptom duration of at least 6 months; schizophrenia, mental retardation, or other mental disorders have been excluded; and among those with no interest or willingness to attend school or work, those who maintain personal relationships (e.g., friendships) have been excluded.

One of the most comprehensive and precise descriptions of *hikikomori* came in 2010 from the MHLW:

> *"Hikikomori* is a psycho-sociological phenomenon, one of its characteristic features being withdrawal from social activities and staying at home almost each day for more than half a year. This occurs among children, adolescents, and adults under 30 years old. Although *hikikomori* is defined as non-psychotic state, it is better to think that patients with schizophrenia may be mixed into this grouping until they receive the diagnosis of psychosis." [Ministry of Health Labour and Welfare (MHLW) 2010].

Between 2003 and 2010, an important shift occurred: The population concerned was first considered as purely non-psychotic, whereas it is now recognized that among individuals in the *hikikomori* situation, there might be found individuals with psychotic disorders such as schizophrenia.

Regarding the psychiatric research into *hikikomori*, two tendencies should be distinguished. The first one (Kinugasa 1998, Hirashima 2001, Suwa et al. 2003, Suwa and Hara 2007) considers a primary *hikikomori* (without mental disorder) and a secondary *hikikomori* (with a mental disorder), but the distribution of this population has not yet been clearly established. On the one hand, the distinction "primary" and "secondary" is a weakness and a paradox of this theory, because the only way for these psychiatrists to recognize an individual who does not belong to a psychiatric field of research, is to create a psychiatric category: primary *hikikomori*. On the other hand, a strength of this theory is that it takes into account that there is effectively a primary social withdrawal without any mental disorder: in other words, it does not over-psychiatrize the *hikikomori* phenomenon.

In contrast, the second tendency does not consider a primary *hikikomori*, but claims every individual in a *hikikomori* situation could be diagnosed with existing DSM-IV-TR categories, with a few exceptions (Kondo et al. 2013). It should also be noted that in the DSM-IV-TR, a "glossary of culture-bound syndromes" mentions an "interpersonal fear disorder" specific to the Japanese: *taijin kyōfushō*. At this point, it's important to understand why *taijin kyōfushō* was considered a "culture-bound syndrome" and why *hikikomori* was not included in the list of "cultural concepts of distress" in DSM-5.

The promotion of hikikomori as a culture-bound syndrome

Concerning the attempts made by some psychiatrists to introduce *hikikomori* into the DSM-5, two questions should be asked: Is *hikikomori* really a mental disorder? Do individuals given the label "*hikikomori*" necessarily have some kind of a mental disorder? Three propositions emerge among psychiatrists: First, *hikikomori* individuals always have a mental disorder already available in DSM-IV-TR or ICD-10. Second, a portion of the *hikikomori* population suffers from some kind of mental disorder, while the rest does not seem to have any mental disorder (it is the distinction between primary *hikikomori* and secondary *hikikomori*). Third, a portion of the *hikikomori* population could be diagnosed with a mental disorder already available in DSM-IV-TR or ICD-10, and the other portion suffers from a new pathology: It could be included in the glossary of culture-bound syndromes.

In a 2010 article, American psychiatrists attempted to provide "evidence of *hikikomori* as a new mental disorder," and claimed that *hikikomori* can "often but not always" be classified in the DSM-IV-TR or ICD-10 (Teo and Gaw 2010). For those patients who cannot be classified, they propose including *hikikomori* among the DSM's list of culture-bound syndromes. This proposition should face a first critique: *hikikomori* cases have been encountered outside Japan: in South Korea (Kim et al. 2008, Lee et al. 2013), Hong-Kong (Wong 2009, Wong et al. 2015), Australia (Kim et al. 2008), United States (Teo 2013, Teo et al. 2015), Spain (Garcia-Campayo et al. 2007, Ovejero et al. 2014), Italia (Sagliocco et al. 2011), Oman Kingdom (Sakamoto et al. 2005), and France (Guedj-Bourdiau 2011, Furuhashi et al. 2013, Fansten et al. 2014). Moreover, a wide group of psychiatrists from diverse countries (Australia, Bangladesh, Iran, India, South Korea, Taiwan, Thailand, United States) testify to the presence of *hikikomori* cases outside of Japan (Kato et al. 2012). Among this group of psychiatrists, some published an article in *The Lancet* where they clearly associated *hikikomori* to depression, or more precisely, a "modern-type depression" (Kato et al. 2011). Another research team offers the position that *hikikomori* could be a severe form of social anxiety disorder (Nagata et al. 2013). Among these psychiatrists, Alan Teo claims he has cured a case of an American *hikikomori* with 25 sessions of cognitive and behavioral therapy, but he simultaneously underlines that his patient had a bipolar disorder with social withdrawal during periods of depression (Teo 2013).

In Japan, a study compiling 337 cases of *hikikomori* found that, from these, only one could not be given a diagnosis using DSM or ICD existing categories (Kondo et al. 2013). In previous investigations, psychiatrists diagnosed *hikikomori* as depression, social anxiety disorder, or mood disorder, and the results of this study divide *hikikomori* population in three main subgroups: schizophrenia, mood, and anxiety disorders (33.3%); developmental disorders (32%); and personality disorders (34.7%). The remaining 0.7% represents an individual impossible to diagnose within existing categories who should be included in a new category inside the glossary of culture-bound syndromes. Finally, a recent study supported *hikikomori* syndrome's similarities to some aspects of personality disorders (Ryder, Sunohara, and Kirmayer 2015).

After examining the above psychiatric data, there seems to be an apparent consensus: outside of Japan, *hikikomori* individuals always have a mental disorder; within Japan, these cases exist but there are also cases suffering from a culture-bound syndrome. Despite this consensus, *hikikomori* was not introduced as a culture-bound syndrome in DSM-5. It is time to show the reasons why it failed, even though the idea of a Japanese culture-bound *hikikomori* remains very popular.

Hikikomori versus taijin kyōfushō

The fifth version of the DSM does not mention *hikikomori* among the culture-bound syndromes, and replaces the glossary of culture-bound syndromes (American Psychiatric Association 1994) with a glossary of cultural concepts of distress (American Psychiatric Association 2013).

Why is it that *taijin kyōfushō*, which reflects a considerably lower number of people as compared to *hikikomori*, appears in the DSM, while *hikikomori* fails to earn the distinction? Is it because the clinical descriptions of the latter are not satisfactory? Or is it because we can find *hikikomori* in many different countries? Let us consider the category of *taijin kyōfushō*.

From 1979 until May 2013, *taijin kyōfushō* was thought of as a culture-bound syndrome (Tanaka-Matsumi 1979, Kirmayer 1991, Maeda and Nathan 1999) and considered similar to social phobias (American Psychiatric Association 2000). Against the idea of *taijin kyōfushō* as a culture-bound syndrome, many articles are strengthening the hypothesis of *taijin kyōfushō* as a social phobia or social anxiety disorder (Kleinknecht et al. 1997, Essau et al. 2011, Essau et al. 2012, Asakura et al. 2012, Nagata et al. 2013), which responds favorably to medication used in these pathologies (Matsunaga et al. 2001, Nagata et al. 2003, Nagata et al. 2006). It is necessary to point out that *taijin kyōfushō* includes the *kanji* "*shō*," which refers to an illness (*byōki*) or a syndrome (*shōkōgun*): undoubtedly, *taijin kyōfushō* is a mental disorder (*seishin shōgai*). Additionally, surprisingly, its Romanization written in the DSM-IV and DSM-5 is incorrect: you may write *kyoufushou* or *kyōfushō*, but never *kyofusho*. With the incorrect orthography of the DSM-IV's "*boufee delirante*" (instead of "*bouffée délirante*"), one might regret the lack of linguistic accuracy of this manual. Moreover, the maintenance of *taijin kyōfushō* in the DSM5's glossary of cultural concepts of distress might seem confounding when we recognize the following: "Similar syndromes are found in Korea and other societies that place a strong emphasis on the self-conscious maintenance of appropriate social behavior in hierarchical interpersonal relationships. *Taijin kyofusho*-like symptoms have also been described in other cultural contexts, including the United States, Australia, and New Zealand" (American Psychiatric Association 2013).

One might see a major problem with maintaining *taijin kyōfushō* as a mental disorder that relates somehow to Japanese culture, while simultaneously recognizing its presence in so many different cultures. Beyond this apparent contradiction, there has been an important transformation of the conceptualization of culture from the DSM-IV to the DSM-5. Despite the fact that these elements could have led the APA to suppress the inclusion of *taijin kyōfushō* in the glossary of culture-bound syndromes and instead include it as a social anxiety disorder, the DSM-5 includes *taijin kyōfushō* in the glossary of cultural concepts of distress, which replaced the glossary of culture-bound syndromes. Among the 25 items in the DSM-IV's glossary of culture-bound syndromes, only 9 remain in the DSM-5 (American Psychiatric Association 2013: 833–837). This means that 14 culture-bound syndromes were suppressed, and are ineligible for being listed in the glossary of cultural concepts of distress (Tajan 2015b). However, this does not mean that cultural elements were suppressed in the DSM-5. For instance, ten pages detail the cultural formulation: It includes an Outline of Cultural Formulation (OCF), a "Cultural Formulation Interview that operationalizes the process of data collection by the OCF," (Lewis-Fernández et al. 2014) and two pages defining cultural concepts of distress (while the glossary of cultural concepts of distress is located in the appendix) (American Psychiatric Association 2013: 749–759; 833–837). To sum up, the DSM-IV includes appendix I, entitled "Outline for Cultural Formulation and Glossary of Culture-bound Syndromes," while the DSM-5 includes a chapter dedicated to cultural formulation in Section III and a distinctive glossary of cultural concepts of distress located in the appendix. Overall, the DSM-5 significantly changed its perception of culture (e.g., distinction between syndrome, idiom, and explanation) and contains more information on culture than did the DSM-IV and the DSM-IV-TR. Compared to the previous versions of the DSM, the APA considered cultural psychiatrists' argument about culture-bound syndromes (Bhugra, Sumathipala and Siribaddana 2007), and one can recognize an advancement of the attitudes toward culture in the DSM-5.

Although *hikikomori* affects hundreds of thousands of individuals in Japan, it does not appear in the glossary of cultural concepts of distress in the DSM-5. I will invoke another reason for this by highlighting a pervasive methodological problem concerning the investigations into the subject of *hikikomori*, and the attempt to describe it as a syndrome.

Fictive cases and typification of hikikomori in psychiatry

Typification, as a research methodology rooted in the Weberian notion of ideal-type, is a way, amongst others, of producing scientific results. However, as it should represent the average image of the individuals investigated, it obviously diminishes the singularity of each subject. In psychiatrists' studies on *hikikomori*, typification is widespread. Saitō Tamaki used typification and was followed by two groups of researchers doing quantitative research by questionnaire: The first one asked if *hikikomori* exists out of Japan (Kato et al. 2012), and the second one asked if *hikikomori* could be a clinical term in psychiatry (Tateno et al. 2012). The purpose of the first article was to understand if and how *hikikomori* is diagnosed and cured outside of Japan.

In order to do so, psychiatrists invented two fictive cases (Mr. A and B), submitted them to their colleagues in Japan, Australia, Bangladesh, Iran, India, South Korea, Taiwan, Thailand, and the United States. The study is based upon the responses of 239 psychiatrists (123 in Japan and 124 in other countries). Their results show that *hikikomori* is seen in each country, predominantly in urban areas: The causes are biopsychosocial, cultural, and environmental. Researchers conclude that *hikikomori* is seen by psychiatrists in a vast variety of cultures.

The first fictitious case, Mr. A is a 15-year-old eldest son who refuses to see the psychiatrist. (Note: For Mr. A and B, I only quote the social history sections.)

> He is the first son, with a younger brother. He is brought up by his father who is a company employee and his mother who works part-time. His father, a salesman, has been transferred every 2–3 years and moved with his whole family, but when he entered junior high school, his father moved by himself, so he now lives with his mother and a brother three years his junior. There was nothing particularly problematic during his development and his school grades were medium, but not bad. He naturally found it hard to make friends and he would prefer reading books rather than sports.
>
> *(Kato et al. 2012: 1063)*

On a superficial level, Mr. A could seem to be representative of *hikikomori* individuals, but on closer inspection several problems become evident. First, many non-*hikikomori* individuals could be described with a similar social history and teenage struggles, and the fragment "family history: none" is questionable. Second, it is often said that *hikikomori* individuals are overwhelmingly elder sons, but the Japanese low fertility rate (1.3 children per family) should be remembered: Deeper investigations on family members and structure (e.g., do they have brothers or sisters?) are needed. Third, the father's professional conditions described here are known in Japan under the terms of *tanshin funin* (posting without family) but it only concerns 3.7% of Japanese families (Holloway 2010: 98). Consequently, the situation described here only corresponds to a small number of cases and is always less than 3.7% of Japanese families. In sociological terms, this case represents an extreme minority of Japanese families and certainly not the majority of familial situations in which we can find a *hikikomori* child: For most of them, the father comes back home every evening (Fansten et al. 2014: 142). Moreover, Yong and Nomura's secondary analysis of the Cabinet Office of the Government of Japan (Director-General for Policy on Cohesive Society)'s (2010) survey "does not support the idea that *hikikomori* is more common in urban areas, has no association between the city size, region, and *hikikomori* was identified. Instead, *hikikomori* was found to be less common in residential areas that have many business and service industries." (Yong and Nomura 2019: 7).

Let us now turn to the second fictitious case, Mr. B, 24 years old:

He is an only child. He is brought up by his parents in a two-bedroom urban apartment. There was nothing particularly problematic during his development until elementary school. In junior high school, he often skipped school and avoided mingling with peers, which he linked to experiences such as being bullied by classmates in elementary school. His academic performance was historically good, and he directly entered a middle-class university of engineering faculty, but 3 years ago (third grade, 21 years old) Mr. B dropped out of university for lack of motivation.

(Kato et al. 2012: 1063)

The second fictive case, Mr. B, better describes an older population of *hikikomori* and does not fall into the stereotype of an Internet addiction that does not correspond to all *hikikomori* situations. A weak point of this case could be illustrated by what has already been underlined in recent investigations (Tajan 2015a, 2015b, 2015c, 2017, Tajan and Shiozawa 2020): Japanese psychiatrists only meet with a subcategory of *hikikomori* cases while most of the withdrawn youth receive support from Non-Profit Organizations' caregivers. Individuals who have met several psychiatrists represent a small proportion of Japanese *hikikomori* cases. In a way, these psychiatrists constructed an ideal-type of *hikikomori*, which only represents a small percentage of individuals in a social withdrawal situation. This is exactly the opposite of what ideal-type should be on a typification's methodology: Ideal-type should represent an average portrait of people excluding the extremes and representing the majority. And what about the mention of "family history: none"? Is it a way for researchers to simplify the questionnaire? How do they take into account the familial dimensions in clinical settings and what the questions they ask are? Despite a good methodology, we cannot conclude anything from the results of this investigation because they only represent a minority of the cases. It should be underlined that this investigation deals with the representation of *hikikomori* among psychiatrists, rather than *hikikomori* outside Japan.

A second article seems more aware of this bias and carefully investigates the opportunity to introduce *hikikomori* as a psychiatric term (Tateno et al. 2012). Researchers openly claim they investigate the *hikikomori* "perception" among health practitioners. A vast study was conducted ($n = 1038$ individuals in total): psychiatrists ($n = 80$), pediatrics ($n = 26$), nurses ($n = 595$), psychologists ($n = 46$), students ($n = 229$), and others ($n = 62$). While it is not possible to detail the complete results of the research, it should be noted that 30% of psychiatrists find the more appropriate category for *hikikomori* to be schizophrenia, while 50% of pediatricians diagnose neurotic disorders or disorders related to stress. Almost all the subjects interviewed tend to disagree with the statement "*hikikomori* is not a disorder." Finding such unanimity on the statement that "*hikikomori* is not a disorder" raises crucial questions. Does commenting "no" to a negative statement correspond to commenting "yes" to a positive statement? Is it exactly the same? In other words, here, does it mean that respondents consider that *hikikomori* is a disorder? If yes, getting to this conclusion through two negations remains, to me, problematic. Moreover, there are translation problems that need to be addressed. Their article, written in English, mentions the word "*disorder*," but the questionnaires were completed by Japanese individuals in Japanese. From which Japanese word comes the term "disorder"? It is not mentioned in the article, but if we refer to the usual translation of "disorder" in DSM, it is obviously "*shōgai*." Yet, *shōgai* in Japanese means both disorder and disability, and if a Japanese read "*hikikomori wa shōgai dewa nai*," of course he/she would not agree. So then, the underlined questions become clear: What is it that these interviewees reject so overwhelmingly? To what do they answer "no"? In other words, it is difficult to conclude anything from results implying a comment of the statement "*hikikomori* is not a disorder," in terms of agreement or disagreement.

Hikikomori is an idiom of distress

Hikikomori is not a syndrome but an idiom of distress (Nichter 1981). These individuals are resistant to psychiatric treatment, and the literature review regarding this insists on possible underlying causes. First, *taijin kyōfushō* has historical significance and is the only Japanese syndrome to be listed in the DSM-5's glossary of cultural concepts of distress; for the APA, it was neither possible to suppress *taijin kyōfushō* nor to add *hikikomori* in the DSM-5. Second, even though *hikikomori* is a much broader category than *taijin kyōfushō*, and an epidemic recognized by the Japanese Ministry of Health, Labour and Welfare, it does not meet the criteria for being considered a syndrome. Also, in the DSM-5, the number of items was reduced and the renewed understanding of culture from the DSM-IV to the DSM-5 should be seen as an advancement of the attitudes toward culture. Third, researchers in psychiatry manipulate an ideal type of *hikikomori* that fits with a minority of *hikikomori* cases. Finally, Japanese psychiatrists only clinically evaluate a minority of *hikikomori* cases.

To sum up, this review of the literature reveals the necessity for the scientific community to abandon considering *hikikomori* as a syndrome. Given the absence of a clinical description in the literature, it should definitely be considered as an idiom of distress. Although my viewpoint differs somewhat from that of the APA, such a statement is consistent with the noninclusion of *hikikomori* in the DSM-5. In further research, *hikikomori* individuals' narratives, the support they receive from nonprofit organizations' caregivers, the relationship with school nonattendance, family and risk factors, and the role of culture should receive closer attention. An investigation focusing on these aspects could contribute to establishing *hikikomori* as an idiom of distress, and improve the delivery of services for socially withdrawn individuals and their families.

Perspectives

The aging of the Japanese population is a demographic bomb that might cause many socioeconomic problems in the near future. The impact of being at stage 5 of the demographic transition (i.e., experiencing loss to the overall population as the death rate becomes higher than the birth rate) is still unknown and its consequences difficult to gauge. Moreover, thousands of individuals who could participate in society and work, are not doing so. These shut-ins and their situation are called *hikikomori* (acute social withdrawal). In Japan, it is now recognized that *hikikomori* affects at least 541,000 individuals between 15 and 39 years old and 613,000 between 40 and 64 [Cabinet Office of the Government of Japan (Director-General for Policy on Cohesive Society) 2016, 2019].

Hikikomori is an epidemic, and, simultaneously, its status of mental disorder is highly criticized (Tateno et al. 2012; Tajan 2015b). Do we have previous examples of an epidemic of a mental disorder the very status of mental disorder of which is highly criticized? Yes, we have: namely, depression. The over-medicalization of sadness was perceived by scholars like Alain Ehrenberg or Jerome Wakefield, and the new definition of depression in the DSM-5 (stipulating a period of 2 weeks of symptoms) confirm their views: In many cases, you simply cannot distinguish depression from sadness or bereavement. It is not the first time an epidemic of a mental disorder seems to relate to historical, social, and cultural factors. A predecessor was hysteria in the second half of 19th century Europe. It is worth reviewing a few of its elements, not only because it was the birth of psychopathological clinics, but also because it introduced psychological trauma as a cause in the development of a mental disorder.

Hysteria, depression, *hikikomori*. The sequence does not have to be taken literally; rather, it has to be understood for heuristic purposes: In the 1870s and 1880s, there was the birth of neurology and the introduction of hypnosis as a psychotherapeutic tool by Charcot, and now, the rise of neurosciences and suggestion through directive therapies. According to Michel Foucault, Hysteria was an ensemble of struggles, inside and outside asylum, against the new apparatus of neurological clinics. (Foucault 2006: 309). He argues that three great maneuvers took place between the hysteric and the neurologist: the organization of the symptomatic scenario, the maneuver of the "functional mannequin," and the redistribution around trauma.

Can we observe these three maneuvers when applied to *hikikomori*? The first maneuver clearly fails. *Hikikomori*, as I have shown throughout this book, resists being a psychiatric category. He is the bad patient and the psychiatrist cannot recognize himself as good (the patient is reluctant to meet a psychiatrist who cannot cure him). The second maneuver also fails because *hikikomori* is not a tool delimiting truth and lie: After all, who really wants to hear what they have to say?

Contrarily, the third maneuver might partially be accurate for *hikikomori* survivors. Can we not notice the subjective importance attributed to trauma related to school, involving parents, teachers, and peers? And a haunting idea related to school, work, or interpersonal relationships in their narratives? Bullying is a trauma, and it triggers social withdrawal (Tajan 2015a). It is the first traumatic dimension of *hikikomori*.

The second one has already been reported as "traumatization" (Murasawa 2012). It is related to the fact that the social isolation endlessly reactivates the trauma, what Saitō calls the vicious cycle of the *hikikomori* system. Consequently, acute social withdrawal constitutes in itself a trauma.

The third one is family trauma. "Trauma" is a word Misaki's father (see Chapter 7) used when he suggested that telling his daughter to leave the house was the most difficult thing he had to do: It broke his heart and, simultaneously, he had to do it to improve the family atmosphere and help his daughter. I also gathered accounts of NPO members having met parents referring to the Japanese economic growth (1955–1973) as a traumatic period, and I feel this aspect should be investigated in light of recent research on trauma and cultural history (Hashimoto 2015).

Although most of the *hikikomori* survivors cannot be diagnosed with PTSD, psychological trauma cannot be reduced to PTSD. Bullying and the abandonment of others leave subjective wounds for decades: In their 40s or 50s, *hikikomori* survivors speak of their teenage years as though they were only yesterday (Tajan 2015c), a distortion of time that is often seen in trauma survivors.

I would suggest that *hikikomori* is a form of passive aggressivity, unknown as such by the subjects themselves, concealed to those who expose their reclusion, despite themselves. Shut-ins fall into the norms of capitalistic societies and are one of their byproducts. Would it be accurate to say that, like Bartleby, they "would prefer not to"? Is it the meaning of their absence of social participation? I would suggest *hikikomori* might be a struggle inside the home and outside social institutions, against the contemporary practices of the mental health field. The shut-in confronts the benevolent caregiver, the volunteer, the psychiatrist, and mirrors their own desire: What do you want from me? If what you want from me is to go back to school or work, why should I do so? What is your desire, as a human being, to participate in society?

References

American Psychiatric Association. 1994. "Outline for Cultural Formulation and Glossary of Culture-Bound Syndromes." In *Diagnostic and Statistical Manual of Mental Disorders (DSM-IV)*. 843–849. Washington DC: American Psychiatric Association.

———. 2000. *Diagnostic and Statistical Manual of Mental Disorders (DSM-IV-TR)*. Washington DC: American Psychiatric Publishing.

————. 2013. *Diagnostic and Statistical Manual of Mental Disorders, 5th Edition: DSM-5 [Paperback].* Washington DC: American Psychiatric Publishing.

Asakura, Satoshi et al. 2012. "Social Anxiety Taijin-Kyōfu Scale (SATS): Development and Psychometric Evaluation of a New Instrument." *Psychopathology* 45: 96–101.

Bhugra, Dinesh, Athula Sumathipala, and Sisira Siribaddana. 2007. "Culture-bound syndromes: a re-evaluation." In: *Textbook of Cultural Psychiatry.* Edited by Bhui Bhugra, 141–156. Cambridge: Cambridge University Press.

Cabinet Office of the Government of Japan (Director-General for Policy on Cohesive Society) 内閣府政策統括官 (共生社会政策担当). 2010. *Wakamono no ishiki ni kansuru chōsa – Hikikomori ni kansuru jittai chōsa* 若者の意識に関する調査・ひきこもりに関する実態調査 (Survey on Youth Consciousness – Survey on *Hikikomori*). https://www8.cao.go.jp/youth/kenkyu/hikikomori/pdf_gaiyo_index.html.

Cabinet Office of the Government of Japan (Director-General for Policy on Cohesive Society). 2016. *Wakamono no seikatsu ni kansuru chōsa hōkokusho* 若者の生活に関する調査 報告書 (Research Survey on Youth's life). https://www8.cao.go.jp/youth/kenkyu/hikikomori/h27/pdf-index.html.

Cabinet Office of the Government of Japan (Director-General for Policy on Cohesive Society). 2019. *Seikatsu Jōkyō ni Kansuru Chōsa* 生活状況に関する調査 (Survey on Living Conditions). https://www8.cao.go.jp/youth/kenkyu/life/h30/pdf-index.html.

Essau, Cecilia A., Satoko Sasagawa, Jungwen Chen, and Yuji Sakano. 2012. "Taijin Kyōfushō and Social Phobia Symptoms in Young Adults in England and in Japan." *Journal of Cross-Cultural Psychology* 43 (2): 219–232.

Essau, Cecilia A., Satoko Sasagawa, Shin.ichi Ishikawa, Isa Okajima, Jean O'Callaghan, and Diane Bray. 2011. "A Japanese Form of Social Anxiety Taijin Kyōfushō: Frequency and Correlates in Two Generations of the Same Family." *International Journal of Social Psychiatry* 58 (6): 635–642.

Fansten, Maia et al. 2014. *Hikikomori, ces adolescents en retrait.* Paris: Armand Colin.

Foucault, Michel. 2006. *Psychiatric Power: Lectures at the Collège de France, 1973–1974.* Basingstoke and New York: Palgrave MacMillan.

Furuhashi, Tadaaki et al. 2013. "État des lieux, points communs et différences entre des jeunes adultes retirants sociaux en France et au Japon (Hikikomori)." *L'Évolution Psychiatrique* 78 (2): 249–266.

Garcia-Campayo, Javier, Marta Alda, Natalia Sobradiel, and Beatriz Sanz Abós. 2007. "A Case Report of Hikikomori in Spain." *Medicina Clinica (Barcelona)* 129 (8): 318–319.

Guedj-Bourdiau, Marie-Jeanne. 2011. "Claustration à domicile de l'adolescent Hikikomori." *Annales Médico-Psychologiques* 169 (10): 668–673.

Hashimoto, Akiko. 2015. *The Long Defeat. Cultural Trauma, Memory, and Identity in Japan.* New York: Oxford University Press.

Hirashima, Natsuko. 2001. "Psychopathology of Social Withdrawal in Japan." *Journal of the Japan Medical Association* 44 (6): 260–262.

Holloway, Susan D. 2010. *Women and Family in Contemporary Japan.* Cambridge University Press.

Kaneko, Sachiko. 2006. "Japan's 'Socially Withdrawn Youths' and Time Constraints in Japanese Society: Management and Conceptualization of Time in a Support Group for Hikikomori." *Time & Society* 15 (2/3): 233–249.

Kasahara, Yomishi 笠原嘉. 1978. "Taikyaku shinkeishō to iu shinkategorii no teishō" 退却神経症という新カテゴリーの提唱 (Proposition of a New Category Called Retreat Neurosis). In *Shishunki no Seishinbyōri to Chiryō* 思春期の精神病理と治療 *(Psychopathology and Treatment of Adolescence)*. Edited by H. Nakai and Y. Yamanaka 中井久夫・山中康裕編, 287–319. Tōkyō: Iwasaki Gakujutsu Shuppan.

Kasahara, Yomishi. 1984. *Apashī shindorōmu — kōgakureki shakai no seinen shinri* アパシー・シンドローム—高学歴社会の青年心理 (Student Apathy Syndrome). Tōkyō: Iwanami Shoten.

Kato, Takahiro, Takaoka Shinfuku, Norman Sartorius, and Shigenobu Kanba. 2011. "Are Japan's Hikikomori and Depression in Young People Spreading Abroad?" *The Lancet* 378 (9796): 1070. http://www.thelancet.com/pdfs/journals/lancet/PIIS014067361161475X.pdf.

Kato, Takahiro et al. 2012. "Does the Hikikomori Syndrome of Social Withdrawal Exist Outside Japan? A Preliminary International Investigation." *Social Psychiatry and Psychiatric Epidemiology* 47 (7): 1061–1075.

Kim, Jinkwan, Ronald M Rapee, Kyung Ja Oh, and Hye-Shin Moon. 2008. "Retrospective Report of Social Withdrawal during Adolescence and Current Maladjustment in Young Adulthood: Cross-Cultural Comparisons between Australian and South Korean Students." *Journal of Adolescence* 31 (5): 543–563.

Kinugasa, Takayuki. 1998. "Social Withdrawal of Young Adult." *Rinshō Seishin Igaku* 27: 147–152.

Kirmayer, Laurence J. 1991. "The Place of Culture in Psychiatric Nosology: Taijin Kyōfushō and DSM-III-R." *Journal of Nervous and Mental Disease* 179: 19–28.

Kitanaka, Junko. 2003. "Jungians and the Rise of Psychotherapy in Japan: A Brief Historical Note." *Transcultural Psychiatry* 40: 239–247.

———. 2012. *Depression in Japan, Psychiatric Cures for a Society in Distress*. Princeton, NJ: Princeton University Press.

Kleinknecht, Ronald A., Dale L. Dinnel, Erica E. Kleinknecht, Natsuki Hiruma, and Nozomi Harada. 1997. "Cultural Factors in Social Anxiety: A Comparison of Social Phobia Symptoms and Taijin Kyōfushō." *Journal of Anxiety Disorders* 11 (2): 157–177.

Kondo, Naoji, Motohiro Sakai, Yasukazu Kuroda, Yoshikazu Kiyota, Yuji Kitabata, and Mie Kurosawa. 2013. "General Condition of Hikikomori (Prolonged Social Withdrawal) in Japan: Psychiatric Diagnosis and Outcome in Mental Healths Welfare Centres." *International Journal of Social Psychiatry* 67: 193–202.

Ministry of Health Labour and Welfare (MHLW) 厚生労働省. 2001. *Jūdai/nijūdai wo chūshin toshita shakaiteki hikikomori wo meguru chiiki seishin hoken katsudō no gaidorain* 十代二十代を中心とした社会的ひきこもりをめぐるちいき精神保健活動のガイドライン (Guidelines for Mental Health Support and Evaluation of Hikikomori in their 10's and 20's). Edited by Jun.Ichirō Itō et al. Tōkyō: Kokuritsu Seishin/shinkei Centre.

———. 2003. *Jūdai/nijūdai wo chūshin toshita shakaiteki hikikomori wo meguru chiiki-seishin hoken katsudō no gaidorain* 十代二十代を中心とした社会的ひきこもりをめぐるちいき精神保健活動のガイドライン (Guidelines for Mental Health Support and Evaluation of Hikikomori in their 10's and 20's – Full version). Edited by Jun.Ichirō Itō et al. Tōkyō: Kokuritsu Seishin/shinkei Centre.

Ministry of Health Labour and Welfare (MHLW). 2010. *Hikikomori no hyōka/shien ni kansuru gaidorain* ひきこもりの評価ー支援に関するガイドラン (Guidelines for Support and Evaluation of Hikikomori). Edited by Kazuhiko Saitō et al. http://www.mhlw.go.jp/stf/houdou/2r98520000006i6f.html.

Lee, Young Sik, Jae Young Lee, Tae Young Choi, and Jin Tae Choi. 2013. "Home Visitation Program for Detecting, Evaluating and Treating Socially Withdrawn Youth in Korea." *Psychiatry and Clinical Neurosciences* 67 (4): 193–202.

Lewis-Fernández et al. 2014. "Culture and Psychiatric Evaluation: Operationalizing Cultural Formulation for DSM-5." *Psychiatry: Interpersonal and Biological Processes* 77 (2): 130–154.

Lock, Margaret. 1995. *Encounters with Aging. Mythologies of Menopause in Japan and North America.* Berkeley, CA: University of California Press.

Macé, Mieko. 2013. *Médecins et médecine dans l'histoire du Japon.* Paris: Les Belles Lettres (Collection Japon).

Maeda, Fumiko, and Jeffrey H. Nathan. 1999. "Understanding Taijin Kyōfushō through Its Treatment, Morita Therapy." *Journal of Psychosomatic Research* 46 (6): 552–530.

Matsunaga, Hisato, Nobuo Kiriike, Tokuzo Matsui, Yoko Iwasaki, and Dan J. Stein. 2001. "Taijin Kyōfushō: A Form of Social Anxiety Disorder that Responds to Serotonin Reuptake Inhibitors?" *International Journal of Neuropsychopharmacology* 4: 231–237.

Morita, Shōma 森田正馬. 1928. *Shinkeishitsu no hontai oyobi ryōhō* 神経質ノ本態及療法 The Nature of Shinkeishitsu and Its Therapy – 2 volumes). Tohōdo shoten 吐鳳堂書店. http://kindai.ndl.go.jp/info:ndljp/pid/1049833.

Murasawa, Watari. 2012. "Saikiteki purosesu toshite no 'hikikomori'" 再帰的プロセスとしての「ひきこもり」 (Social withdrawal as a reflexive process). *Shinri kagaku* 33 (1): 61–74.

Nakamura, Karen. 2013. *A Disability of the Soul: An Ethnography of Schizophrenia and Mental Illness in Contemporary Japan.* Ithaca: Cornell University Press.

Nagata, Toshihiko, Takenori Nakajima, Alan R. Teo, Hisashi Yamada, and Chiho Yoshimura. 2013. "Psychometric Properties of the Japanese Version of the Social Phobia Inventory." *Psychiatry and Clinical Neurosciences* 67: 160–166.

Nagata, Toshihiko, Jun Oshima, Akira Wada, Hisashi Yamada, Toshiya Iketani, and Nobuo Kiriike. 2003. "Open Trial of Minalcipran with for Taijin Kyōfushō in Japanese Patients with Social Anxiety Disorder." *International Journal of Psychiatry in Clinical Practice* 7: 107–112.

Nagata, Toshihiko, Irene Van Vielt, Hisashi Yamada, Kōhei Kataoka, Toshiya Iketani, and Nobuo Kiriike. 2006. "An Open Trial of Paroxetine for the 'Offensive Subtype' of Taijin Kyōfushō and Social Anxiety Disorder." *Depression and Anxiety* 23: 168–174.

Nagata, Toshihiko, Hisashi Yamada, Alan R. Teo, Chiho Yoshimura, Takenori Nakajima, and Irene Van Vielt. 2013. "Comorbid Social Withdrawal (hikikomori) in Outpatients with Social Anxiety Disorder: Clinical Characteristics and Treatment Response in a Case Series." *International Journal of Social Psychiatry* 59 (1): 73–78.

Nichter, Mark. 1981. "Idioms of Distress: Alternatives in the Expression of Psychosocial Distress. A Case Study from South India." *Culture, Medicine & Psychiatry* 5 (4): 379–408.

Ovejero, Santiago, Irene Caro-Cañizares, Victoria de León-Martínez, and Enrique Baca-Garcia. 2014. "Prolonged Social Withdrawal Disorder: A Hikikomori Case in Spain." *International Journal of Social Psychiatry* 60 (6): 562–565. https://doi.org/10.1177/0020764013504560.

Ryder Andrew G, Momoka Sunohara, and Lawrence J. Kirmayer. 2015. "Culture and Personality Disorder: From a Fragmented Literature to a Contextually Grounded Alternative." *Current Opinion in Psychiatry* 28 (1): 40–45.

Sagliocco Giulia, et al. 2011. *Hikikomori e adolescenza. Fenomenologia dell'autoreclusione*. Milano: Mimesis.

Saitō, Tamaki 斎藤環. 1998. *Shakaiteki hikikomori — owaranai shishunki* 社会的ひきこもり—終わらない思春期 (Social Hikikomori – Adolescence without End). Tōkyō: PHP Shinsho.

———. 2002. *"Hikikomori" kyūshutsu manyuaru* 「ひきこもり」救出マニュアル (Rescue Manual for Hikikomori). Kyoto: PHP kenkyūjo.

———. 2003. *OK? hikikomori OK!* OK? ひきこもり OK! Tokyo: Magajinhausu.

———. 2006. *Sentō bishōjo no seishin bunseki* 戦闘美少女の精神分析 (Psychoanalysis of the *Beautiful Fighting Girl*). Tokyo: Chikumashobō.

———. 2010a. *Hikikomori kara mita mirai* ひきこもりから見た未来 (Future Seen through Hikikomori). Tokyo: Mainichi shinbunsha.

———. 2010b. *Hakase no kimyō na seijuku sabukaruchā to shakai seishin byōri* 博士の奇妙な成熟　サブカルチャーと社会精神病理 (Subculture and Social Psychopathology). Tokyo: Nippon hyōronsha.

———. 2012a. *Hikikomori wa naze "naoru" no ka? seishin bunseki teki apurōchi* ひきこもりはなぜ「治る」のか? 精神分析的アプローチ (Why should we cure hikikomori? Psychoanalytical Approach). Tokyo: Chikumashobō.

———. 2012b. *Ikinobiru tame no rakan* 生き延びるためのラカン (Lacan for Survival). Tokyo: Chikuma shobō.

———. 2013. *Hikikomori: Adolescence without End*. Translated by Jeffrey Angles. Minneapolis: University Of Minnesota Press.

Saitō, Tamaki, and Hiroki Azuma. 2011. *Beautiful Fighting Girl*. Minneapolis: University Of Minnesota Press.

Sakamoto, Noriyuki, Rodger G. Martin, Hiroaki Kumano, Tomifusa Kuboki, and Samir Al-Adawi. 2005. "Hikikomori, Is It A Culture-Reactive or Culture-Bound Syndrome? Nidotherapy And A Clinical Vignette from Oman." *International Journal of Psychiatry in Medicine* (35): 191–198.

Suwa, Mami, and Koichi Hara. 2007. "Hikikomori among Young Adults in Japan. The Importance of Differential Diagnosis between Primary Hikikomori and Hikikomori with High-Functioning Pervasive Developmental Disorders." *Iryō fukushi kenkyū* 3: 94–101.

Suwa, Mami, Kunifumi Suzuki, Koichi Hara, Hisashi Watanabe, and Toshihiko Takahashi. 2003. "Family Features in Primary Social Withdrawal among Young Adults." *Psychiatry and Clinical Neurosciences* 57: 586–594.

Tajan, Nicolas. 2015a. "Adolescents' School Non-Attendance and the Spread of Psychological Counselling in Japan." *Asia Pacific Journal of Counselling and Psychotherapy* 6 (1/2): 58–69.

———. 2015b. "Social Withdrawal and Psychiatry: A Comprehensive Review of Hikikomori." *Neuropsychiatrie de l'Enfance et de l'Adolescence* 63 (5): 324–331.

———. 2015c. "Japanese Post-Modern Social Renouncers: An Exploratory Study of the Narratives of Hikikomori Subjects." *Subjectivity* 8: 283–304.

————. 2017. *Génération hikikomori*. Paris: L'Harmattan (Collection Japon).

Tajan Nicolas, and Meiko Shiozawa. 2020. "Hikikomori wo saikōsuru – kaigai, tokuni furansu no jirei 「ひきこもり」を再考する—海外、特にフランスの事例" (Rethinking Hikikomori – Examples from France and Abroad), *Kyōku to Igaku* 教育と医学. 3/4: 54–61.

Tanaka-Matsumi, Junko. 1979. "Taijin Kyōfushō: Diagnostic and Cultural Issues in Japanese Psychiatry." *Culture, Medicine and Psychiatry* 3: 231–245.

Tateno, Masaru, Woo Park Tae, Takahiro Kato, Wakako Umene-Nakano, and Toshikazu Saito. 2012. "Hikikomori as a Possible Clinical Term in Psychiatry." *BMC Psychiatry* 12: 169.

Teo, Alan R. 2010. "A New Form of Social Withdrawal in Japan: A Review of Hikikomori." *International Journal of Social Psychiatry* 56 (2): 178–185.

————. 2013. "Social Isolation Associated with Depression: A Case Report of Hikikomori." *International Journal of Social Psychiatry* 59 (4): 339–341.

Teo, Alan R., and Albert R. Gaw. 2010. "Hikikomori, A Japanese Culture-Bound Syndrome of Social Withdrawal? A Proposal for DSM-5." *The Journal of Nervous and Mental Disease* 198 (6): 444–449.

Teo, Alan R., Kyle Stufflebam, Somnath Saha, Michael D. Fetters, Masaru Tateno, Shigenobu Kanba, and Takahiro A. Kato. 2015. "Psychopathology Associated with Social Withdrawal: Idiopathic and Comorbid Presentations." *Psychiatry Research* 228 (1): 182–183.

Uchida, Chiyoko. 2010. "Apathetic and Withdrawing Students in Japanese Universities – With Regard to Hikikomori and Student Apathy." *Journal of Medical and Dental Sciences* (57): 95–108.

Ueyama, Kazuki, Kosuke Tsuiki, and Nicolas Tajan. 2010. "Hikikomori nitsuite" ひきこもりについて (About *Hikikomori*). Video-recorded interview.

Wong, Victor. 2009. "Youth Locked in Time and Space? Defining Features of Social Withdrawal and Practice Implications." *Journal of Social Work Practice* (23): 337–352.

Wong, Paul WC, Tim MH Li, Melissa Chan, Y Law, Michael Chau, Cecilia Cheng, KW Fu, John Bacon-Shone, and Paul SF Yip. 2015. "The Prevalence and Correlates of Severe Social Withdrawal (Hikikomori) in Hong Kong: A Cross-Sectional Telephone-Based Survey Study." *International Journal of Social Psychiatry* 61 (4): 330–342.

Yoneyama, Shoko. 2000. "Student Discourse on Tōkō Kyohi (School Phobia/ Refusal) in Japan, Burnout or Empowerment?" *British Journal of Sociology of Education* 21 (1): 77–94.

Yong, Roseline, and Kyoko Nomura. 2019. "Hikikomori Is Most Associated with Interpersonal Relationships, Followed by Suicide Risks: A Secondary Analysis of a National Cross-Sectional Study." *Frontiers in Psychiatry* 10:247.

4 Mental health surveys on *hikikomori*

Epidemiological and psychological data

Epidemiological surveys

Three epidemiological surveys have already been mentioned in the previous chapter, and each one offers the following conclusions: the condition of *hikikomori* is reduced to depression (Kato et al. 2011, 2012), to social anxiety disorder (Nagata et al. 2013), or divided into three subcategories: schizophrenia, mood disorder, anxiety disorder; developmental disorders; and personality disorders (Kondo et al. 2013). The following epidemiological research provides further insight into the *hikikomori* condition.

Between 2002 and 2006, a group of researchers participated in the World Mental Health Survey Japan (WMH-J) under the auspices of the World Health Organization (WHO). They conducted 4134 face-to-face interviews using a standardized questionnaire with people over 20 years of age (Koyama et al. 2010). Two sets of questions were asked: the first was about the *hikikomori* experience of the respondents themselves (1660 people between the ages of 20 and 49 years), and the second about the *hikikomori* experience of the children of these people. The results are as follows. Of the 1660 people surveyed, 1.2% experienced a *hikikomori* period in their lives and of this group, 54.5% had a history of psychiatric pathology. Of all respondents (4134), 0.5% reported that they have had at least one child *hikikomori,* allowing the authors to advance the figure of 232,000 people at the national level. The average age of initiation of *hikikomori* is 22.3 years with a peak between 15 and 19 years of age. The reported average withdrawal time was 1 year, and for half of the cases, the withdrawal period was less than 1 year. Of these cases, 78% reported that they had experienced distress caused by concern and irritability, and 75% saying they have never been violent during this period of withdrawal (Koyama et al. 2010: 72). Although it underestimates the number of people involved, this survey is important for several reasons. First, the cohort was large, and the instruments used were standardized. Also, it considers people over 39 years old. Second, it does not see the phenomenon in purely psychiatric terms: 45.5% of cases have not experienced psychiatric pathology, and the study questions the fact that *hikikomori* may be a culture-bound syndrome. Finally, the authors take precautions with their projected minimum of 232,000 cases and recognize six limitations (Koyama et al. 2010: 73) which suggest improvements for future research.

Data from the 2002 to 2006 WMH-J survey noted above also have been the subject of a study on the association of family factors with *hikikomori* risk (Umeda, Kawakami, and The World Mental Health Survey Group 2002–2006. 2012). Data for 708 people between the ages of 20 and 49 were examined. It appears that *hikikomori* is triggered most often in families where parents have a high level of education. The presence of the mother's panic disorder is considered a risk factor for children who develop *hikikomori*.

Another epidemiological survey on *hikikomori* and student apathy is worth mentioning here (Uchida 2010) because of its size, which included 390,526 students – 249,337 men (64%) and 141,189 women (36%). The data was collected by health professionals from 74 Japanese national universities (out of a total of 83 Japanese national universities in 2005) from students enrolled on April 30 of each academic year between 1985 and 2005. The survey shows a steady and significant increase in the number of apathetic students over this period. Fourth-year students (the last year of the Bachelor's degree in Japan), and especially male science students, are considered a high-risk population.

In addition to the results mentioned before, a survey conducted by Saitō et al. (MHLW 2010) provides particularly detailed data relative to age distribution, age of onset, and age at first diagnosis among the *hikikomori* population. With regard to age distribution, an average age of just above 32 years (32.6) with 16% between 21 and 25 years old; 18% between 26 and 30 years old; 31% between 31 and 35 years old; and 34% over 36 (only 1% between 16 and 20, and 0% are under 15).

With regard to age of onset, Saito et al. (2008) found that the average age of onset is about 20 years (20.3) with 19% under 15 years old; 38% between 16 and 20 years old; 21% between 21 and 25 years old; 21% between 26 and 30 years old; and 1% between 26 and 30 years old (0% are over 36).

Finally, with regard to age at first diagnosis, the average age is a little more than 27 years of age (27.3) with 19% under 15 years old 19% between 16 and 20 years old; 29% between 21 and 25 years old; 27% between 26 and 30 years old; and 6% between 31 and 35 years old (0% are over 36 years old).

Investigations about hikikomori individuals' parents

Various investigations have been conducted on *hikikomori* individuals' parents (Koshiba 2007, Koyama et al. 2010). Japanese researchers first noted greater psychological distress among parents with a *hikikomori* child compared to parents who do not have *hikikomori* children (Kobayashi et al. 2003). They highlighted the fact that support relieves family anxiety and helps parents to see their *hikikomori* child more positively (Narabayashi 2003). Also, 20% of *hikikomori* individuals whose parents received support from mental health professionals started social activities 1 year after the start of support (Kurita, Kiba, and Hayashi 2004).

Ueda (2010) trained five parents during a 3-day *hikikomori* parent workshop. Three of the five parents had a child who had withdrawn for less than 5 years; these parents managed to implement behavioral support skills. The other parents who had a *hikikomori* child who had withdrawn for more than 5 years were unable to incorporate behavioral support skills and only paid attention to what their child could not do. This article presents an interesting initiative, but the limited and heterogeneous sample of the study does not produce significant results. Nevertheless, the general idea is quite right: the more time passes, the more difficult it is for parents to see their withdrawn child in a positive light.

Another *hikikomori* parent study is Funakoshi's doctoral thesis, which focused on the difficulties faced by the parents of *hikikomori* people (2011). It is composed of a qualitative study in which 18 parents and 3 counselors were interviewed in order to know the process by which "they themselves find the answers to their child's problems" (Funakoshi 2011: 28). This allows the researcher to suggest clinical improvements in supporting families. Then, a quantitative study of 176 parents and 55 couples describes, by means of standardized scales, the differences of parental difficulties. The results show that fathers are almost two times less likely than mothers to receive support; the researcher concludes that they need more support. This study illustrates one fact: support for *hikikomori* people occurs in the vast majority of cases, first in consultation with the mother, and to a lesser extent (one case out of two in this study) in consultations with both parents. In the vast majority of cases, it is only in the second instance that the *hikikomori* subject himself will participate in a consultation, most often with his mother also present. For more details of testimonials from parents, the reader might refer to Rubinstein (2016), which provides accounts collected through self-help groups for parents of *hikikomori* people.

Qualitative surveys on hikikomori themselves

In 2006, Ishikawa Ryoko argued that the confusion between *hikikomori* and NEET would have negative effects on the *hikikomori* themselves and, in fact, deplores the treatment of *hikikomori* within a support system for NEETs. These negative effects were confirmed in the conclusion of a series of interviews with young people in associations that help them: "Those who consider themselves *hikikomori* see themselves as inferior and withdraw from relationships with others, because, although they have difficulties to work, they are overly concerned about the idea that working is natural for an adult."(Ishikawa 2006: 45). Ishikawa (2006: 46) insists that "their self-esteem cannot be restored immediately even if they participate in a support group." She adds that *hikikomori* people ask questions like "Why do we have to work? What do I want to do? Who am I?" And must first return to their personal history and go through a moment of psychological elaboration to return to society. In this sense, the measures with regard to the NEETs who commit them to first insert themselves at the workplace, would not be adapted to *hikikomori* people who would first wish to question the meaning of work. In other words, the fact that *hikikomori* people are involved in a system of assistance for NEETs would lead them to give up their efforts.

In a completely different way, a study done in Japan by two American psychologists (Krieg and Dickie 2013) tried to think of *hikikomori* in light of the concept of attachment. Twenty four *hikikomori* individuals aged 14–32 years participated in the study (14 men, 10 women). They were met via a group therapy center – a *hikikomori* day care center and a Christian support group. A control group consisted of 59 people (27 men, 32 women) aged 18–24 years. All participants resided in the Kantō region. The results suggest *hikikomori* people have a greater incidence of ambivalent attachment, report more rejection by their parents and peers (bullying), and express a shy temperament. In other words, they found that "shy temperament and parental rejection predicted ambivalent attachment that when coupled with peer rejection, predicted *hikikomori*." (Krieg and Dickie 2013: 61) They, therefore, call for greater attention to the insecure attachments of late childhood and early adolescence.

Psychologist Morisaki Shima, meanwhile, tried to understand *hikikomori* from the point of view of *hikikomori* subjects themselves. To do this, she studied three autobiographies, including those of Ueyama (2001), Katsuyama (2001), and Moroboshi (2003). It focused on two aspects: the relationship of the *hikikomori* subject with the society from which he retires, and the relationship of the *hikikomori* subject with the home from which he withdraws. According to her, they are afraid to work in society, but at the same time they internalize the values that they should work. They find themselves in a negative spiral where they are ashamed of themselves because they do not work, and subsequently find it even more difficult to participate in social life. "As they are in a negative spiral because of the negative message they receive from society, *hikikomori* can be thought of as an illness of social relationships" (Morisaki 2012: 287). According to her, the *hikikomori* phenomenon questions our social values: it invites us to think how to respond to the message sent by those who opt to withdraw themselves from society, and in doing so potentially improve the way we live as a society.

In his 2012 study, Itoh Kohki also relied on the autobiographies of the three authors mentioned before. He also studied that of Hayashi (2003) and … his own (Itoh 2010). It highlights the problem of aging *hikikomori* people and the impossibility for parents, once they retire, to provide for themselves. There is great concern about their future after their parents' death, including the possibilities of suicide or becoming homeless. Social programs are geared toward social participation: increasing social and communication skills, psychotherapy, vocational training, and employment assistance. Programs are public or private and take place in mental health centers, clinics, schools, or NPOs. In the short term, this allows social participation, but in the medium and long term, their fundamental problems remain unresolved. For Itoh Kohki, one can observe a problem related to vertical structures of seniority in *hikikomori* accounts. For example, Moroboshi Noa describes difficulty in adapting to relationships with colleagues in the work-place. He did not get along with his supervisor or other employees, especially those who were younger than him: when they did not respect him, his pride was abused. In their accounts, one observes a critique of seniority whose val-ues they have internalized. There is also the problem of "a gap in the resume" (employment or education) identified by Ueyama Kazuki, Hayashi Kyoko, and Itoh Kohki. Finally, problems of communication, particularly love, sexu-ality, and difficulties in finding a partner were also common (I will comment further on when I discuss Ueyama Kazuki and Mr. Onishi).

Two additional surveys must be mentioned. From the study of 12 clin-ical cases, Murasawa (2012) highlights how a *hikikomori* mentality could be constructed from "traumatization" (the individual reconstructs a trau-matic experience through a repetition of memory) and stigma (the self is repeatedly damaged through an internal persecutory gaze). Okabe et al.'s (2012) study presents questions about *hikikomori*'s internal experience in semi-structured interviews conducted with nine young people. The initial idea of these researchers is that *hikikomori* subjects think they should be "normal" and that this causes many conflicts at home. Their conclusions are that *hikikomori* subjects are able to free themselves from the idea that they must be "normal", but only under specific circumstances.

Works by a Japanese–French research team

Works by the Japanese–French *hikikomori* research team have brought new ways to understand Japanese *hikikomori* cases through a comparison with their French counterparts. Furuhashi et al. (2013) studied five Japanese and four French cases. The insights of the study are as follows:

> It seems that in Japan we enter a *hikikomori* state following difficulties encountered on the way to one's ideal, and that in France, we enter a *hikiko-mori* state following a "concrete problem" (specific failure in the affective and sexual domains, drugs, delinquency, etc.). In Japan, the avoidance of a disorder or a failure plays an important role in the causes that lead to the state of *hikikomori*, and in turn, the prolongation of the state of *hikiko-mori* results in a breakdown of relations with society, whereas in France, a "concrete problem" or failure is in themselves the causes that lead to the state of *hikikomori* (Furuhashi et al. 2013: 258).

Specifically, the entry into the *hikikomori* state is accompanied by ruptures, failures, and troubles in France, while Japanese subjects avoid a break, a failure, or a disorder. Indeed, these researchers find:

> …concrete problems in French *hikikomori* who seem to deviate from the mainstream of society following a breakup or failure in the emotional

or sexual areas. On the other hand, Japanese *hikikomori* preemptively avoid these problems. For example, students who wish to remain students: they seem to try to avoid deviating from their path (Furuhashi et al. 2013: 259).

They add that the transition to adulthood corresponds in France during high school to university, whereas in Japan, it is during the passage from university to employment. The Franco-Japanese study also shows that, contrary to what has been argued previously (Ishikawa 2006), the adoption of the term NEET can favor the professional reintegration and social participation of *hikikomori* subjects. Yet, there are other aspects that are not covered by Furuhashi et al., for instance, the results of the study do not make it possible to draw conclusions about internet addiction among *hikikomori* individuals. Further, the article mentions the possibility of different types of *hikikomori* (narcissistic, schizoid, and avoiding). However, the insistence on the role played by *seken* as "a notion rooted in the psychic structure of the Japanese" (Furuhashi et al. 2013) is likely to promote a culturally determinist approach of *hikikomori*.

The Japanese–French collective volume entitled *Hikikomori, these withdrawn teenagers* (Fansten et al. 2014) presents the phenomenon of Japanese social withdrawal which worries a number of professionals and families in France. The collaboration was unprecedented in its inclusion of sociologists, anthropologists, psychologists, psychiatrists, and psychoanalysts from both countries. The coauthors are members of a French-Japanese team that has been researching social withdrawal of young people since 2009, and the book benefits from contributions from a school doctor, C. Guigné, and two psychiatrists working on these issues in France, M.-J. Guedj-Bourdiau and S. Tisseron.

The foreword to this volume is written by sociologist A. Ehrenberg, who places the *hikikomori* problem within the transformations of autonomy and the pathologies of the ideal. The introduction then provides an excellent synthesis of the issues and elements of the *hikikomori* debate. Next, in the first part of the book, "Obstacles, suspensions and passages from the threshold of childhood to adulthood" six chapters in length present the views of a sociologist (Ms. Fansten, Associate professor in sociology at Paris University) and an anthropologist (C. Figueiredo, Associate professor in education sciences at Paris University), a school doctor (C. Guigné), a psychiatrist (K. Suzuki, Professor at Nagoya University), a specialist in educational sciences and Japanese studies (C. Galan, Professor at Toulouse university), Japanese social anthropologists (J. Teruyama, Assistant Professor at Tsukuba University, and S. Horiguchi, Associate Professor at Temple University Japan Campus). This first part concludes by tracing the history of the concepts of autonomy and autarchy (P.-H. Castel, CNRS-EHESS Senior Researcher).

The second part of the Japanese–French collective volume "Stories, experiences and interpretation of withdrawal" is composed of five chapters and focuses on the psychiatric, psychological, and psychoanalytic aspects of social withdrawal in France and Japan. We note in particular the contribution of S. Tisseron who deploys his thesis of a double psychological and social disarticulation, as well as that of M.-J. Guedj-Bourdiau concerning home confinement of young people in France, which formulates hypotheses and proposals supported by several clinical cases. Second, the psychiatrist T. Ogawa (Nagoya University professor and psychoanalyst, member of the executive committee of the Japanese society of psychoanalysis affiliated with the IPA) develops his conception of a *hikikomori* as a manifestation of a pathological narcissism and passive aggression due to a failure of the containing function in childhood. The notion of "refusal" inherent in this condition is presented according to a triple approach (phenomenological, anthropological, psychoanalytic) developed by the psychiatrist N. Pionnié-Dax (Head of Department of infantile-juvenile psychiatry, Paris Erasmus Hospital), which concludes the work.

Hikikomori, these withdrawn teenagers (Fansten et al. 2014) is the first book to bring together French and Japanese researchers from different disciplines to reflect on the problems of contemporary youth. It is also the first comprehensive French study of the *hikikomori* phenomenon in Japan, while bringing comparative examples of similar cases in France. Finally, very little work on the field of "youth, mental health and society in Japan" was available in French; this multidisciplinary book came at the right time to fill this gap. It is not my ambition to give an exhaustive account of each chapter, although each deserves a detailed analysis of its contributions and limitations. I would rather mention the one written by a French psychoanalyst (N. Vellut, psychologist at the CNRS) and a Japanese psychiatrist (T. Furuhashi, Associate professor at Nagoya University), saluting their having not given up on the extreme difficulty of Franco-Japanese comparisons in this field. One of the positive aspects of their contribution is to refute some extremely tenacious ideas in popular representations of *hikikomori* that, for example, skew fictional vignettes produced by psychiatrists themselves (Kato et al. 2012). Thus, the authors show, contrary to the published scientific literature in French or English, that in the vast majority of Japanese families where there is a *hikikomori* child, the father is present at home and works (which is different from the French cases). With the difficulties of separation between parents and children as well as fraternal rivalries, these authors indicate avenues for clinical research on the family factors associated with the *hikikomori* phenomenon. In addition, they formulated the following statement, which reveals different expressions of the pathologies of the ideal:

> While the young French withdraw after a failure in relationships, young Japanese withdraw when a failure, either with their school or with other students, seems possible. On the Japanese side, it is the forecast or the possibility of even relative failure that is significant.
>
> *(Fansten et al. 2014: 150)*

Overall, advances in this exploratory research could help shape the assumptions of future epidemiological research involving a larger sample. The novelty of this type of project, combined with the complexity of Franco-Japanese comparisons, is likely to inspire new insights and perhaps extend the scope of comparison to other countries.

2016 Cabinet office survey

Introduction

First reports from the Ministry of Health, Labor, and Welfare were published in 2001 and 2003, but the 2010 report is considered a milestone in *hikikomori* studies (MHLW 2001, 2003, 2010). Also, in 2010, a shorter survey was published by the Cabinet Office of Japan (2010). We discuss the latter survey below, which estimates the *hikikomori* population. Here, I present a synthesis of the youths' life survey published by the Cabinet Office of Japan in September 2016. I include details concerning questions such as "What applies to me?" (III-8) and "daily life habits" (III-9). This 169-page survey is descriptive. It presents data about the phenomenon while never discussing, providing statistical analysis, or interpreting the results. In the present synthesis, I present the survey while remaining faithful to its descriptive spirit before comprehensively assessing it.

The survey was published in September 2016 and is entitled *"Wakamono no seikatsu ni kansuru chōsa hōkokusho,"* which in English is *"Research Survey of Youth's Life"* (Cabinet Office 2016). Although the survey is dedicated to *hikikomori*, the term *hikikomori* is surprisingly not mentioned in the title. It starts by describing the results of the first investigation in 2010. At the time, the Cabinet Office (2010) formed a team of psychiatrists and clinical psychologists to produce a report entitled *"Investigation on Youths' Consciousness (Investigation on Hikikomori)"*. The target of the investigation was a cohort of five thousand individuals between 15 and 39 years old, nationwide. In Japan, individuals in this age range are classified as *"wakamono"* meaning "youth": in Western industrialized countries, it would encompass emerging adulthood and young adulthood (Arnett, Žukauskienė, and Sugimura 2014). Questionnaires were distributed to (randomized distribution) and collected from the home. In total, valid questionnaires completed by 3287 individuals (65.7%) were collected. Among them, the *hikikomori* group was composed of 59 individuals (1.79%). Based on demographic estimates of the Ministry of Internal Affairs and Communications (2008), the *hikikomori* corresponded to 696,000 individuals nationwide. In addition, the investigation included items such as "I understand the feeling of being *hikikomori,"* and those who responded affirmatively were numerous, representing what was then considered the affinity group, estimated at 1.55 million individuals nationwide. Individuals belonging to the affinity group are not *hikikomori* themselves.

Following the 2010 results, a similar investigation was conducted by the Cabinet Office to research the actual conditions of withdrawal. I present the principal results, which were made public in September 2016. The report explains the necessity of actively supporting youth who are struggling in their social life and researching their actual condition. The survey underlines the difficulty of understanding the relational mechanisms that are so challenging for troubled youth, especially those who are *hikikomori*.

Overview of the survey

The purpose of the investigation was to determine the number of individuals experiencing *hikikomori*, to identify the nature of appropriate assistance, to understand the onset and character of the youths' difficulties and to promote the implementation of an assistance network in every region nationwide. The target of the investigation was 15- to 39-year-old individuals and their families living in 198 municipalities nationwide. Auto-questionnaires were distributed (randomized distribution) to 5000 individuals (90.3% live with one or several members of their family). The investigators distributed and collected the questionnaire at home from December 11 to 23, 2015.

A first portion of the investigation allowed the identification of a group of "*hikikomori* in the broad sense" (*Kōgi no hikikomori gun*), based on precise inclusion and exclusion criteria. The aim was to focus on whether autonomy was acquired, an important issue in terms of Japanese youth policy (Toivonen 2008). Individuals who responded to Q20 with number 5, 6, 7, or 8 noted below and to Q22 with its below-noted response were included in the group of *hikikomori*:

Q20: "In what circumstances do you go out?" (*Fudan dono kurai gaishutsu shimasu ka)*

5. I only go out for my hobbies.
6. I go out in the neighborhood, to the convenience store, etc.
7. I leave my room, but not the house.
8. I rarely leave my room.

Q22: "How long have you experienced this condition?"

Those who responded "more than 6 months" were included as *hikikomori*.
Individuals who responded as follows to Q23, Q13, and Q18 were excluded:

Q23: "What triggered your current state?" Those who selected "disease" and responded "schizophrenia" or gave the name of a physical disease, "pregnant"; "other" or wrote that they work at home, gave birth, or took care of their children's education were excluded.

Q13: "Are you currently working?" Each individual among those who stayed home and who responded "housewife/husband" or "cleaner" was excluded.

Q18: "State what you often do when you are at home." Individuals who responded doing domestic tasks or helping with their children's education were excluded.

Consequently, those who gave responses 6, 7, or 8 to Q20 stated previously were defined as *"hikikomori* in the strict sense" (*Kyōgi no hikikomori*). Those who responded 5 (I only go out for my hobbies) to Q20 are defined as "quasi-*hikikomori"* (*jun hikikomori*). The group defined as *hikikomori* in the broad sense is composed of the sum of individuals defined as *hikikomori* in the strict sense and quasi-*hikikomori*. Among over 3000 valid questionnaires (62.0%) collected, nearly 50 (1.57%) satisfied the definition of *hikikomori* in the broad sense. According to demographic estimates of the Ministry of Internal Affairs and Communications (2015), the population aged 15–39 is 34,450,000 people, while the estimated number of individuals with *hikikomori* in the broad sense, is estimated, based on the present survey, as 541,000.

Additionally, individuals who feel sympathy for, or those who understand *hikikomori*, and those who think they might want to withdraw were extracted and defined as an affinity group (*shinwa gun*), as follows. Those who responded to Q32 (what applied to me) "agree" or "rather agree" (to at least one the four items), 13–16 below, comprise the affinity group.

13. I understand the feelings of those who shut themselves in at home or in their room and do not go out.
14. I already thought about shutting myself in at home or in my room.
15. If there is an unpleasant event, I do not want to go out.
16. If there's a reason, I think it is normal to shut myself in at home or in my room.

Individuals in the group *hikikomori* in the broad sense are excluded from the affinity group. According to the representative sample of the present survey, the estimated number of individuals in the affinity group is 1656,000 nationwide.

The general group identified as *hikikomori* is composed of the total number of respondents (3104) minus the group with *hikikomori* in the broad sense (49 individuals), and the affinity group (150 individuals), i.e., 2905 individuals.

Results

Concerning gender, the group with *hikikomori* in the broad sense is 63.3% men and 36.7% women. In the affinity group, 40.7% are men and 59.3% are women. In the general group, 48.0% are men and 52.0% are women. (Note: Graphs and tables were prepared by the authors. They were not included

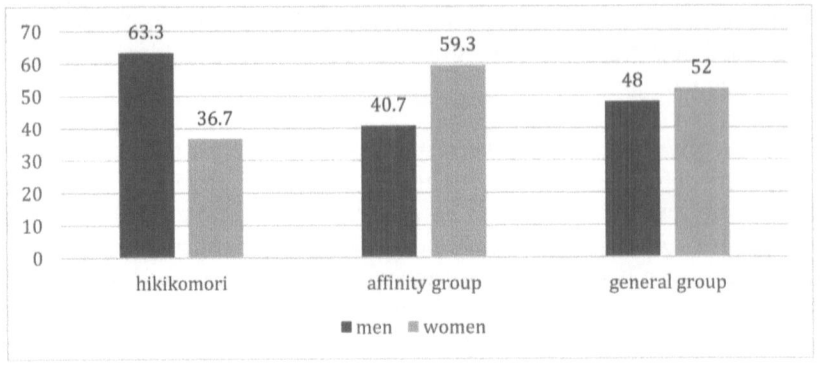

Chart 4.1 Gender

in the survey of the Cabinet Office and were made to present the data in a comprehensive manner.)

With regard to age, the group classified as *hikikomori* in the broad sense comprised individuals aged 15–19 (10.2%), 20–24 (24.5%), 25–29 (24.5%), 30–34 (20.4%), and 35–39 (20.4%). The affinity group comprised individuals aged 15–19 (27.3%), 20–24 (24.7%), 25–29 (21.3%), 30–34 (18.0%), and 35–39 (8.7%). The general group comprised individuals aged 15–19 (18.1%), 20–24 (16.8%), 25–29 (17.2%), 30–34 (22.0%), and 35–39 (25.8%).

Concerning education, the percentage of those who responded "I am currently studying" was 24.4% in the general group, 33.3% in the affinity group, and 10.2% in the group with *hikikomori* in the broad sense. The percentage of those who responded "I already graduated" was 71.7% in the general group, 62.0% in the affinity group, and 63.3% in the group with *hikikomori*

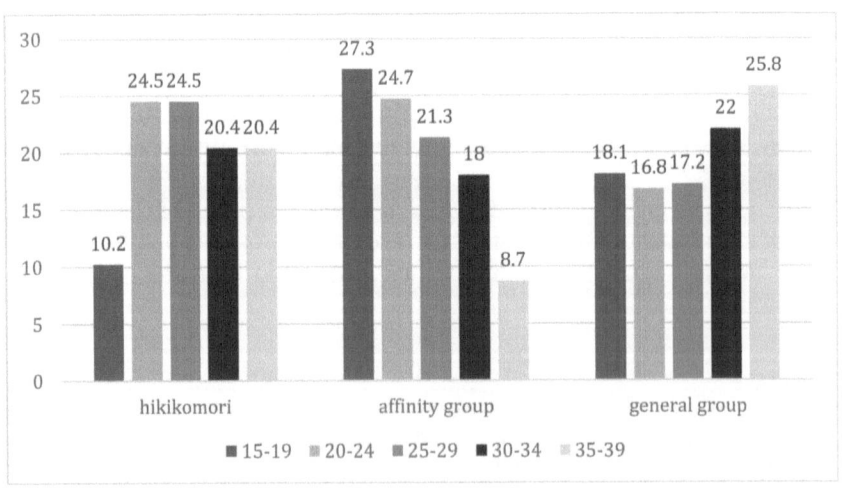

Chart 4.2 Age

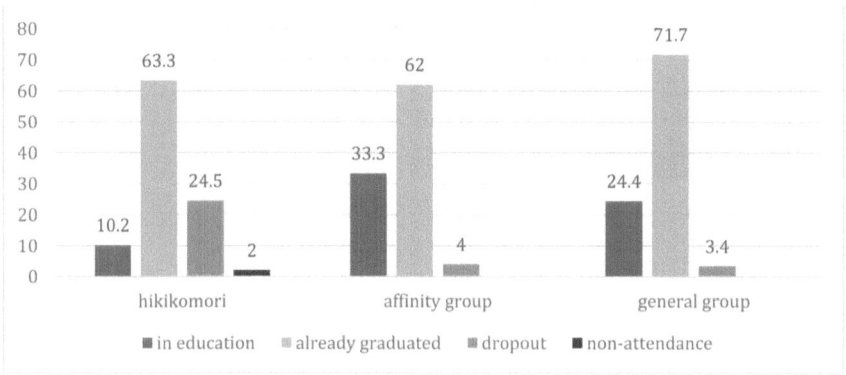

Chart 4.3 Education

in the broad sense. The percentage of those who responded "I dropped out" was 3.4% in the general group, 4.0% in the affinity group, and 24.5% in the group with *hikikomori* in the broad sense. The percentage of those who responded "I am temporarily not attending school" was 2.0% in the group with *hikikomori* in the broad sense.

Concerning their current employment status, 43.2% of those in the general group responded "I am working." The percentage of those who responded "housewife/husband" or "assistance in domestic tasks" was 7.4% in the general group. The percentage of those who responded "student" was 32.0% in the affinity group; the percentage of those who responded "I am registered in a part-time work agency, etc., but I do not work at the moment" was 8.2% in the group with *hikikomori* in the broad sense. The

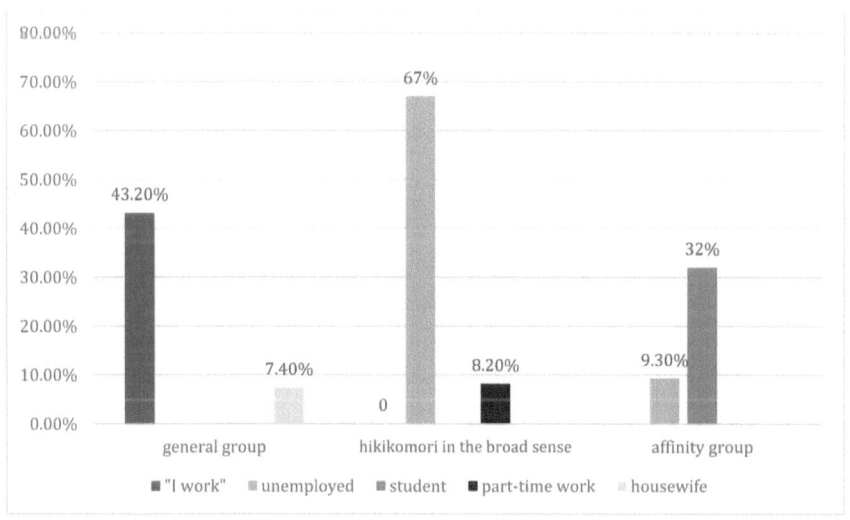

Chart 4.4 Work

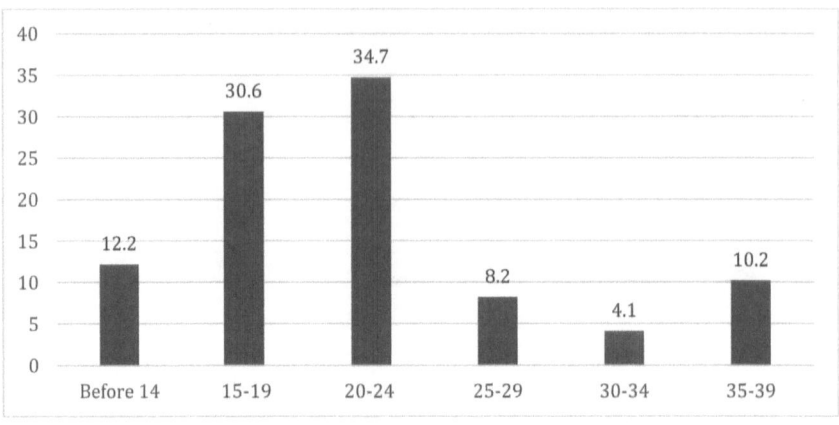

Chart 4.5 The age when *hikikomori* begins

percentage of those who responded "currently unemployed" in the group with *hikikomori* in the broad sense was 67.3% and was 9.3% in the affinity group.

When those in the group with *hikikomori* in the broad sense were asked about their approximate age when their current situation started, 12.2% responded "before 14," 30.6% "between 15 and 19," 34.7% "between 20 and 24," 8.2% "between 25 and 29," 4.1% "between 30 and 34," and 10.2% "between 35 and 39."

When asked about the duration of withdrawal, for those in the group with *hikikomori* in the broad sense, 12.2% reported "from 6 months to 1 year," 12.2% "1–3 years," 28.6% "3–5 years," 12.2% "5–7 years," and 34.7% "more than 7 years."

When 49 individuals in the group with *hikikomori* in the broad sense were asked what triggered their current state, nine individuals responded "school non-attendance" or "I did not adapt to the workplace;" eight reported "my job-seeking activities failed" or "my human relationships were bad," seven said "illness," three said "I failed the exam," and two responded, "I did not

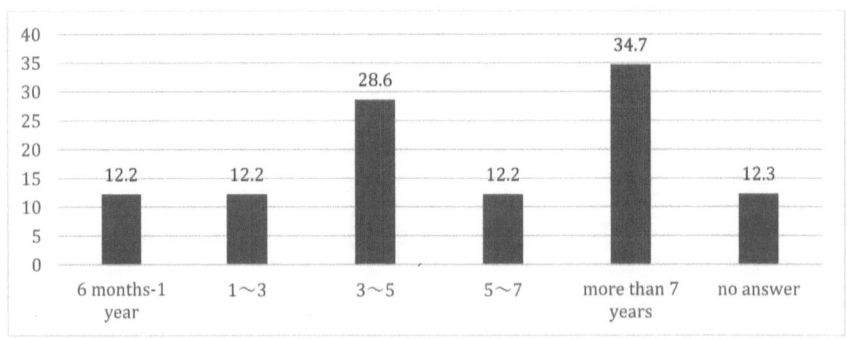

Chart 4.6 Duration of *hikikomori*

adapt to the university." Among the 15 individuals who responded "other," the following responses were given: "apathy," "no specific reason," "because I am inside," "I never really thought about it," "the company moved its services," and "I wanted to do what I wanted." Many did not give a specific response.

Results are detailed in Table 4.1 for Q32, "What applies to me?" and Q34, "Habits of daily life".

Regarding Q34-3 "In the morning, I wake up at a fixed time.", 44.9% disagreed with this statement in the *hikikomori* group in the broad sense, whereas 39.3% in the affinity group and 22.7% in the general group disagreed.

Table 4.1 Agreement (%) with statements for Q32 "What applies to me?" and Q34, "Habits of daily life"

Questions (statements)	Groups		
	Group with hikikomori *in the broad sense*	Affinity group	General group
Q32-1, "If someone criticizes my defects or failures, it makes me very upset."	67.3	78.7	49.5
Q32-2 "When I am with people, if they make fun of me or do not treat me well, it makes me feel anxious."	55.1	66.7	31.2
Q32-3 "It's a source of anxiety? when someone around me thinks I am weird."	51.0	63.3	25.2
Q32-4 "It depresses me if another person points out my errors and faults."	49.0	76.0	42.2
Q32-7 "With people I meet for the first time, I can immediately talk to them."	32.7	42.7	57.1
Q32-8 "I am preoccupied by not being able to communicate well with others."	57.1	70.7	40.3
Q32-9 "I hardly can express my emotions."	53.1	64.0	41.1
Q32-10 "When there is a problem with people around me, I don't know how to solve it."	63.3	57.3	25.7
Q32-12 "As for my daily life, I don't like people who intervene."	69.4	85.3	75.1
Q34-1 "As for my personal things, my parents take care of them."	67.3	55.3	37.4
Q34-2 "As for meals and cleaning, my parents take care of it."	67.3	60.7	43.6
Q34-5 "I live with a day-night inversion."	36.7	18.7	9.5
Q34-8 "There are many days when I don't speak to anyone."	32.7	16.7	3.8
Q34-9 "It bores me to speak to people."	44.9	42.7	12.7
Q34-10 "I can't trust anybody among my past acquaintances and relatives."	30.6	23.3	7.6
Q34-11 "I think my mental state is not healthy."	40.8	50.0	14.1
Q34-12 "I often think about my current situation."	79.6	77.3	53.3

Concluding remarks

In the 2010 survey, the estimated *hikikomori* population was 696,000; in the 2016 survey, their number was estimated at 541,000, which suggests a decrease in the *hikikomori* population. However, according to the 2010 survey, 23.7% of those belonging to the category *hikikomori* were between 35 and 39 years old. As this group was older than 39 in 2015, they represent an aging *hikikomori* population that was not included in the 2016 survey. Nevertheless, the aging of this population is a great problem in contemporary Japanese society. Regarding the duration of the withdrawal, the comparison of the two surveys' results shows a lengthening of the withdrawal: 34.7% were *hikikomori* for more than 7 years in 2016, while only 16.7% were in 2010. The phenomenon has, thus, accelerated in the last 6 years of survey-taking.

Again, the 2016 survey does not include those who are above 39 for reasons of age. In this respect, it would be necessary to take into account the *hikikomori* population between 40 and 50 years old. In fact, researchers, clinical practitioners, social workers, and parents have been concerned for many years about the aging of the *hikikomori* population. The absence of consideration of individuals above 39 is one of the reasons we conclude, along with other experts (Kato et al. 2017), that 541,000 is an underestimation of the phenomenon. Other reasons might be cited as well. For instance, 38% of the questionnaires were considered invalid. It is highly unlikely that current *hikikomori* individuals would not be in this group. As some of them are distressed, their responses could easily become invalid.

In addition, the criteria defining the affinity group seem questionable. We understand why it is interesting to distinguish an affinity group from the *hikikomori* group, but some members of the affinity group may themselves be *hikikomori*. One approach could be to consider the affinity group as an "at-risk group." The affinity group represented 1.55 million individuals in 2010 and would be composed of 1.65 million individuals today. In fact, the group at risk of becoming *hikikomori*, those who are struggling at school or work, never stops increasing. This group is highly visible in Q32 where one observes hypersensitivity and communication problems in interpersonal relation settings. It would be possible, and important, to better support these individuals in school, work, and medical settings. In fact, no one previously paid attention to the affinity group. Since the survey showed that it was a hypersensitive population, measures should be taken to support this suffering population. Alternatively, nothing indicates that this affinity group is a real "at-risk group." We would rather consider that, although they cognitively feel close to *hikikomori* individuals, or share the same ideas, the very fact they have not developed this behavior should lead us to question the "protecting" factors they might benefit from, environmental factors such as family. Sociological, anthropological, and psychological reflections could focus on why they are not *hikikomori* and what kind of strategies they developed to cope with their problems. Additionally, men represented 66.1% of *hikikomori* individuals in the 2010 survey, and 63.3% in the 2016 survey, which is a slight decrease. Given that women in the affinity group of the 2016 survey represent 59.3%, one could not reasonably claim that *hikikomori* is essentially a problem among men.

In terms of the daily life of *hikikomori*, responses to Q34 show that the level of autonomy is low, and the rhythm of daily life is disturbed. This is a consequence of social withdrawal and, simultaneously, one could think that it is also a risk factor. In a society where the birth rate is constantly declining, strong parental intervention might cause problems in terms of youth autonomy. In the future, it would be important to focus on developmental mechanisms of *hikikomori* and to facilitate autonomy from childhood to prevent codependency (child–parent). Here, a few remarks are necessary to explain why and how the declining birthrate is related to codependency. When several children are present in the family, like earlier Japanese families, the time spent by a parent with each child, individually, is lower compared with families in which there is only one child.

With the decline of natality and the increase of families with a single child, certain expressions appeared such as *boshi kapuseru* (mother child capsule) and *mama tomo* (mother friend). *Boshi kapuseru* designates a phenomenon in which the mother is isolated from her own family and the local community alone with her child. In this situation, Japanese psychiatrists, nurses, and social and clinical practitioners found that it became difficult for mothers to separate from their child. For instance, they might tend to do many things for the child. This problem of codependency could be explained in various ways. The model of the housewife raising the child and the father as the breadwinner (Lock 1995) is weakening in Japan, because increasing numbers of mothers work part-time. However, it does not mean that they are financially autonomous (in this sense the model might just have transformed while not fundamentally changing the structure of gender inequality). Also, the model of the mother housewife/father breadwinner is still very strong compared to other countries, and women are still expected to quit work during pregnancy (while there are maternity leave opportunities, it is an open secret that women are strongly discouraged from asking their employers for it – with exceptions – such as civil servants). Notably, there is a generation of mothers who, despite receiving a university education, stay at home to raise the children. For those with a university education who might work part-time, salary inequality with their husband is significant, and they fail to fulfill their professional goals. In this context, codependency appears. In extreme cases, the "mother–child capsule" is combined with strong gender inequality, sometimes contributing to child neglect and abuse. Another phenomenon known as "*mama tomo*" (mother–friend) describes mothers constantly comparing their child to other children, and comparing children among themselves. The spread of this competitive mindset, which aims at reinforcing social and academic success, may also contribute to the creation of codependence.

Overall, the survey is highly informative. However, additional statistical and qualitative analyses remain to be conducted. The increasing number of articles on the topic from diverse epistemological backgrounds with diverse methodologies have created confusion concerning the definition, the epidemiological scope, and the severity of designated behavioral disorders. The present section seeks to better define the problem and the characteristics associated with social withdrawal and to facilitate investigations and international exchanges on a phenomenon that seems to extend to other industrialized societies.

2019 Cabinet office survey

Introduction

As we have seen previously, in 2010, the Cabinet Office presented the results of a survey entitled "Survey on Youth Consciousness – Survey on *Hikikomori*" (*Wakamono no ishiki ni kansuru chōsa – Hikikomori ni kansuru jittai chōsa*). Curiously, the word *hikikomori* did not appear in the title of their subsequent 2016 survey, "Research Survey on Youth's life" (*Wakamono no seikatsu ni kansuru chōsa hōkokusho*), even though the investigation focused exclusively on this phenomenon. Would the *hikikomori* phenomenon be so shameful that one should exclude its name in a report specifically targeting it? The 2019 survey interests us here because, in the same logic, it is entitled "*Survey on Life Conditions*" (Cabinet Office 2019).

According to the 2016 survey, it appeared that the total number of *hikikomori* individuals had dropped since 2010. This suggestion was immediately refuted by the persons concerned, their families, and the associations which had been warning for years about the aging of this group. Those who were between 35 and 39 years old in 2009 were simply excluded from the evaluation. That is, by 2015, they were older than 39, and their numbers were not replaced in the survey group by an equivalent number of adolescents. Consequently, one cannot truthfully speak of any decrease in the *hikikomori* population that can be linked to the success of support measures in this domain. On the contrary, one can observe a failure of the measures taken to combat the social isolation of youngsters, one of the consequences of which is that the withdrawn population is now older. This is referred to in Japan as "the 80–50 problem." Today, many parents of *hikikomori* individuals are around 80 years old, and their withdrawn children are in their 50s. In other words, many of those we were talking about in the late 1990s and 2000s never came out of their isolation. What we did not know until 2019 was whether those individuals were numbered in the tens of thousands or in the hundreds of thousands. One consequence of this situation is that, their parents having aged or died, their households are increasingly falling into poverty. It is within this context that the Cabinet of Japan was urged to produce another survey, the results of which were published in 2019.

Overview of the survey

The target of the investigation was 40- to 64-year-old individuals and their families living in 198 municipalities nationwide. Auto-questionnaires were distributed (in a randomized distribution) by investigators and were collected from respondents' homes between December 7 and 24, 2018. The number of valid questionnaires collected was 3248 (65% of those distributed). Overall, methods used were similar to those employed in the 2016 survey. The main differences were the age range of the participants and the absence of an affinity group in the 2019 study. The 2019 survey is especially interesting when its findings are compared with those from the 2010 and 2016 surveys. After defining the groups, I will highlight some of these comparisons as I detail the results.

The first part of the investigation was intended to determine who, among the participants, belonged to the group of *"hikikomori* in the broad sense" (*Kōgi no hikikomori gun*), based on precise inclusion and exclusion criteria. The following questions were designed to identify this group:

Q19: "In what circumstances do you go out?" (*Fudan dono kurai gaishutsu shimasu ka).* Those who gave one of the following responses were included in the group of *hikikomori*:

5. I only go out for my hobbies.
6. I go out in the neighborhood, to the convenience store, etc.
7. I leave my room, but not the house.
8. I rarely leave my room.

More specifically, those who gave responses 6, 7, or 8 to Q19 previously were defined as *"hikikomori* in the strict sense" (*Kyōgi no hikikomori).* Those who gave response 5 were defined as "quasi-*hikikomori"* (*jun hikikomori).*

Q20: "How long have you experienced this condition?" Those who responded "more than 6 months" were included as *hikikomori*. Individuals whose current state had been triggered by an illness, such as schizophrenia or a physical disease; those who were pregnant or had recently given birth; those who worked from home; and those who were taking care of their children's education were excluded.

Q12: "Are you currently working?" Those who stayed home, but who described themselves as a "housewife/husband" or "cleaner" were excluded.

Q17: "State what you often do when you are at home." Individuals who responded that they did domestic tasks or helped with their children's education were excluded.

The group defined as *hikikomori* in the broad sense comprised the sum of individuals defined as *hikikomori* in the strict sense and those defined as quasi-*hikikomori*. According to demographic estimates of the Ministry of Internal Affairs and Communications (2018), the population aged 40–64 is 42,350,000, of which the estimated number of individuals with *hikikomori* in the broad sense is 613,000. Of those, the estimated number who would be defined as "*hikikomori* in the strict sense" would be 365,000, with 248,000 considered "quasi-*hikikomori*." Results of the survey would also suggest that 26,000 *hikikomori* never leave their rooms at all, which represents 4.2% of the estimated 613,000 *hikikomori* population (which reflects 0.06% in the general population). In contrast, an estimated 274,000 *hikikomori* do leave home at times, based on those *hikikomori* respondents who agreed with the statement, "I usually stay at home but go to a convenience store in my neighborhood." The second largest group was the "quasi-*hikikomori*" group, based on those respondents who agreed with the statement, "I usually stay home but only go out for my hobbies."

Results

In this survey, the group classified as *hikikomori* in the broad sense was composed of 76.6% men and 23.4% women. It appears that the male *hikikomori* population is higher in the 40–64 age range (76.6%) compared to the 15–39 group (63.3%). Note: Charts and tables have been prepared by the author. They were not included in the survey by the Cabinet Office but have been designed to present the data comprehensively here.

The distribution of ages in the group classified as *hikikomori* in the broad sense was as follows: 40–44 years old (25.5%), 45–49 (12.8%), 50–54 (14.9%), 55–59 (21.3%), and 60–64 (25.5%). The following is the age distribution of the group "other than *hikikomori* in the broad sense": 40–44 (18.2%), 45–49 (22.1%), 50–54 (20.5%), 55–59 (18.1%), and 60–64 (21%).

Results on livelihood showed that 29.8% of *hikikomori* individuals relied on their own financial resources, 34.1% on the resources of their parents, and 17.6% on those of a spouse.

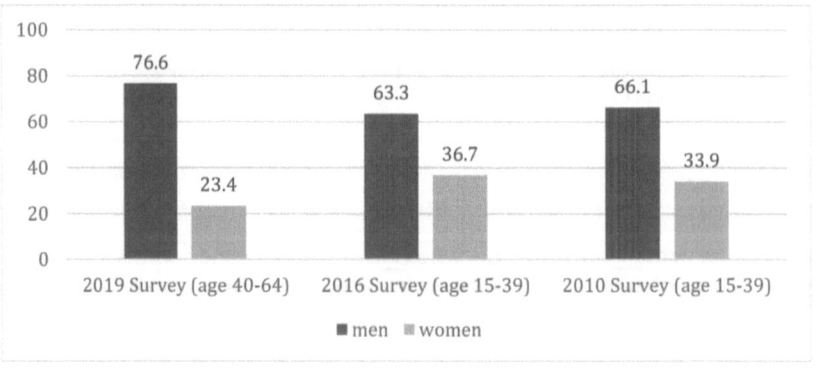

Chart 4.7 Gender

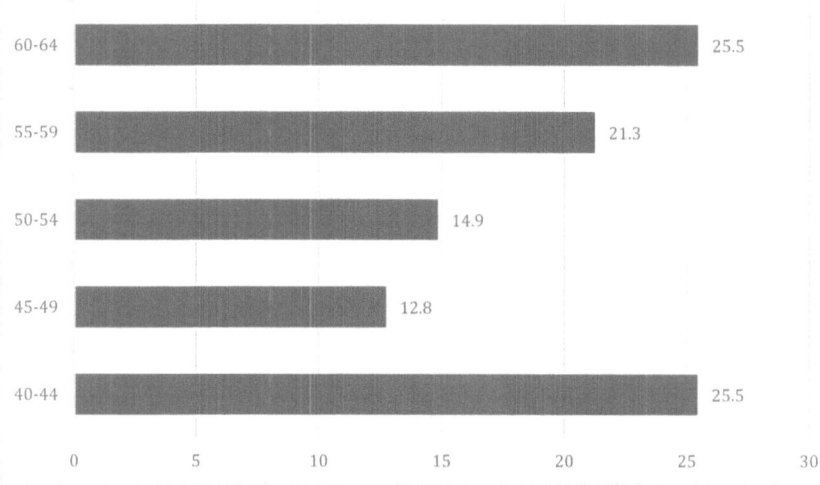

Chart 4.8 Age

The prevalence of hospitalization or outpatient care for reasons of mental illnesses was higher among the *hikikomori* group aged 40–64 (31.9%) than among the general group, i.e., those who were not classified as *hikikomori* (5.6%). In the 2016 survey, the prevalence of hospitalization or outpatient care for reasons of mental illnesses was also higher among the *hikikomori* group aged 15–39 (18.4%) than in the general group (4.5%).

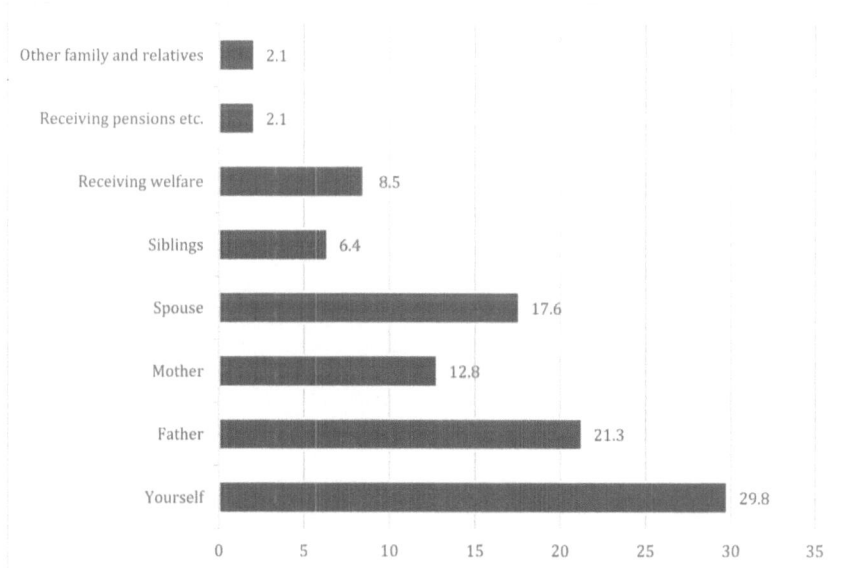

Chart 4.9 Livelihood

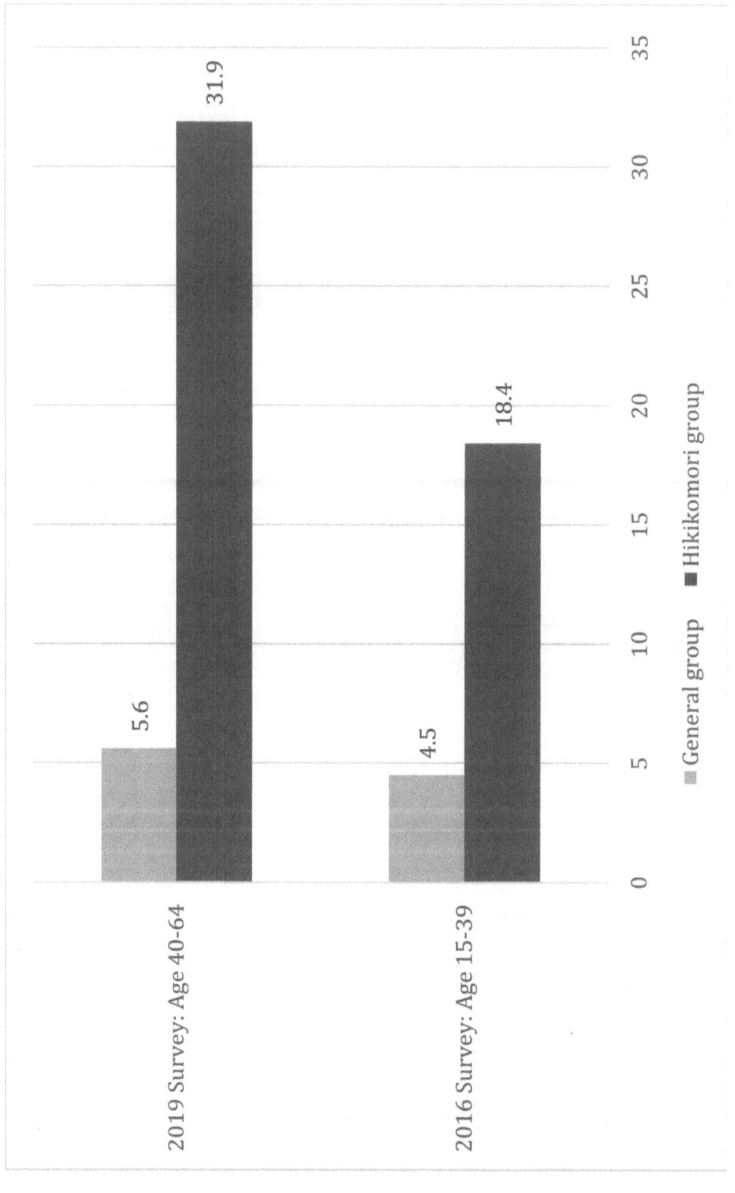

Chart 4.10 Prevalence of mental illnesses (outpatient care/hospitalization)

When comparing the population aged 15–39 to the population aged 40–64, it appears that the mental condition of shut-ins deteriorates more quickly than the general group.

In the *hikikomori* group, 76.6% of individuals were unemployed at the time of the survey, whereas 73.9% had at some time worked as regular employees (Cabinet Office 2019: 31).

With respect to the activities that the two groups engaged in at home, the most common was watching television: 82.5% in the general group and 74.5% in the *hikikomori* group. This was followed by using the internet: 43.3% in the general group and 29.8% in the *hikikomori* group. It appears

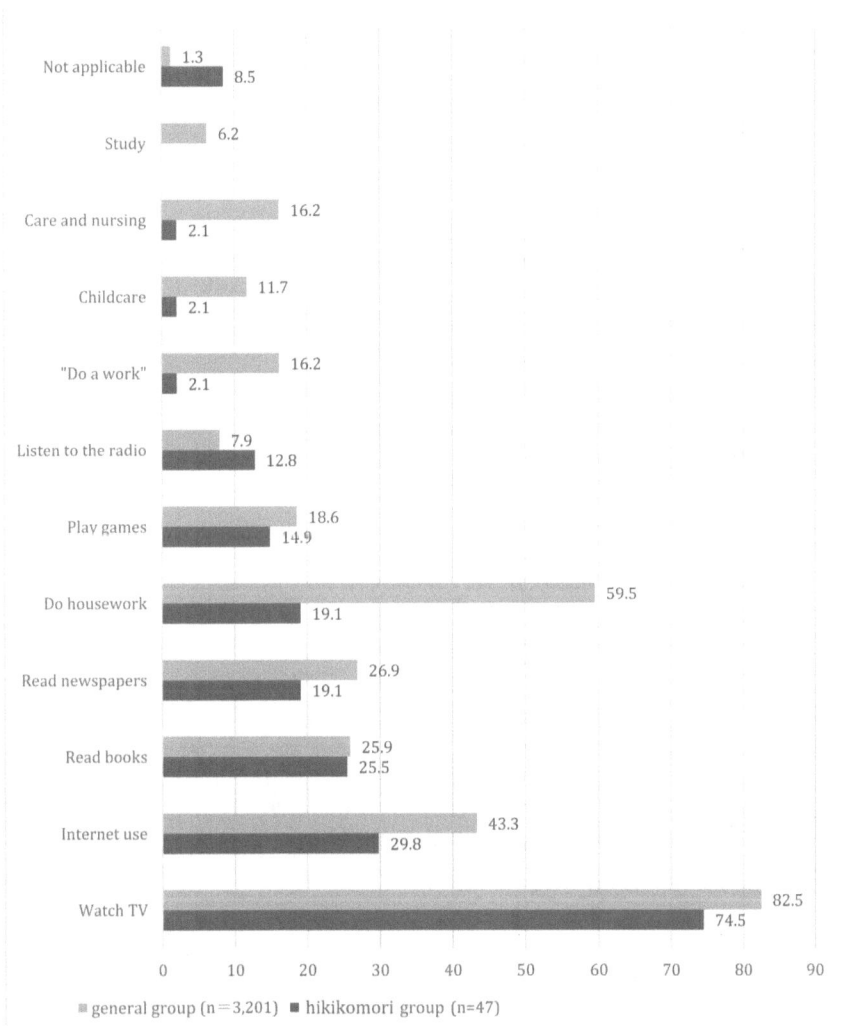

Chart 4.11 What I often do at home (Q17)

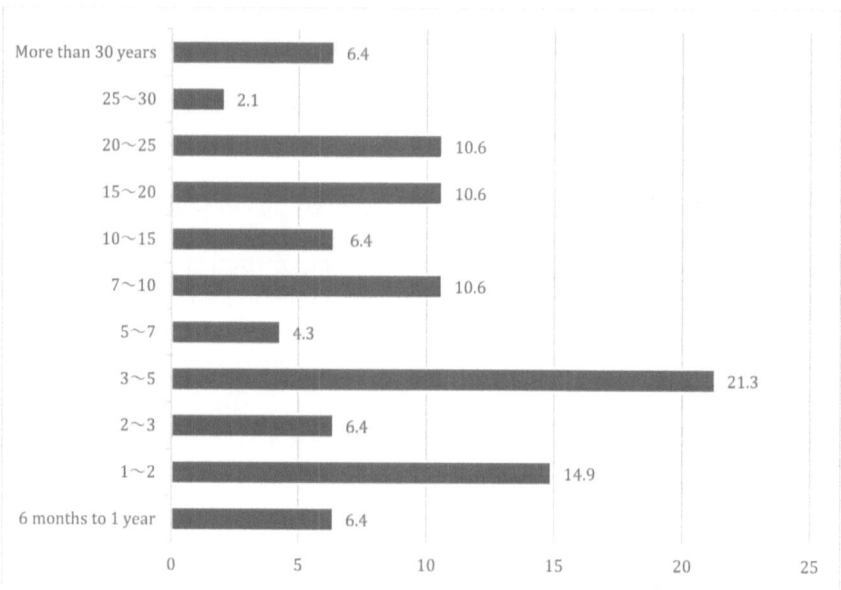

Chart 4.12 How long have you been in the current state? (Q20)

that individuals in the *hikikomori* group aged 40–64 used the internet less often than those in the general group.

By comparison, let us examine those aged 15–39. Watching television and using the internet were also the most popular activities done at home for this group. The proportion who watched television was 75.7% in the general group and 61.2% in the *hikikomori* group. For those who used the internet, it was 59.2% in the general group, and 59.6% in the *hikikomori* group (Cabinet Office 2019: 43). It appears that individuals in the *hikikomori* group aged 15–39 used the internet as much as the general group.

When asked about the approximate duration of their current state, *hikikomori* individuals responded as follows: 6 months to 1 year – 6.4%; 1–2 years – 14.9%; 2–3 years – 6.4%; 3–5 years – 21.3%; 5–7 years – 4.3%; 7–10 years – 10.6%; 10–15 years – 6.4%; 15–20 years – 10.6%; 20–25 years – 10.6%; 25–30 years – 2.1%; and more than 30 years – 6.4%.

Finally, regarding the question, "How did you get into the current state of *hikikomori*", 17 *hikikomori* individuals responded "retirement", 10 "human relationships were bad", 10 "illness", and 9 "did not adapt to the workplace" (other responses are not detailed here).

Discussion

The 2019 report provides us with unprecedented insights into an older population of *hikikomori* individuals and, simultaneously, raises new issues.

Now that we have data about shut-ins aged between 15 and 64, we can assess many of the stereotypes regarding social isolation in Japan.

The first insight gleaned from the survey is that only 4.2% of the *hikikomori* (0.06% of the total respondents) never leave their room in this older age group. This means that, in Japan, although most of those regarded as *hikikomori* usually stay at home, those in this older age bracket, at least, also sometimes go to a convenience store in the neighborhood. At the same time, "quasi-*hikikomori*" individuals usually stay at home and only go out for a hobby. The *hikikomori* subject who never goes out does exist but does not represent the vast majority of those surveyed.

A second finding reveals the significant rate of hospitalization or outpatient care for reasons of mental illnesses among the *hikikomori* group aged 40–64 (31.9%) that is consistent with existing data on the consequences of social isolation: the more one stays socially isolated, the more one's mental health condition declines. In this respect, the results are striking, not only when comparing the older and younger *hikikomori* populations, but also when the *hikikomori* population is compared to the general population. Generally, the mental condition of shut-ins is shown to be more vulnerable to deterioration.

Third, the data shows that excessive use of the internet among the *hikikomori* population is largely an inaccurate stereotype. Within the 15–39 age group, there was simply no significant difference between the proportion of individuals who used the internet in the hikikomori group (59.2%) and in the general group (59.6%) (Cabinet Office 2019: 43). Those aged 40–64 who used the internet formed a smaller percentage (29.8%) than those in the general group (43.3%). Overall, watching television was the most common activity at home for both groups, in both the 2016 and 2019 studies.

Fourth, it was found to be common for the state of *hikikomori* to last for years, and even decades, which confirms previous data on the issue.

A fifth finding is that one-quarter of the 2019 survey's targeted age group (40–64 years of age) was female, compared to one-third reported in earlier surveys for a younger cohort of roughly equivalent size. The decline in the number of female *hikikomori* revealed in this survey still requires explanation. Possible hypotheses include their successful occupational integration into part-time or full-time jobs; the onset of mental disorders needing hospitalization; and/or difficulty in gathering questionnaires from women in this age group. This last hypothesis falls into the hidden population category: the possibility that the older female *hikikomori* population is not reported, or is hidden, out of a sense of shame. This would explain why they were not represented among the valid questionnaires returned. Finally, a fourth hypothesis is that women may recover from the *hikikomori* condition more successfully than men (Yong and Nomura 2019: 7). Not only the decline in women in this older age group, though, but also the increase of *hikikomori* males that underlies this finding—and which reflects a large influx of males—is of interest and will be discussed next.

The 2019 survey, with its focus on the population aged 40–64, produced results that, despite being widely expected, were disturbing, nonetheless. Namely, when 17 of the 47 respondents in the *hikikomori* group (36.17%) stated that they got to their current state because of retirement, we have no other choice than to be very careful interpreting the data. It seems that the study of *hikikomori* never stops playing tricks on those who engage in it. It was only to be expected that, in a survey of those aged 40–64, we would likely gather responses from individuals who had worked all their life, and who had become socially isolated after retirement. This raises many issues, including the following: an adolescent aged 15 who has dropped out from junior high school the year before does not have anything in common with a 64-year-old salary man who has retired the year before. However, in the logic of the Cabinet Office surveys, they could both be considered as having been *hikikomori* in the strict sense, for the period of 1 year. Obviously, it is unlikely that the general public would consider them as *hikikomori* in the same way, or as sharing anything in common. They would perhaps not consider themselves *hikikomori* either. For instance, the adolescent might attribute his situation to bullying at school, and the adult to just feeling blue for a few months.

Nevertheless, what emerges here is the need to provide an appropriate response to social isolation across people's lifespan. The associated distress does not seem to have been addressed by ministries of health and local initiatives, a topic I will discuss further in Chapter 7.

References

Arnett, Jeffrey, Rita Žukauskienė, and Kazumi Sugimura. 2014. "The New Life Stage of Emerging Adulthood at Ages 18–29 Years: Implications for Mental Health." *Lancet Psychiatry* 2014(1): 569–576

Cabinet Office of the Government of Japan (Director-General for Policy on Cohesive Society) 内閣府政策統括官 (共生社会政策担当). 2010. *Wakamono no ishiki ni kansuru chōsa – Hikikomori ni kansuru jittai chōsa* 若者の意識に関する調査・ひきこもりに関する実態調査 (Survey on Youth Consciousness – Survey on *Hikikomori*). https://www8.cao.go.jp/youth/kenkyu/hikikomori/pdf_gaiyo_index.html

———. 2016. *Wakamono no seikatsu ni kansuru chōsa hōkokusho* 若者の生活に関する調査 報告書 (Research Survey on Youth's life). https://www8.cao.go.jp/youth/kenkyu/hikikomori/h27/pdf-index.html

———. 2019. *Seikatsu Jōkyō ni Kansuru Chōsa* 生活状況に関する調査 (Survey on Living Conditions). https://www8.cao.go.jp/youth/kenkyu/life/h30/pdf-index.html

Fansten, Maia et al. 2014. *Hikikomori, ces adolescents en retrait*. Paris: Armand Colin.

Funakoshi, Akiko. 2011. "Hikikomori seinen no oya ga idaku kon.nankan nikansuru kenkyū" ひきこもり青年の親が抱く困難感に関する研究 (Study of Parental Difficulties in Families With Hikikomori Syndrome Children (Social Withdrawal)). Thèse de doctorat, Tōkyō: Université de Tōkyō.

Furuhashi et al. 2013. "État des lieux, points communs et différences entre des jeunes adultes retirants sociaux en France et au Japon (Hikikomori)" (Current Situation, Commonalities and Differences Between Socially Withdrawn Young Adults (Hikikomori) in France and Japan). *L'Évolution Psychiatrique* 78 (2): 249–266.

Hayashi, Naomi. 2003. *Hikikomori nante, shitakunakatta* ひきこもりなんて、したくなかった (I did not want to become hikikomori). Tōkyō: Bungeishunju.

Ishikawa, Ryōko. 2006. "'Hikikomori' to 'nīto' no kondō to sono mondai: 'hikikomori' tōjisha e no intabyū kara no shisa" 「ひきこもり」と「ニート」の混同とその問題:「ひきこもり」当事者へのインタビューからの示唆 (Confusion of the Concepts of "Hikikomori" and "NEET": Seen from the Perspective of People Who Regard Themselves as "Hikikomori"). *The Journal of Educational Sociology* 79: 25–46.

Itoh, Kohki 2010. Hikikomori no jibunshi: Hikikomori genshou no syakaigaku-tekikousatsu (Autobiography of hikikomori: Sociological analysis of hikikomori phenomenon). unpublished B.A. thesis Kwansei Gakuin University.

Itoh, Kohki. 2012. "Difficulties Faced by Hikikomori: From the Life History in Autobiographies and Private Papers." *Kwansei Gakuin Sociological Review*: 137–141.

Kaneko, Sachiko. 2006. "Japan's 'Socially Withdrawn Youths' and Time Constraints in Japanese Society: Management and Conceptualization of Time in a Support Group for Hikikomori." *Time & Society* 15 (2/3): 233–249.

Kato, Takahiro, Takaoka Shinfuku, Norman Sartorius, and Shigenobu Kanba. 2011. "Are Japan's Hikikomori and Depression in Young People Spreading Abroad?" *The Lancet* 378.

Kato, Takahiro, Masaru Tateno, Takaoka Shinfuku, Daisuke Fujisawa, Alan R. Teo, Norman Sartorius, Tsuyoshi Akiyama, and Ishida Tetsuya. 2012. "Does the Hikikomori Syndrome of Social Withdrawal Exist Outside Japan? A Preliminary International Investigation." *Social Psychiatry and Psychiatric Epidemiology* 47 (7): 1061–1075.

Kato, Takahiro, Alan Teo, Masaru Tateno, M. Watabe, H. Kubo, and Shigenobu Kanba. 2017. Can Pokémon GO Rescue Shut-ins (*hikikomori*) from their Isolated World? *Psychiatry & Clinical Neurosciences* 71: 75–76.

Katsuyama, Minoru 2001. *Hikikomori karendā* ひきこもりカレンダー (Hikikomori Calendar). Bunshun nesuko.

Kobayashi Seika, Koji Yoshida, Hirobumi Noguchi, Toru Tsuchiya, and Junichiro Ito. 2003. "Research for Parents of Children with Social Withdrawal." *Seishin Igaku* 45 (3): 749–756

Kondo, Naoji, Motohiro Sakai, Yasukazu Kuroda, Yoshikazu Kiyota, Yuji Kitabata, and Mie Kurosawa. 2013. "General Condition of Hikikomori (prolonged Social Withdrawal) in Japan: Psychiatric Diagnosis and Outcome in Mental Health Welfare Centres." *International Journal of Social Psychiatry* 67: 193–202.

Koshiba, Yoriko. 2007. "A Study of Family Functioning in Hikikomori." *Journal of Health Science of Hiroshima University* 6 (2): 95–101.

Koyama, Asuka, Yuko Miyake, Norito Kawakami, Masao Tsuchiya, Hisateru Tachimori, Tadashi Takeshima, and The World Mental Health Japan Survey Group 2002–2006. 2010. "Lifetime Prevalence, Psychiatric Comorbidity and Demographic Correlates of 'Hikikomori' in a Community Population in Japan." *Psychiatry Research* 176 (1): 69–74.

Krieg, Alexander, and Jane R. Dickie. 2013. "Attachment and Hikikomori: A Psychosocial Developmental Model." *International Journal of Social Psychiatry* 59 (1): 61–72.

Kurita Inuki, Kiyoko Kiba and Midori Hayashi. 2004. "The Process of the Parents Group (hokuriku Kai) for Hikikomori (social Withdrawal) - the Support Process and Its Role -." *Hokuriku Kōshū Eisei Gakkaishi* 30 (2): 87–91.

Lock, Margaret. 1995. *Encounters with Aging. Mythologies of Menopause in Japan and North America*. Berkeley, CA: University of California Press.

Ministry of Health Labour and Welfare (MHLW) 厚生労働省. 2001. *Jūdai/nijūdai wo chūshin toshita shakaiteki hikikomori wo meguru chiiki seishin hoken katsudō no gaidorain* 十代二十代を中心とした社会的ひきこもりをめぐるちいき精神保健活動のガイドライン (Guidelines for Mental Health Support and Evaluation of Hikikomori in their 10's and 20's). Edited by Jun.Ichirō Itō et al.

———. 2003. *Jūdai/nijūdai wo chūshin toshita shakaiteki hikikomori wo meguru chiiki-seishin hoken katsudō no gaidorain* 十代二十代を中心とした社会的ひきこもりをめぐるちいき精神保健活動のガイドライン (Guidelines for Mental Health Support and Evaluation of Hikikomori in their 10's and 20's – Full version). Edited by Jun.Ichirō Itō et al. Tōkyō: Kokuritsu Seishin/shinkei Centre.

———. 2010. *Hikikomori no hyōka/shien ni kansuru gaidorain* ひきこもりの評価ー支援に関するガイドラン (Guidelines for Support and Evaluation of Hikikomori). Edited by Kazuhiko Saitō et al. http://www.mhlw.go.jp/stf/houdou/2r98520000006i6f.html

Morisaki, Shima. 2012. "Kankei no yamai toshite no hikikomori – hikikomori tōjisha hon no bunseki o tooshite" 関係の病としてのひきこもりーひきこもり当事者本の分析を通して (Hikikomori as Illness of Relationship: Through Analysis on Autobiographical Works by Hikikomori). *Kyōto daigaku daigakuin kyōikugaku kenkyūka kiyō* 58: 275–287.

Moroboshi, Noa 2003. *Hikikomori sekirarara* ひきこもりセキララ (Frankly hikikomori). Tōkyō: Sōshisha.

Murasawa, Watari. 2012. "Saikiteki purosesu toshite no 'hikikomori'" 再帰的プロセスとしての「ひきこもり」 (Social withdrawal as a reflexive process). *Shinri kagaku* 33 (1): 61–74.

Nagata, Toshihiko, Hisashi Yamada, Alan R. Teo, Chiho Yoshimura, Takenori Nakajima, and Irene Van Vielt. 2013. "Comorbid Social Withdrawal (hikikomori) in Outpatients with Social Anxiety Disorder: Clinical Characteristics and Treatment Response in a Case Series." *International Journal of Social Psychiatry* 59 (1): 73–8.

Narabayashi, Riichirō 2003. "Helping Families with 'hikikomori'." *Seishin Igaku* 45: 271–277.

Okabe, Akane, Hidemitsu Aoki, Hirokazu Hukaya, and Mao Saito. 2012. "Hikikomoru wakamono no katari ni miru 'futsū' he no toraware to kattō — hikikomoru wakamono e no intabyū chōsa kara —" ひきこもる若者の語りに見る"普通"への囚われと葛藤—ひきこもる若者へのインタビュー調査から— (Lived Experience of Hikikomori and Their Conflicts). *Ritsumeikan Ningen Kagaku Kenkyū* 25: 67–80.

Rubinstein, Ellen. 2016. "Emplotting Hikikomori: Japanese Parents' Narratives of Social Withdrawal." *Culture Medicine & Psychiatry* 40(4): 641–633.

Saitō, Tamaki 斎藤環. 1998. *Shakaiteki hikikomori — owaranai shishunki* 社会的ひきこもり—終わらない思春期 (Social Hikikomori – Adolescence without End). Tōkyō: PHP Shinsho.

———. 2013. *Hikikomori: Adolescence without End*. Translated by Jeffrey Angles. Minnesota University Press.

Tajan, Nicolas. 2015a. "Adolescents' School Non-Attendance and the Spread of Psychological Counselling in Japan." *Asia Pacific Journal of Counselling and Psychotherapy* 6(1/2): 58–69.

———. 2015b. Social Withdrawal and Psychiatry: A Comprehensive Review of Hikikomori, *Neuropsychiatrie de l'Enfance et de l'Adolescence* 63 (5): 324–331.

———. 2015c. "Japanese Post-Modern Social Renouncers: An Exploratory Study of the Narratives of Hikikomori Subjects." *Subjectivity* 8: 283–304.

———. 2017. *Génération hikikomori*. Paris: L'Harmattan.

Tajan Nicolas, and Meiko Shiozawa. 2020. "Hikikomori wo saikōsuru – kaigai, tokuni furansu no jirei 「ひきこもり」を再考する—海外、特にフランスの事例" (Rethinking Hikikomori – Examples from France and Abroad), *Kyōku to Igaku* 教育と医学. 3/4: 54–61.

Tajan, Nicolas, Yukiko Hamasaki, and Nancy Pionnié-Dax. 2017. "Hikikomori: The Japanese Cabinet Office's 2016 Survey of Acute Social Withdrawal." *The Asia-Pacific Journal* 15 (1): 1–11.

Tateno, Masaru, Woo Park Tae, Takahiro Kato, Wakako Umene-Nakano, and Toshikazu Saito. 2012. "Hikikomori as a Possible Clinical Term in Psychiatry." *BMC Psychiatry* (12): 169.

Teo, Alan R., and Albert R. Gaw. 2010. "Hikikomori, a Japanese Culture-Bound Syndrome of Social Withdrawal? A Proposal for DSM-5." *The Journal of Nervous and Mental Disease* 198 (6): 444–449.

Toivonen, Tuukka. 2008. "Introducing the Youth Independence Camp. How a New Social Policy Is Reconfiguring the Public-Private Boundaries of Social Provision in Japan." *Sociologos* 32: 42–57.

Uchida, Chiyoko. 2010. "Apathetic and Withdrawing Students in Japanese Universities - with Regard to Hikikomori and Student Apathy-." *Journal of Medical and Dental Sciences* (57): 95–108.

Ueda, Yoko. 2010. "Katei ni oite oya wa 'hikikomori' hon'nin ni taishite dō taiō sure ba ii no ka" 家庭において親は「ひきこもり」本人に対してどう対応すればいいのか (How Parents Support Hikikomori Children at Home: The Results of a Parents' Workshop). *Ritsumeikan Ningen Kagaku Kenkyū* 21: 147–161.

Umeda, Maki, Noriko Kawakami, and The World Mental Health Survey Group 2002–2006. 2012. "Association of Childhood Family Environments with the Risk of Social Withdrawal ('hikikomori') in the Community Population in Japan." *Psychiatry and Clinical Neurosciences* 66: 121–129.

Ueyama, Kazuki. 2001. *"Hikikomori" datta boku kara* 「ひきこもり」だった僕から (From me, who was *hikikomori*). Tōkyō: Kōdansha.

Yoneyama, Shoko. 2008. "The Era of Bullying: Japan Under Neoliberalism." *The Asia-Pacific Journal: Japan Focus* 1-3-09.

Yong, Roseline and Kyoko Nomura. 2019. "Hikikomori Is Most Associated with Interpersonal Relationships, Followed by Suicide Risks: A Secondary Analysis of a National Cross-Sectional Study." *Frontiers in Psychiatry* 10: 247.

5 NPO support toward *hikikomori* youths

Introduction

Among anthropological works on youths' social withdrawal, Lock's (1986) article on school refusal is an important marker. The 1980s saw school refusal (*tōkō kyohi*), school phobia (*gakkō kyōfu*), and absenteeism (*futōkō*) as concerns; however, it was not until the early 2000s that we observed the proliferation of articles on *hikikomori* and *futōkō*.

Previous anthropological investigations

Ogino Tatsushi (2004)

Ogino (2004) was the first to publish an English language social science article on *hikikomori*. Two years of participant observation in a free school with 45 young people allowed him to describe *hikikomori* group efforts, and to interpret the relationships between group characteristics and the integration process. In particular, he highlighted the way in which *hikikomori* people appropriate and use the categories that define them. The author names this "managing categorization." This term was coined to describe how *hikikomori* people remain vague about the categories that designate their social status as well as the roles involved in this status: the term "indicates a tendency not to define who they are and what they definitely have to do." (Ogino 2004: 124). This recourse to a flexible use of categorization is mobilized by *hikikomori* subjects themselves but also by members of support groups and non-governmental organization (NGO) teams. Ogino (2004: 124–126) observed it in group activities, where the avoidance of the names of disorders, the sidelining of health professionals, incentives for not behaving as a member of the team were present, and rigid rules about where or when a young person should do something were absent. One of the founders of this association said, "Professionals who smell like professionals such as psychiatrists, therapists, certified clinical psychologists, health visitors and school teachers, are not suitable to contact the members."(Ogino 2004: 125). The reason given is that professionals imply the idea of abnormality to *hikikomori* subjects and worsen their withdrawal. We will find again the same type of argument in the founder of Newstart: this position is far from being peculiar to the nonprofit organizations (NPOs).

According to Ogino, the flexible use of categorization facilitated participation in social activities. He describes a time when few support systems were in place and where two conceptions of psychiatrists dominated: that of Saitō (1998), as we have seen, that accentuates the omnipotence of *hikikomori* subjects through the notion of denial of castration and that of Kanō and Kondo, *hikikomori* as a narcissistic pathology. Ogino (2004: 122) embraces the latter when he writes that *hikikomori* subjects' "pride is too high to endure damage to dignity or self-image in ordinary human relations." Based on a field survey in the FSW alternative school, famous for its effectiveness among *hikikomori* subjects, Ogino's "managing categorization" has, thus, become a cornerstone in his understanding of the *hikikomori*.

Ogino recorded 20 hours of interviews with the leader of FSW, many interviews took place, sometimes informally. As researcher, he stayed 42 days with the young people, including a stay of two consecutive weeks. He was first considered a guest and researcher, then a roommate and caregiver. He was also referred to as a teacher/master (*sensei*). The FSW, based in Tōhoku, has existed since April 1997 and was created by two women in their forties. The place, originally intended for disabled, elderly, or children not going to school, has eventually come to focus on under-18s recluses at home. In 2001, thanks to paid volunteering activities, young members joined the team which had until then been limited to the two founders.

The researcher's fieldwork began in August 2001 at FSW; the association gained further popularity after several televised appearances of one of its founders in 2002. In 2003, the team consisted of ten people including five former users of FSW. In 2001, it welcomed 15 users, and the following year they were already 40, then 60 at the time of writing the article. Eighty percent of them are male: 25% are teenagers, 50% are in their 20s, and 25% are in their 30s. Very few had gone to university, and the vast majority of them dropped out of high school (Ogino 2004: 123). The typical support process begins with an interview with the mother, followed by a home visit. After 6 months, the young person consults one of the founders in her office, and then thinks for 3 months about his participation in FSW. Once admitted, they are often withdrawn from collective activities and do not want to talk with other recluses. They begin by discussing their hobbies with team members, then join activities with peers and people living "in society," to begin an occupational integration through part time jobs. Obviously, it is not always that simple, and some are unsuccessful. Flexibility, epitomized in the phrase, "managing categorization," is key throughout this process. For example, a young woman who, after a stay at FSW, had "relapsed" but returned for a second stay after she was able to verbalize that at the time, she did not want to consider herself a *hikikomori* and thought she was different from other members.

It is common for parents, as soon as their child joins FSW, to force him to try to find a job when they are still unable to do so, resulting in another withdrawal period (Ogino 2004: 123). Living in FSW is also an opportunity for some to experience a place in a group where they are not subject to bullying: sharing conversations about hobbies or sharing the anxieties of members between themselves produce positive effects. A form of competition can also occur, which can increase the self-confidence of some, but accentuates the feeling of inferiority among others. Of the 45 members observed by Ogino Tatsushi, this type of support was ineffective for more than one in ten users (13.3%), while for all others, personal changes were significant. However, if some manage to return to high school, attend university, work part time or become a member of the team, very few manage to work full time (Ogino 2004: 127).

As Ogino notes, there is frequent apprehension among *hikikomori* when they accidentally cross a former classmate or someone who asks him what he does in life. Where he should be able to present himself as a member-of-society (*shakaijin*), he struggles – just like his parents – to say that he is *hikikomori*. However, there is potential for the word *hikikomori* to allow him to join a community, with possible positive effects. Some parents feel a heavy sense of shame and hide the situation by saying that their child works part time (Ogino 2004: 129). A method is used: faced with the multiple concerns that the postponement of a task implies (which may result in not doing the scheduled task at all), one of the founders may ask the *hikikomori* person to do something right away. This approach can result in successfully getting the *hikikomori* to take action; however, no deep reflection is engaged in this process. Feelings of inferiority have been widely observed in the *hikikomori* population since the first investigations (Saitō 1998, Kondō 2001), resulting in negative perceptions of self (Ogino 2006: 19). Consequently, we can see that since the beginning of *hikikomori* studies, there has been debate as to whether *hikikomori* should be given medical recognition as a pathology or whether the preservation of "normality" via a flexible use of categorization was more important (Ogino 2004: 130; Futagami 2012).

Kaneko Sachiko (2006)

Much like Ogino's work, Kaneko (2006) has contributed significantly to elucidating the *hikikomori* phenomenon. Kaneko studies the testimonies of those who have experienced *hikikomori* (*hikikomori keikensha*) and conducted an ethnographic survey of support groups. Her work first highlights the presence of a *hikikomori* industry (*gyōkai*) – Internet forums, TV shows, articles, anime, manga, novels – with more than 100 support groups since 2002 (Kaneko 2006: 234), and which has increased significantly since then. According to her, when the Japanese are led to explain the causes of social withdrawal, answers are highly varied: not only education, new technologies, nuclearization of the family, *amae*, collectivism, changes in society but also staying at home for psychological and economic reasons, the fact that society allows it, etc. As this anthropologist asserts, saying that *hikikomori* comes from the middle class implies that this situation could potentially affect all Japanese families, because it is popular to self-identify as middle class in Japan. Under age 18, one speaks of *futōkō* (school nonattendance) rather than *hikikomori*, and in accordance with what has already been highlighted by the Ministry of Health, Labor and Welfare (MHLW 2003), it is often the parents who seek help. Her field survey began in July 2003 and ended in July 2004: she regularly participated in the activities of a group, named by her "group A" and conducted research interviews with those who were engaged in the *hikikomori* industry. As part of her investigation of *hikikomori* autobiographies, she noticed that these writings are structured in the same way: before, during, and after the *hikikomori* period. The following excerpts of an interview with Mr. Suzuki illustrate this.

First, concerning the period prior to *hikikomori* up until primary school, Mr. Suzuki had experienced much emotional pain; he could not trust anyone, not even his parents who were always fighting with each other; he could not accept them as they were: "My mother always complained to me about my father who had a short temper. Often, after dinner, I would listen to my mother's complaints, and when doing so, I saw myself as playing the 'supporter' role for my mother." (Kaneko 2006: 237). So he suggested his mother to divorce his father, but she had a particularly traumatic answer for him: if she were to divorce, she would take his sister and leave him with his father. "I thought I had always hated my father, but it was after my father passed away that I became *hikikomori*. This happened when I was in my late twenties. I have never wanted to become an adult because I could not respect my parents. This was why I went to university so that I could delay becoming an adult for as long as possible." (Kaneko 2006: 237). The story continues with the postgraduate period: "I had no choice but to start a full-time job. This was at a time when there were no such things as *furītā*. (...) I felt as if my life was over, and that I was going to hell. I escaped from such feelings by intoxicating myself with alcohol. As I thought the environment was to blame, rather than myself, I kept on changing jobs in a continuous, but unsuccessful search for my place of belonging (*ibasho*)." This situation lasted several years "and when my virtual enemy – my father – died, I completely lost vitality and became *hikikomori*." (Kaneko 2006: 237).

Concerning his period of social withdrawal, he indicates that he had plenty of time to think about the reasons that had brought him to this situation. He was just getting out of bed to eat and was not bathing. "When I was in the worst condition, I went into the kitchen after my mother went to bed, and had the meal by myself. I lost contact with most friends, though there were a few friends who regularly tried to reach me. The more I failed to respond to them, the more I lost touch with the outside world." Yet it was necessary:

> I needed to continue this life for a while in order to recharge myself with the energy I had lost through almost thirty years of life. After a year of *hikikomori* and recharging myself, I could go out and start working. But after a year, my energy ran out, and I became *hikikomori* again. Life during the second *hikikomori* period was much the same as the first, and I gradually regained my energy.
>
> *(Kaneko 2006: 238)*

Finally, during the post-withdrawal period, "After finding places for counselling and self-help groups on the Internet, I was able to get out of the second *hikikomori* period. It was in January that I heard of a psychiatrist at a local health centre, and started seeing the psychiatrist who I now see regularly for counselling. I learned about group A from the psychiatrist (...) Since then, I have been going to group A on a regular basis." (Kaneko 2006: 239). Group A., unlike other groups, does not force the professional integration of young people and their acquisition of punctuality: it welcomes all those who call themselves *hikikomori*. It is structured like many NPOs that I will discuss later, with a common space where one can socialize, computers are available, as well as televisions, video games, and sofas. It is spread over two floors with spaces designed to be alone. Six counselors (*kaunserā*) come every week and are employed part-time: the first consultation is free but the following sessions cost 1000 yen for an individual interview and 3000 yen for a family interview. It is not uncommon to observe that some wait up to 2 years between the first telephone contact and the arrival to group A, which is open from 11 am to 10 pm and welcomes between 10 and 20 people a day. It is considered a free space where the members of the team also socialize with young people, outside of sports activities or leisure (tennis, cultural events, fireworks, etc.). Some job search activities are planned as well as a monthly parent group (Kaneko 2006: 240–245).

At the end of her 2003–2004 survey, Kaneko Sachiko argues that *hikikomori* is an act of withdrawal from the spatial and temporal constraints inherent in Japanese society. In this sense, this phenomenon illustrates the pressures in terms of performance and social role under which the Japanese are subjected. *Hikikomori* subjects embody, in a certain way, elements rejected by Japanese society: the absence of work or too much slowness for certain tasks, a "disordered" life and lack of punctuality. The recent analyses of this author offer an excellent synthesis of the history and social context in which the *hikikomori* phenomenon has developed and introduces another aspect: the increase of the influence of *hikikomori* parents association – *Zenkoku Hikikomori KHJ Oya no Kai* – which contributed in August 2008 to deciding the allocation of

500 million yen by the Ministry of Health, Labor and Welfare for young people with *hikikomori* (Horiguchi 2012). (Note: for sociological works, see Ishikawa et al. 2008.)

Others

As Saitō Tamaki, Horiguchi Sachiko, and Andy Furlong note, media interest has increased following various crimes committed by people in social withdrawal: "One popular approach has been to suggest that conservative Japanese families have become somewhat dysfunctional and encounter problems in trying to prepare their children for modern social and economic contexts (Furlong 2008: 314)." In other words, the phenomenon is seen as partly related to the overprotection of children and difficulty with adapting to our modern times. Furlong takes up the work of Inui (2005) to emphasize that the youth labor market changed dramatically during the 1990s. In 1992, over one and a half million jobs were available for high school students and graduates. This number decreased to only 600,000 in 1995, and 200,000 by 2003. For Furlong, the increase in the *hikikomori* population is related to "changes in the labor market and the types of support provided by the family and the state." (Furlong 2008: 320–322).

This evolution has also favored the emergence of a category of young people who do not work, do not pursue studies, and are not in training: *nīto*. This popular term today originates from NEET, assigned to young people who are Not in Employment, Education or Training. In 2006, between 520,000 and 2500,000 people aged 15–34 were considered *nīto* (Toivonen 2012). This category is of interest to us in which one might consider *nīto* as partially encompassing some *hikikomori* individuals that are included in its definition. In addition, after being out of their isolation, the former *hikikomori* are often called *nīto* until they find a job, training, or resume studies. As Finnish researcher Tuukka Toivonen notes, the figure of 2.5 million people comes from the Ministry of Health, Labor and Welfare (MHLW) which, in 2002, includes women who produce domestic work and who raise children (between age 15 and 34). We might, therefore, consider that the number of *nīto* is likely overestimated, with agreed estimates for 2005 being roughly 640,000 individuals (Toivonen 2011: 414). Much like *hikikomori,* there was a dramatic increase in newspaper articles about *nīto* between 2003 and 2007 (Toivonen 2011: 422), which may suggest that there has been a period in the newspapers when the subject of *nīto* exceeded *hikikomori*.

In an article combining sociology and psychology, Toivonen affirms with Uchida Yukiko and Vinai Norasakkunkit that part of the current Japanese youth (including *hikikomori* and *nīto*) are unable to conform: "... such youth who deviate from typical Japanese motivational patterns, but have not necessarily become more Western. This poses serious problems in an interdependence-oriented culture, but the paralysis of this group seems

to be an outcome of labor market change rather than a psychopathology."
(Toivonen, Norasakkunkit, and Uchida 2011: 1).

Toivonen and Miller's investigations

Totsuka Yacht School (Miller)

From its founding in 1976 until 2007, Totsuka Yacht School (TYS) has reha-
bilitated over 600 troubled youths, bringing them together around nautical
activities. However, the history of this NGO has been plagued with extreme
events. In 1980, one of the youths, Mr. Yoshikawa, was repeatedly thrown into
the ocean and died as a result of shock. In 1982, another, Mr. Ogawa, received
115 strokes (feet, fist, with weapons, beaten with bamboo, thrown into the
water and fire giving rise to burns) resulting in his death. In March 1983, a
student armed with a knife took a hostage at TYS. In August 1983, returning
from a training camp in Kagoshima, two schoolboys jumped from the ferry
and drowned: they wanted to avoid the anger of Mr. Totsuka and his coaches.
In October of the same year, six coaches were charged with manslaughter. The
trial of Mr. Totsuka would last about 20 years. In 1997, after several appeals,
the Nagoya court sentenced him to 3 years in prison and 3 years on parole: the
decision stated, "training methods neglected human rights and had nothing
to do with education" (Miller and Toivonen 2010: 6). It was not until March
2002 that Mr. Totsuka and other coaches were jailed, as school activities continued. Mr. Totsuka was released from prison in 2006. On October 19, 2009,
an 18-year-old girl allegedly undergoing corporal punishment committed suicide by throwing herself from the top of the institution's building. The authorities did not register any complaints from the family. On January 9, 2012, a
21-year-old man also jumped from the roof of the TYS building (Kyodo 2012).

Corporal punishment has been banned from public schools since the
Meiji era, but debate around these issues is still in the news. As such,
Mr. Totsuka's statements can be considered extreme. For example, "*taibatsu*
is 'good' and should be used to help teachers combat the 'collapse of the
classroom' (*gakkyū hōkai*). Mr. Totsuka insists that words would not work
with emotionally disturbed children – that they 'need' *taibatsu* – emphasizing
that such children must experience a 'high quality of unpleasantness' in
order to learn and grow. Finally, he claims that if *taibatsu* is done for the
sake of the child, it is right to employ it." (Miller and Toivonen 2010: 7).
According to him, the ruin of Japanese education is linked to "a feeble
brainstem" (it is obviously referring here to the part of the brain of the same
name). If he started his yacht school, it is to take care of children with emotional problems and a feeble brain stem. He continues:

> children whose instinct has not been adequately trained through the
> use of *taibatsu* will not be able to function properly in society. He adds
> that, as the brain stem governs the physical and mental spirit (*seishin*),

and as the spirit is made up of reason and instinct, in order to train the instinct, the brain stem must be trained by 'tricking' it using a 'high quality of unpleasantness', and this in turn will create a 'correct spirit'.
(cited by Miller and Toivonen 2010: 8)

The principle of his method is very simple. Simply stated, if the educator physically scares the child, the child will say to himself that he should not do what he has done because he risks being punished, and after a while, he avoids punishment. The underlying theory is that of conditioning and, the method, behaviorist. For Mr. Totsuka, corporal punishment should be used with all children as soon as possible, and ideally from the age of 3.

Psychologists, psychiatrists, and psychoanalysts would spot here paranoid features (delusion of persecution, megalomania), and perversion (humiliation of the children). Arguments in favor of paranoid traits (megalomania) are supported by the assertion that he can "save Japan" if given a chance (Miller and Toivonen 2010: 7). Also, we observe the dimension of paranoiac innocence and a feeling of persecution: according to him, the prosecutors have given him an unfair trial, and he complains of being a media scapegoat. Although he is responsible for several children's deaths in his school, he claims he is the victim of the Other and seen as someone who is bad and incapable. For example, psychologists neglect instinct, whereas intellectuals blindly accept the American mind (*seishin*) while forgetting the Japanese spirit (*seishin*). He asserts that Eastern philosophy is superior in all respects to American philosophy: the great principles of Buddhism are sufficient to cover the basics of life, and Japanese "emotionalism" requires punishment, contrary to Western rationalism. With regard to education, Mr. Totsuka thinks that the university is neglecting real life, that the Minister of Education is irresponsible, and that teachers' unions are responsible for the decline in education in Japan. In particular, he argues that public schools fail because they do not use corporal punishment. Finally, he maintains that children and adults are not equal, and, therefore, should not have the same rights. He thinks that his method of rehabilitation is the only one that is intrinsically Japanese. He calls for the liberalization and privatization of education and titles the chapter of a 2003 book "Just let me run one elementary school!" If one considers his remarks, and the number of dead children and adolescents (six) on his hands, one can hope that he will never be given more responsibilities.

This school uses coercive and disciplinary methods including solitary confinement practices. His motto could be "*taibatsu wa kyōiku, taibatsu wa naosu,*" "corporal punishment is education, corporal punishment heals (repairs)." TYS is not representative of NPOs and NGOs that support *hikikomori* individuals, but it has not been closed. Like corporal punishment (*taibatsu*), it is a scandal, but it still exists today.

Another NPO from Aichi prefecture named *Ai mentaru sukūru* created in 2001 also proceeds with coercive methods: enter the room of the *hikikomori* subject by scolding him, even screaming, to force him into the institution where he will be locked up and will have to explain his attitude. The director of this NPO was sentenced after the death of a young person, but she nonetheless gained popularity among those who consider *hikikomori* people as parasites (Furlong 2008). The young person in question was 26 years old: he died on April 18, 2006 after being taken from his home in handcuffs and brutalized by the staff of the association. The director of this NPO, Ms. Sugiura Shoko, told the police that she had only tried to prevent him from being aggressive and did not intend to kill him (Kyodo 2006).

I will not examine here the coercive methods of her older sister, Ms. Osada Yuriko, popular in the 1990s and 2000s for her television shows. But a detour through these practices of "alternative education," allowed in Japan in the form of *juku* or through a status of NPO/NGO, suggests that Japanese law hardly prevents individuals from using dangerous methods when working with children. While public schools' rules are extremely strict and restrict the use of corporal punishment by teachers today, there is more flexibility in private institutions (Maisterra 2013). Corporal punishment is a very sensitive subject in public education, but it is not sufficiently "scandalous" in Japanese society to prevent associations such as those of Mr. Totsuka from existing. TYS was even supported by one of the most powerful Japanese politicians of the 2000s: the former governor of Tōkyō Ishihara Shintarō.

K2 International (Toivonen)

K2 International is aimed at *futōkō*, *nīto* and *hikikomori* people. The space is located on the ground floor of a building in Yokohama City in a large apartment consisting of a living room, an office for the team, and an activity room (sports, music). Most of the 25 young people surveyed by Tuukka Toivonen are about 25 years old, but the age of the persons accommodated ranges from 13 to 34 years old. The young people live in shared rooms and the staff of 10 is mainly composed of women. K2 was originally an educational subsidiary of the Pacific Marine Project Yacht Company and was known as the International Columbus Academy. In this context, teenagers in school refusal (*tōkō kyohi*) left for a period of 1–2 months to sail in Micronesia. This program had to stop after 1 year of existence (1989–1990), but one of its employees, Kanamori Matsuo, decided to continue it. In 1991, supported by parents and some psychiatrists in the city of Yokohama, he created a NPO that later expanded to Japan, New Zealand, and Australia. The founder is Kanamori Matsuo, a Korean *zainichi* trained in performing arts, and who also has experience in business. The other leader in this group is a Japanese woman of about 35, Iwamoto Mami, who was elected Woman of the Year by Nikkei Woman for her work with youth (supportive, job-oriented activities, and management). She worked in a security company in the past. This association trained more than 700 young people by 2010 (Miller and Toivonen 2010: 12).

The year 1992 marked the opening of a first restaurant for K2 and, in 1993, a franchise in New Zealand. Between 1993 and 1998, six boat trips and four expeditions took place. In 2005, K2 was recognized as the "*juku* for youth autonomy" as part of the government's youth autonomy support program, and Iwamoto Mami became the director. For Kanamori Matsuo, the children welcomed are not sick: "They are in a state resembling that of an empty car battery. Hence, they must first be re-charged – not through disciplinary training or persuasion, but through complete relaxation in nature." (cited by Miller and Toivonen 2010: 12). In this association, it is thought that the origin of the malaise of these children lies on the side of the parents and society. Kanamori Matsuo criticizes the superficiality of current social relations, referring to the lost educational and supportive role played by local communities of the past. Today, parents raise their children alone and this is problematic: keeping problems inside the family continues. If Iwamoto Mami can criticize certain Japanese traditions, Kanamori Matsuo criticizes public schools that stress children, favor the "white-collars" to the detriment of technicians and artisans, and neglects minorities for the benefit of the majority. For him, these conditions produce young people who are unable to build relationships of trust and seek help when they are in trouble. All young people in K2 start with a strong sense of inferiority, a negative image of themselves, and feel that others do not need them. According to him, "white-collar" fathers would be responsible for the state of this youth because they neglected the education of their child, giving rise to an imbalance between the maternal (*bosei*) and paternal (*fusei*) types of education. The weakness of the paternal principle (*fusei genri*) causes, according to him, difficulty for the young to behave in a more difficult world than that of the maternal home. Kanamori Matsuo also deplores the bursting of the economic bubble in the early 1990s which was the cause of the increase in the number of *furītā*.

Joining these NGO activities costs participants around 630,000 yen for the first 3 months and then 500,000 yen per month: given this rate, low-income and single-parent families cannot participate. The assistance offered by K2 is carried out through experiential learning, community life (without parents), and occupational integration (resume writing, interview techniques and oral communication, volunteering). A phase centered on fun activities is also provided. For Kanamori Matsuo, sailing and staying on deserted islands stimulates the unconscious, develops an ability to cooperate with others to survive, and fosters the communication skills necessary for teamwork. These expeditions disrupt these young people's malaise and restore their mental and physical health. K2 has links with social work and mental health networks and organizes events in the local community around women with young children. Overall, these programs suggest that it is not the young people, but society that is sick.

It should be noted that an incident occurred on February 26, 2003, which caused the death of a 22-year-old in New Zealand. Accused of failing to comply with security rules and labor rights violations, K2 was forced to leave the country. New K2 students were charged. In reality, they were exasperated by a boy in their group with autism (Asperger syndrome), who kept firing and stealing objects. He was, therefore, beaten during an inter-rogation that went wrong. Four young people were sentenced to 6 months to 3 years' imprisonment; the charges were dropped for the remaining five who refused to return to New Zealand. The youth's parents did not sue K2, and the event made little news in the media, compared to those involv-ing the TYS. Finally, note that if Kanamori Matsuo criticizes corporal punishment (*taibatsu*), it does not condemn it completely and speaks of *sukinshippu*: it is a neologism passed in the current language composed of "skin" associated with "kinship." It refers to a parent–child communi-cation (skin to skin), soft proximity between two people, through touch. According to him, *sukinshippu* would be a form of friendly physical con-tact, which allows one to build positive links between the team and the youths. According to Kanamori Matsuo, it would be difficult to explain to Westerners and is an important part of Asian cultures. Unlike Kanamori Matsuo, Iwamoto Mami completely rejects corporal punishment (Miller and Toivonen 2010: 18).

Youth autonomy juku (Toivonen)

As seen in the framework of K2 International, some associations were part of a government program for youth autonomy. This had already been the subject of a previous survey conducted by Tuukka Toivonen in 2008. According to him, the prevention of the risk of social exclusion in Japan should be private: it is up to individuals and their families, rather than the state or public institutions. Since 2003, a program has been launched to stimulate the independence of young people: *wakamono jiritsu chōsen puran*. As part of this program, youth job spots were developed between 2003 and 2007, and job cafés for *furītā*. Aimed at NEETs, the youth sup-port center (*wakamono sapōto sutēshon*) was created in 2006 and welcomes 10,000 young people per year (Toivonen 2008: 41). This researcher specifi-cally described *juku* for youth autonomy (*wakamono jiritsu juku*) launched in July 2005 and focused on some of those who are socially excluded. It consists of support, and daily training of 3 months oriented toward employment; a little less than 2000 young people a year are welcomed. The young people live 3 months in one of thirty *juku* spread over the territory. The directions and activities of these places are divided into three: *seikatsu kunren, shūrō taiken*, and *shūgyō kunren*. Behind the *seikatsu kunren*, there is the idea that these young people have irregular life rhythms and have difficulty developing daily life habits. The *shūrō taiken* is made up of agri-cultural activities, nursing, or work in restaurants or bakeries. The *shūgyō kunren* brings together the same activities with a basic skill learning class and English.

Participants are in their 20s or 30s; most have only lived with their parents, so *juku* is the first experience of parental separation over a long period with people outside of the family on a daily basis. The priority of *juku* is to help them gain employment, and, therefore, economic independence. The registration fee is 280,000 yen for households earning over 4 million a year, and 210,000 yen for those earning less. The project hosts half as many participants as had been expected for several reasons. First, for many families, it is too expensive. Then, some young people fear switching overnight into a community life and are wary of the discipline of *juku*. Participating in it also awakens the idea of a possible stigma for young people and their families. Finally, there is the selection process: the eligible persons, according to the youth autonomy *juku* assistance center (*wakamono jiritsu juku shien sentā*), are those who have completed the period of compulsory education, and who have been outside of training, education, and employment for at least one continuous year without seeking employment. In addition, they must have already gone through a job search process in the past, not be married, and be under 35 years of age. It is, therefore, a small, well-defined subcategory of long-term *nīto* that is concerned. In fact, these criteria make it possible to include a certain number of *hikikomori* people. After the launch of the program, the organizers realized that half of the people interviewed had mental health issues, but the project was not designed for this population (Toivonen 2008: 49). Subsequently, from 2007 on, they have rejected applicants with a mental condition that requires treatment by professionals.

While this *juku* received some media coverage, it was less popular among participants, prompting questions from researcher Tuukka Toivonen. In the course of his interviews with several ministerial officials, he noticed that the main reasons are economic: they argue that if nothing is done for them, they will become dependent on social benefits, and this will be too costly for taxpayers. So why did they decide to charge tuition fees and to restrict the selection criteria to such an extent that the project receives half as many participants as had been projected? This researcher cites four reasons. First, *nīto* are not perceived as a population that must receive financial support from the state, but rather they are seen as spoiled children who spend their time having fun. Second, the money required is legitimate because it corresponds to accommodation costs. Third, the Ministry of Economy opposes granting more money for various reasons, including the notion mentioned before that they do not deserve public support. Finally, in the Japanese public social security system, people who have already worked for a few years are preferentially treated. It is clear from this researcher's investigation that these projects are marked by a certain ambiguity and ambivalence toward these young people. Although they encounter difficulties, a number of them are quite capable of understanding the logic of the institutions offering to support them. This ambivalence is particularly visible for the female population, but in this case, is more a reflection of inequality between men and women. In fact, only 23% of the participants are women in these assistance programs, partly because parents are less likely to see their daughter's unemployment as a problem. In addition, the gendered nature of the juku's activities affects participation rates: "farm work, waste collection, cleaning, etc., may seem too 'masculine' to many women, although there are now some organisations that provide 'female-friendly' work sites such as bakeries and restaurants. [*Juku*] themselves may be more hesitant to actively recruit women as it is generally harder to find work for them in the Japanese labour markets." (Toivonen 2008: 50).

My investigations in nonprofit organizations

NPOs related to Buddhist schools

In some prefectures, religious movements have seized the opportunity to create NPOs to help *hikikomori* people. I visited one of them in a medium-sized town in G. prefecture, thanks to an informer: a retired teacher who is a member of a Zen Buddhist school. (I met this former teacher, Mr. Sano, thanks to a common acquaintance.) Indeed, while I needed help to translate the written account of a former *hikikomori* (Mr. Onishi), a colleague had referred me to Mr. Sano's son. It was during our meeting that Mr. Sano's son informed me of his father's activities, and that he allowed me to meet him. It was done a few weeks later in a restaurant at the H train station, where we got to know each other and agreed to a future stay in G. prefecture.

I had arrived at the appointment with Saitō Tamaki's book, "Lacan to survive," which provided an opportunity to discover Mr. Sano's and my shared knowledge of Lacan and his famous statement (appearing in *The Direction of Treatment and the Principles of Its Power)*: "the desire of man is the desire of the Other" – even though, as I indicated earlier, this quote is not translated by Saitō Tamaki in a manner consistent with Jacques Lacan's original meaning. Here, my interlocutor understands that the *hikikomori* cannot get out of their isolation if nobody wants them outside: the *hikikomori* subject is not in a position to desire ... so we have to go find them, want them, and hence the need for home visits. Mr. Sano is, therefore, involved in helping these young people in a network that has been woven around their social withdrawal. He is called by families for home visits in order to get young people out of their isolation. He can then direct them to two NPOs in the city.

The first, the NPO P., proposes a free space where they can arrange a personal place (*ibasho*), a place where they can come at any time to converse with peers or members of the NPO, read (manga, books, newspapers), go on the Internet, or look for a job. My informant had organized a collective meeting in NPO P. with young people, and two members of the NPO. During this meeting, I met five people, three of whom had already met a psychiatrist and had a psychiatric diagnosis. The first of those three, Mr. Ando, a young man with massive earrings, declared himself a little later in our discussion as having schizophrenia (*tōgō shicchōshō*). His withdrawal period was marked by staying at home with his sick grandmother while his parents were working. He is currently employed in a nursing home. The second, Ms. Kojima, is a young woman who describes a period of 1 year in which she stayed in bed continuously, watching television: she says she is interested in medical things and advises me of a medical television drama series. My informant interrupts the conversation to say (in English) that she had gone through a period of depression. Third, Mr. Takagi, a young man very eager to question me, claimed his diagnosis of schizophrenia from the first, and, showing off his medication, ingested them greedily a few inches from my face while talking to me about his passion for books. The following two people did not meet a psychiatrist and did not have a psychiatric diagnosis. Mr. Endo is interested in horse racing and works part time carrying heavy loads (i.e., storekeeper). The last individual, Mr. Chiba, describes a withdrawal period that started during high school and then lasted 10 years. He has also done small jobs; today is luckily his day off. After having attended this NPO for a while, he no longer comes; it is the first time that the others have met him. Before Mr. Sano and I went to the second association for dinner, he told us he was going to join us for the meal, but he did not come.

The name of the second NPO, C., is a neologism composed of words referring to the Buddhist universe and the culture of another prefecture. This association offers agricultural work and is located in a "True Pure Land" (*jōdo shinshū*) Buddhist Temple. It is located on the outskirts of the city near a river, behind dikes, and other houses and fields. The important figure of the temple – who had also contributed to the making of films on the history of Japan – had just given way to the new leader Mr. Taniguchi, a married man in his forties and father of two children. This young priest of *jōdo shinshū* is responsible for the temple but also acts as coordinator of the NPO for rehabilitation through agricultural work, by employing former *hikikomori*. He lives in a house next to the temple with his wife and two children. In another house adjacent to the temple is a shared house hosting several people in separate rooms. In the temple on the ground floor is a large kitchen, a large collective room, a living room, and a room containing funeral urns.

In the kitchen, I meet three young men on their return from the fields. They left their withdrawal period to engage in agricultural activities and sales of their products (e.g., edamame beans) at markets. I learned very little about their experience, but did learn that none had ever met with a psychiatrist. Mr. Goto said he had always been bullied (*ijime*) when he was at school; he was often in the nurse's office and finished high school with difficulty. The youngest, Mr. Hirano, is 19 years old, and has just come out of his *hikikomori* period (a few weeks ago). He is a turbulent boy who used to get into trouble, fight, and then withdraw at home. The third, Mr. Iwasaki, was quite interested in meeting with a foreigner (he asked me several questions) but, unfortunately, I did not have the chance to discuss his experience in more detail with him. However, I systematically questioned my interlocutors about their use of the Internet in order to identify possible Internet addiction. None of the three youths of the NPO C. testified to any intensive Internet use. Moreover, none of the five people of the NPO P. were engaged in any online games (such as Massively Multiplayer Online Roleplaying Games MMORPG), although some may play from time to time on a family video game console. I also met a former *hikikomori*, Mr. Arai, with whom I had a more in-depth interview. I will discuss this in the next chapter.

An ordinary NPO in the H. city

The NPO A., located in the city of H., offers a space open to the public, including a place where one can arrange a personal place for oneself that produces a sense of belonging (*ibasho*), similar to NPO P. that I mentioned before. This NPO is very small with only one permanent employee and some volunteers. Mr. Wada, the leader of this NPO, had a 10-year withdrawal period between the age of 19 and 29. He says he only went out monthly with his mother to go to the doctor to renew his prescription of psychotropic drugs (anxiolytics, antidepressants). In this period of his life, he experienced a lot of anxiety and left the house with great difficulty. According to him, many *hikikomori* people go out once a month to go to the doctor to renew their psychotropic prescription. Today, Mr. Wada is the manager of a small NPO related to the social services of the city.

I attended one of the meetings of this NPO in a social center, and afterward helped with some gardening at the center, attended by a young *hikikomori* man, Mr. Kinoshita, who had managed to come out for the occasion. It is important to note that the premises of the NPO A., like the social center of F., are located in one of the neighborhoods inhabited by *zainichi* Koreans, discriminated communities (*burakumin*), and poor people. I also went to a temple of a *jōdo shinshū* school located in another district to clean the graves after Ōbon (day of the dead). I cleansed the sanctuary with a man, Mr. Onishi, still *hikikomori* but outside for the purpose of our meeting. He was very late, and Mr. Wada had to phone him, and leave him a message before he finally arrived. He was interested in talking to a stranger and the fact that there are *hikikomori* people in France. He also enjoyed spending a friendly moment with the family managing the temple around *takoyaki* (octopus fritters very popular in Japan). The association also organized a job fair (*jobu saron*); a café (twice a month) where the theme was bread making, counseling sessions, and farm work. I participated in a meeting of volunteers within the NPO but gradually lost contact with Mr. Wada and did not continue my work with them. It seems appropriate to explain this point.

My informant had organized the first meeting with Mr. Wada. The latter wanted us to meet in a neutral place, outside of his NPO, and demanded that I pay his transportation costs as well as the rental of the room where we would meet. In other words, he clearly had some reservations about me.

We had to meet halfway between the town of H. and my informant's home. Our meeting was unusual from the beginning and marked by mistrust of the coordinator of this NPO. Nevertheless, after 4 hours of reflection and exchanges, Mr. Wada allowed me to participate in the activities of his association. During this meeting and afterward, he remained quite negative, saying he was alone in his NPO, having few financial means and did not look favorably on the visits of his supervisory authorities (H. city's social services). While we expected to meet again with my informant 1 year after our first meeting, Mr. Wada's behavior was erratic, accepting the meeting but not answering emails the days that preceded it, and eventually provoking my informant's anger. This association was poorly organized, perhaps, mixing *hikikomori* subjects with other kinds of troubled youth such as those who might have been bullies during junior high school. For *hikikomori* subjects, this was like mixing them with the very same people that had harassed them previously. Contact with Mr. Wada broke because of a misunderstanding that made it difficult for me to return to his NPO. Consequently, I did not get any additional information from Mr. Wada but translated certain elements of the account of a person in social withdrawal, Mr. Onishi, who had kindly written in the gazette of the NPO. I will mention it in the following chapter, devoted to *hikikomori* subjects' accounts.

Hikikomori parents' association

Mr. Yamamoto (born in 1935 or 1936) was 77 years old at the time of our exchanges. I contacted him when he had just retired from the *hikikomori* parents' association in which he had played a central role. I complied with his wish for an email questionnaire in Japanese rather than an in-person interview. We had regular internet correspondence from December 2012 to January 2013 and met on January 9, 2013 at X. University, and then again on July 13, 2013 at H. University. At the time of our conversation on January 9, he gave me particularly informative documents related to the association.

The full name of the national association is *"Zenkoku KHJ Hikikomori Oya no Kai."* *Zenkoku* indicates the national character and *Oya no kai* refers to the parents' association. KHJ is, according to Mr. Yamamoto, more difficult to explain. "K" is the capital letter of *kyohaku shinkeishō*, which would mean obsessive-compulsive disorder (in reality the correct translation is obsessional neurosis); "H" is the capital letter of *higai nenryo* which accentuates the idea of a persecution complex, and "J" is the capital letter of *jinkaku shōgai* meaning "personality disorder." For the founder of the NPO Okuyama Masahisa (deceased in 2011), the *hikikomori* condition was considered to be related to neurosis in its pathological sense, but, according to Mr. Yamamoto, it has since been thought that social withdrawal may be linked to developmental disorders and schizophrenia. A large number of people in the movement wanted to remove the initials KHJ, but Mr. Okuyama persisted, and the use of "KHJ meeting" and "KHJ family" continued. It should be noted that this recognition of psychiatric pathologies among the withdrawn population raises the question of the prevention of these disorders during childhood and adolescence, especially in schools (see Chapters 1 and 2).

This NPO is widespread in Japan, bringing together 40 groups from the north (Hokkaidō) to the south (Okinawa), as well as 15 subgroups. Its goal is threefold: get together to avoid isolation, to talk to each other and support each other; learn from each other about the characteristics of the problem and invite speakers; and, promote more assistance from the government and pressure politicians and senators to build an appropriate legal system. The rise of this NPO and the audience it has received at the political level is dependent on the mobilization of parents and the charismatic presence of its founder, Mr. Okuyama Masahisa. As a teenager, he had to undergo leg amputation because of osteogenic sarcoma. Then, suffering from cancer of the lung and gallbladder, he had half his stomach removed. According to Mr. Yamamoto, "the pathological *hikikomori* of his son began when he was 55, and as he knew that many people were in the same pathological condition, he decided to create an NPO." Okuyama Masahisa died at the age of 66 during a recurrence of his lung cancer.

Mr. Yamamoto became involved in KHJ in 2002 and was a particularly active member because of his administrative and communication skills. He was a key player in the movement, and his departure from KHJ was partly due to his age, and partly due to the difficulty of bearing the death of his leader and friend. He also considered the production of the 2010 MHLW guidelines a sufficient achievement. The meetings of Nagoya (2006), Hiroshima (2008, 2009), and Tōkyō (2010) attest to close collaboration between the parents' association and the ministerial authorities, and some psychiatrists like Kondo Naoji and the psychologist Sakai Motohiro (Sakai et al. 2004, Kondo et al. 2013). It should be noted that there is no financial relationship between the MHLW and KHJ, other than the reimbursement of transportation expenses at meetings. Also, psychiatrist Saitō Tamaki may have had some influence on the general perception of the *hikikomori* phenomenon, but he would not – according to Mr. Yamamoto – have participated in the development of the 2010 guidelines. Why does Mr. Yamamoto not recognize that Saitō (2013: 7) was actually involved in the development of these guidelines? Is it because Saitō Tamaki criticized the guidelines afterward? Or is it because of a personal conflict that Mr. Yamamoto erased, or denied, his participation in the development of ministerial guidelines?

According to Mr. Yamamoto, the 2010 guidelines significantly accentuated the perception of *hikikomori* as an illness. He says that more than 80 people have collaborated with the latest 2010 guidelines, and the psychiatrist associated with KHJ did show certain documents of the NPO to the research teams. Indeed, the NPO has a section of medical treatment occupied by Professor N., a psychiatric specialist in psychosomatic medicine. Mr. Yamamoto hopes that one day we will be able to describe, by name, the nature of the illness so that it may be included in the DSM® or the International Classification of Diseases in the future.

My questions also focused on the popular notion of *tōjisha* in Japan, that is, the legal and cultural self-determination of the "concerned party" (McLelland 2009). *Tōjisha* has become a central concept in debates around minority groups in Japan, originally stemming from the terms used in legal battles over sexual minorities in the 1970s which have now become common vernacular for the affected parties in activist circles. Applied to the situation of *hikikomori, tōjisha* only describes the person in a *hikikomori* situation excluding the family and parents. The term "double-*hikikomori*" is also used to refer to the situation of a family "hiding" the fact that a person affected by social withdrawal is present at home. In this sense, the fact that the family hides the *hikikomori* compounds its situation of seclusion. These situations of double-*hikikomori*, where one sees the level of social communication collapse completely, are unfortunately common: "it is a deep tragedy. At home, there is a person concerned, and the brother cannot get married," Mr. Yamamoto writes. Sometimes the *tōjisha* (in other words, the children of members of this parents' association or those of their generation) come to the meetings that are organized for them, the "youth meetings" (*wakamono no kai*). Places where young people can interact exist in the KHJ network at the national level. *Hikikomori* subjects coming out of their isolation, to go to places that their parents created for them, and where they are present, is a valuable initiative. However, in my opinion, if *hikikomori* subjects must become autonomous and go toward more independence, places for the young people organized by the parents might achieve the opposite, i.e., lead to more dependence. These young people are dependent on their parents and, by staying in the family home, locking themselves in their room, they flee. The actions to be taken should be more on the side of a separation, than on the side of maintaining a dependence outside the walls of the home.

Finally, according to Mr. Yamamoto, "there is a gap between the recognition of parents and that of children. My feeling is that 1/3 of them recognize it, 1/3 of them deny it, and the last third do not really know. There is an unconscious stigma." The formation of a group of *tōjisha* would be necessary but, according to him, difficult to achieve. As we have seen with the works of Kaneko (Horiguchi) Sachiko, and as we will see in the next chapter, a group of *tōjisha* existed for more than 10 years and includes some parents, but is a relatively small group. Let us move on to a famous NGO near Tōkyō: Newstart, and then focus on NPO M.

Newstart and the NPO M.

Newstart

Newstart was created by Futagami Nōki. Born in 1943 in Korea, he was repatriated at the end of the Second World War at the age of two and a half: "I was a refugee. In a sense I remained a displaced refugee and have identified with social refugees, on a journey that has brought me through

63 years." (Futagami and Asano 2006: 2). As a teenager, he was expelled from high school while in first class and describes himself at the age of 17 as a "high-school dropout refugee." He nevertheless managed to enroll at Waseda University but did not attend classes. Indeed, he opened a *juku* which he directed from the age of 19 to 35. Since he was the first to create a *juku* in Matsuyama City, the business flourished. But with 3000 students, he had become a businessman and it bothered him deeply. So he gave it up and decided to leave the city of Matsuyama to live in the place where he knew the fewest people: Chiba prefecture. He was then, in his own words, a "refugee-*nīto*" at 35 years old. He did not know what to do and lived with his family on his savings. In 1993, at the age of 50, he saw a report broadcast by NHK television about an integrated community in Tuscany. On a farm, four families had started a vineyard and produced olive oil while working with people with mental disorders. He went to stay a month and started an exchange project with Japan. Over the next 6 years, eight groups of seven people were sent. It was a small project, expensive for each participant: 1 million yen for 2 months. The idea of creating an integrated community in Chiba came to him after his stay in Italy, when parents who took back their child called him to tell him they were reclusive again. When I visited it, Newstart hosted some 60 current and former *hikikomori* people, with full-time staff and international volunteers. They were not qualified professionals (psychologists, psychiatrists, social workers, etc.) because, for the founder, those who experienced personal hardships would be more effective, as he stated "a wife who has left her home, a woman who fled domestic violence, a former president who had to disappear when his company went bankrupt—are more useful than professionals as staff members." (Futagami and Asano 2006).

Several associations I have mentioned have a charismatic leader with strong opinions (Mr. Totsuka, Mr. Kanamori, and later the leaders of associations M. and U.). Futagami Nōki is another example. According to him, there are two categories among those who are *hikikomori* or *nīto*. Some are between 30 and 40 years old and are victims of the bursting of the economic bubble. Others dropped out of high school or university, "unable" to find a job. After several years, they would be in a state of "stupor," and would struggle to make a new start. When politician Asano Shirō asked Futagami Nōki if society plays a greater role in the creation of these problems than characteristics of individuals themselves, he replied in the affirmative: "young people today are more decent as human beings, in a way, than people of our generation who had such strong material and financial desires. They look at their fathers, who have worked hard, built a house, and reached economic independence, but they aren't happy at all, and they say, 'I don't want to end up like that.' Where they might want to choose a more human, slow way of living, the structure of society hasn't changed at all from the impoverished value system of our generation." This leads them to despair of a society where one kills oneself at work without any satisfaction.

Unable to go anywhere, they become social refugees. "Young people who have been raised in affluence are looking for work that helps make the world a better place and ways of working that allow them to enjoy life, rather than working long hours and earning a high salary. [...] I can't help but feel that for the Japanese, language has caused a kind of autointoxication, and that communication is inadequate throughout the society." (Futagami and Asano 2006: 6–7).

Sixty percent of Newstart's revenue comes from parents and the remaining 40% from commercial activities: a bakery, a restaurant, a café, a day center for the elderly and young children, and a computer shop. Of note is assistance by women available for hire who are getting paid to support shut-ins, i.e., rental sisters (*rentaru oneesan*), a peculiarity of Newstart. According to sociologist Andy Furlong, an organization like Newstart has some good points, but he sees a certain danger because of the lack of employee training and the presence of rental sisters who are "unable to control relationships or deal with the issue of transference." (Furlong 2008: 318). Indeed, these rental sisters are an unusual apparatus: during my visit, the rental sister of a former *hikikomori* had just started a romantic relationship with him, which was considered progress. In other words, there are no guidelines for caregiver–patient relationships regulated by a code of ethics. Let us remember a figure: 6 months of home visits would be necessary to get the young person out of seclusion and then a period of 15 months would be required to gain autonomy. Let us also remember the international dynamic. International volunteers can work on a voluntary basis (free accommodation), for a stay of several weeks. Thus, an Italian photographer, Pierfrancesco Celada, was able to produce a photographic report, and a team of two French filmmakers (Dorothée Lorang and David Beautru) made a documentary film.

NPO M.

No researcher – of any discipline or nationality – has conducted or published research on the association M., which I investigated between the months of April and August 2012. I met the leader Mr. Murata and spoke with him for 3 hours in the presence of my informant, a former *hikikomori*. He introduced me to Mr. Murata and arranged the appointment. Subsequently, I participated in two half-day luncheon meetings with former *hikikomori* hosted at the NPO, some former *hikikomori* who became employees and who came back for the occasion, some parents, staff, and family members. I took part in a full 4-day trip with some members of the NPO and former *hikikomori*. Finally, I attended a session at their "university." The NPO M. was created in the year 2000, and has gradually set up a system of support for families and care of *hikikomori-nīto* people. One of the first actions toward the shut-ins is to make a home visit (*katei hōmon*). Then, when he comes out of his isolation, the *hikikomori* subject becomes *nīto*, and can be hosted in one of the places available to the NPO: a house shared by four ex-*hikikomori* and an ex-*hikikomori* who became a member of the team; two apartments occupied by three ex-*hikikomori* for one, and two ex-*hikikomori* for the other and, in addition to these three shared houses, two separate individual apartments.

In total, the NPO hosts 11 people who have experienced social withdrawal. The team consists of seven to eight employees, whose work is divided into several activities: home visits, a group for parents, individual interviews and interviews with parents, support of youth daily, and cooperation with an external team who takes care of their reintegration. A café run by the NPO employs former *hikikomori* and hosts the "university" every month. This is not really a university, but similar to the French "*café philo*," a place where social issues are discussed with guests. Let us now describe in more detail how this association developed the support intended, not to former *hikiko-mori*, but to *hikikomori* subjects themselves during their isolation period.

It all starts with the parents' decision to contact the NPO M., usually following an advertisement in the newspapers or via their website. They are then invited to an informational meeting with other parents and can participate in a regular support group. As part of an interview, parents can take a package of several sessions that stipulates that a member of the NPO will make home visits according to a specific methodology. First, it is necessary to agree to an oral contract with the family, without the child, because the motto of this association is to open the family (*kazoku wo hiraku*). The meaning of this expression refers, on the one hand, to the need to restore a failing intrafamilial communication and, on the other hand, to the possibility of a "double-*hikikomori*" that I mentioned earlier: the young person becomes *hikikomori* and the family hides this situation from the surroundings and the neighborhood, hence the need to "open up" to others in order to get out of this situation. Then, a member of the team sends letters about *hikikomori* by presenting himself: it is generally a post-card (*hagaki*), without envelope, so that the *hikikomori* person sees directly the written characters, which would dissuade him from throwing it away. Then a letter contained in an envelope informs him of an upcoming phone call. When the call happens, the parent passes it on to the child who, in 90% of the cases, rejects it. Again, a postcard is sent and informs him of a visit. On D-Day, almost all refuse to open the door. Those who answer do so to state their opposition. Some leave home before the appointment time. In one case, a girl was absent because she had started working. In general, the visitor speaks behind the door and hands over his business card. From then on, between 30% and 40% begin to change, between 20% and 30% become violent, and the rest remain silent. Those who start to change start by hav-ing their hair cut, going out shopping, tidying up their room, and washing themselves. (After a long period of isolation, some have dental problems because of their prior lack of proper hygiene.) In some cases, they open the door themselves, or wait in the living room at the time of the appoint-ment. In other cases, they loudly knock behind the door. More rarely, they open the door and push the visitor, but when there is violence, it is mostly directed against the parents.

The arrival of a stranger causes, in two-thirds of the cases, an imbalance of the family life: either positive changes happen, or intrafamilial violence manifests itself. Sometimes, the role of the visitor is oriented toward a progressive referral to a psychiatric hospital, and when the violence is terrible, he invites the parents to call the police whose intervention has the effect of stopping the violent actions toward them. According to Mr. Murata, 10% have a diagnosis of schizophrenia and 30 to 40% of cases have consulted a psychiatrist. It is very important to mention it because it refutes the idea that psychiatrists always meet *hikikomori* people. With 12 years of experience in dealing with these young people, Mr. Murata says that 60–70% have never met a psychiatrist. This is corroborated by the work of the Nagoya University psychiatric research team, which also supports the view that they would meet only some of them (Suzuki 2009: 5).

Part of the research in clinical psychology is focused on improving interviewing techniques. In this context, I wanted to know the questions asked during the interviews with the parents. For Mr. Murata, the conversation is limited to "how they got married, how they found a job," and their current social situation. For more information, I have drawn on some lessons from French clinical practice: I mentioned the presence, in some cases, of trans-generational trauma related to World War II or the Algerian war (Halfon, Ansermet, and Pierrehumbert 2000, Guyotat 2005). These points can emerge in the French consultations; I ask if this is the case in their interviews. Mr. Murata and my informant, on the other hand, do not question parents about their own childhood even though Mr. Murata raises the issue that parents often attribute traumatic value to what they experienced during the period of high economic growth (*kōdo keizai seichō*), between 1955 and 1973. But what is it exactly? Are social workers trained to deal with these issues? Could the clinical approach increase the effectiveness of these NPOs while shedding new light on the complexity of the *hikikomori* phenomenon? In this respect, family mechanisms that contribute to children becoming socially withdrawn deserve further research. As part of my participation in the activities of NPO M., I dealt with these issues in a specific way: I accompanied some team members and some former *hikikomori* subjects on a group trip to Seoul, among their South Korean counterparts.

University of the people

The decision to go to Seoul with M. members was made very quickly during a *nabe no kai*. *Nabe no kai* is a friendly meeting organized around a Japanese hotpot. At the end of the meal, while everyone was caught up in various discussions, Mr. Murata informed my table neighbor of the trip to South Korea and, as I was next to him, invited me too. I agreed right away, "Oh? Really?" Mr. Murata was surprised. Did he expect me to accept on the spot?

Maybe not. Nevertheless, the trip being organized, it was necessary to act quickly and, therefore, a quick response was timely. The trip to South Korea was an opportunity for me to spend 4 days in a community of *furītā, nīto* and ex-*hikikomori* of Japanese and South Korean nationality.

We left on Wednesday morning, spent three nights in Seoul and came back on Saturday night. The first day, we arrived at our accommodation, a youth center in Seoul. The men slept in a large common room, women and children in an adjoining room. Three other rooms were empty including a meeting room, and a desk with computers. There were no showers and we went to the public baths every morning. All meals were taken outside. The Japanese team consisted of 13 people. The current leader Mr. Murata, his wife and their two children (2 and 5 years old); Ms. V., who supports migrant children, and who is also a member of the women's movement against nuclear energy (she takes part in many events such as those, weekly, in front of a regional electricity company); Ms. Y. director of short films; Mr. Maeda, Lecturer in social sciences at a local university and a specialist in new religions (Aum, Moon, etc.); Mr. Kinoshita currently studying sociology and a former *hikikomori*; and Mr. Matsui, a former *hikikomori* currently living in one of the shared houses of the NPO. The entire group lived in the social center and was joined by older people in various activities. The separation into two subgroups was made necessary because of the disability of the founder. This group consisted of the founder, his wife, their daughter (present to help his father with his mother), and another community member in his 70s who had authored several books. These people know each other because they regularly participate in the University of the People, organized in a café belonging to the NPO. The ex-*hikikomori* individuals work there and manage this café offering a panoramic view of the city. The NPO M. and the South Korean association U. are linked through the University of the People, and I attended, in Seoul, a Japanese–Korean event gathering a community around young people who are not "in the society."

On the first day, at the end of the afternoon, we joined the café belonging to association U. and then had dinner together. It was an opportunity for both the Japanese and South Koreans to get to know each other or to meet again. The next day was devoted to a full study day at the U. association's main office, with four conferences of Japanese members, two South Koreans' conferences, and a debate.

We can isolate some common points between the two associations as follows. First, these are two NPOs that provide support to young people who are not working (Korean and Japanese *nīto*), do not want to work, or have lost their jobs. Second, these young people are considered to be on the margins of their respective societies. Third, each NPO includes a café and collective accommodation (shared houses for Japanese and community buildings for South Koreans). Fourth, there is, in both cases, a charismatic figure whose history is extraordinary: on the one hand, the birth in Korea and then the tormented childhood of the founder of the NPO M. in the post-World War II context; on the other, the revolutionary commitment of the leader of the association U. and his imprisonment. And finally, the idea of "sharing": anti-capitalism and the University of the People for the Japanese; and militant activism and reflections on communism, revolution, and human, and social sciences among South Koreans.

It is on this last point that one of two differences lies. The first is summed up by the question of one of the South Koreans during this day: "which texts do you refer to? What are you studying at the University of the People?" The response of the Japanese and Mr. Maeda was: "in fact, it's not really a university," it's a time when, in a café, you can discuss different topics by eating, drinking and where people are invited to give a lecture followed by a debate. The second difference is that South Koreans do not help *hikikomori* people by doing home-visits. In other words, they do not exactly deal with the same population. The targeted Japanese population experience significant hardships and require assistance that would be provided by professionals paid by the State in the West (psychologists, psychiatrists, social workers, social workers, educators, etc.). In Japan, the support provided by NPOs is carried out by a staff of nonprofessionals (who nevertheless often have a bachelor degree like Mr. Murata), but Japanese NPOs "exclude" psychiatrists.

In the South Korean association U., as in NPO M., it is, therefore, the idea of the "sharing" which prevails. In NPO M., this idea refers to anti-capitalism, the questioning of work and the meaning of work. The original Newstart project was influenced by integrated communities inspired by Italian democratic psychiatry applied to the urban environment. In NPO M., this idea of an integrated community is coupled with the idea of "opening the family." However, at the level of the population supported, they must always face people who, if they want to work, work more slowly (and do not necessarily want to work full time) – hence, a need for a suitable workplace. For South Koreans this question does not arise. There are people who have worked before, but who have lost their jobs: for example, a young man experienced an existential crisis (without reporting depressive symptoms) that led him to association U. via a criticism of the current South Korean society. In another case, a young woman described herself as a single mother, unemployed, and in great trouble. The French word *précariat* is common in the vocabulary of the South Koreans of Association U., who have read seminar works of Michel Foucault, Jacques Lacan, Gilles Deleuze, Felix Guattari, Slavoj Žižek, among others. Students also join the association U. because of political convictions that separate them from the rest of the students and the South Korean population; they are neither conservatives nor liberals, nor do they wish to join a particular political party. On the other hand, they carry out actions for the union of the different political parties of the South Korean Left. Despite the energy they have exerted thus far, they have not succeeded, but they pursue an activism quite risky for themselves, insofar as they often have confrontations with the police.

In summary, in association U. as in NPO M., the political dimensions of protest and activism (communist, Marxist, revolutionary, anti-capitalist, ecologist, anarchist) are strong and gather around the idea of "sharing." Activism is claimed, on a regular basis in association U., unlike in NPO M. where it is more discreet. Also, we see that the links with South Korea occupy a particular function for the Japanese: this trip is a source of inspiration for the members of association M. and fosters an imaginary space that allows them to link to a common past and shared future.

During the last day, some members of the Japanese team gave different interviews. The afternoon was devoted to a discussion in another café (less markedly ideological, which is not affiliated with the Association U., but is part of the same network), and oral presentations of the operations of alternative collective housing for young people with limited financial means. After going to public baths, I was alone with two young men at breakfast. I had heard that Mr. Kinoshita was a student in sociology and learned at that time that he had gone through a period of social withdrawal. When we were talking, he emphasized the communication problems *hikikomori* people may have and then addressed the other young man: "*Matsui san wa hikiko-motteta?*" In other words, he asked him if he had experienced a *hikikomori* period. Mr. Matsui answered positively to this question. Several remarks are necessary.

First, this question is very ordinary, and I had certainly already had the opportunity to hear it. Yet in this context, it took a different meaning: "Have you ever gone through this? Did you also have this experience of having withdrawn from the world at some point in your life?" In a sense, the experience of social withdrawal represents a sidelining of the world, of society. The situation of *hikikomori* is presented as a test to which the person concerned survives, without ever being able to consider it as belonging to the past. This withdrawal is never truly voluntary, individuals are necessarily pressed into it; the situation of withdrawal represents a possible solution for a given moment. However, what can temporarily be considered as a solution is transformed after a few months and often for several years, into a dead end from which it is impossible to go out alone. All the *hikikomori* subjects for whom home visits are made were not able to get out of their isolation. We saw that at NPO M., they represented about a third of the cases. An additional difficulty is that you cannot predict in advance who will come out and who will not go out. For example, it cannot be said in advance that only people without a psychiatric diagnosis will go out. It is quite possible that some people with autism or schizophrenia come out (I have met them), and others who do not have psychiatric pathologies remain there. It is easy to understand how social withdrawal may coincide with a psychotic onset, which is true in some cases. But for other cases, social withdrawal may just as well be a way to protect against such an onset, or a coping strategy of subjects within a neurotic structure.

I should add that none of the people I met testified that *hikikomori* is a "social phobia," both on the side of the caregivers and on the side of the former *hikikomori*. This does not mean that such cases do not exist. In fact, three groups among people with *hikikomori* constitute a hidden population: the first group consists of certain people for whom a diagnosis of social anxiety disorder or social phobia could be made; the second group consists of people with *taijin kyofushō*; and the third consists of people who have an addiction to the Internet and especially online games. Recognizing these aspects of the wider phenomenon is important for treatment purposes. When someone who carries the diagnosis of social phobia is properly treated, the diagnosis could become obsolete after a few sessions. Beyond these psychiatric diagnoses (social anxiety syndrome, social phobia, *taijin kyofushō*), psychoanalytic orientations also help us use treatments that consider structural hypotheses (psychosis, neurosis, perversion) and the way a subject make social bonds via his or her symptom. As for addiction to the internet, it necessarily affects *hikikomori* individuals who are "serial gamers," those who spend their lives in MMORPGs. As we have seen, this image only represents a part of *hikikomori* in Japan: it is a hidden population within the socially withdrawn population. Finally, in South Korea we know that the proportion of internet addicts and serial gamers among the socially withdrawn population is very large, more significantly so than in Japan (Sungwon 2012, Lee et al. 2013).

Discussion

"They told us that you were an anthropologist"

Before concluding this chapter on associations that support *hikikomori*, an element is useful for understanding my position. When I was talking, drinking a glass of *makkori* (a South Korean alcohol made from fermented rice), I heard with great surprise a person from association U. announcing to me, "They told us that you were an anthropologist." My first reaction was to burst out laughing: how many times had I introduced myself to the Japanese NPO members as a "psychologist doing a Ph.D. thesis in psychology"? Probably a dozen times, specifying my interest in Lacanian psychoanalysis and anthropology. And had I not introduced myself to the people of the association U., a few hours before in the same way? I interpreted this sentence as an incentive to clarify my position.

My presence in the activities of NPO M. could be likened to the fieldwork (*fīrudowāku*) of anthropologists. In Japan, it seems difficult to imagine a psychologist participating in activities in this way, being with the people concerned, "on an equal footing," one could say. It seems that for the Japanese (and also the South Koreans), I do not fall into the category of what they call "psychologist." Indeed, psychologists are strongly influenced by North American psychological theories and practice (i.e. cognitive and behavioral therapies). In addition, certified clinical psychologists (*rinshō shinri shi*) have a defined place in the organization of work which restricts their field of action (see Chapters 1 and 2). A comparative question then emerges. Do the Japanese imagine "clinical practice" as comparable to that conceived by European psychiatrists and psychologists?

In the West, two representations are popular. On the one hand, the representation of the psychologist in a network of partners, and on the other hand, the representation of the psychologist practicing within the framework of an individual private practice. These two representations contribute – with that of the psychiatrist, the psychoanalyst, and the psychotherapist – to a global representation of what we do when we go see a "shrink": adults, teenagers, and children talk about difficulties (professional, academic, personal, love, family). In addition, the clinical practice of French psychologists and child and adolescent psychiatrists (which is my background) is strongly marked by psychoanalysis which assumes two basic concepts: the unconscious and transference. But in Japan, clinical psychologists are, as we have seen, of recent creation (Kitanaka 2003, Satō 2007, Grabosky, Ishii, and Mase 2012), and psychiatrists are still strongly stigmatized (Sartorius 2010). They are mostly associated with extreme mental illnesses experienced as highly and irreparably pathological (Kitanaka 2012). Yet many students and academics know the names of Sigmund Freud and Jacques Lacan. They may have an intellectual or even philosophical knowledge of psychoanalysis, but this knowledge has not yet reached widespread dissemination among psychologists, psychiatrists, and their patients. More specifically, this knowledge of psychoanalysis has not yet managed to make the clinic a source of education, hence the lack of interest in it outside literary circles (French and English), or psychoanalytical associations.

After this overview of different associations helping *hikikomori* people, many questions emerge. These questions could be approached from a historical, sociological, or anthropological point of view. As part of my Ph.D. thesis in psychopathology defended in 2014, I have privileged issues relating to identity and identification. The approach of these questions is conditioned by my positionality. In the field of educational sciences, the foreign researcher may be a teacher, in a Japanese school. In this way, he or she participates "from the inside" in a concrete project with the children, and with colleagues, which allows the collection of data (Rohlen 1983, Letendre 1995, Cave 2007, Lévi-Alvarès 2007). If they are sociologists or anthropologists and interested in issues involving youth or mental health, it will be difficult for them to occupy a similar place. In these fields, they conduct surveys, observe and perform fieldwork at a given time, and conduct semi-structured interviews (Ogino 2004, Kaneko 2006, Borovoy 2008, Horiguchi 2011, 2012, Toivonen 2008, 2012, Miller 2012). But what about a clinical psychologist?

In a sense, the position of a foreign clinical psychologist in Japan could resemble that of an anthropologist to the extent that both remain "on the threshold" of Japanese society. They are part of it, but in a place that remains marginal. Even for the most important works in the anthropology of mental health in Japan (Kitanaka 2012, Nakamura 2013), one realizes that a field, although led by a Japanese person in a care team, still holds to a position that differs greatly from the clinical psychologist: the anthropologist does not cure, he or she does not offer a therapy or counseling services. Yet, as a foreign psychologist, I was in a similar position. In this sense, and as part of an ethnographic survey conducted in the field of mental health, fieldwork sets limits to the participation of the anthropologist or psychologist; fieldwork necessarily places the researcher in a group, at the margin. He or she is, in a way, "excluded on the inside" observing from the threshold (*genkan*).

As for *hikikomori* subjects, they can be said to be "included outside": they are outside the society (*shakai*) but they are inside the "world" because they cannot escape *seken*. The *hikikomori* subjects are not "in" the Japanese society. This way of thinking about the situation of socially withdrawn youths is quite widespread among the Japanese. Whoever graduated from high school or university "enters society" with the first job. He or she is no longer a college student, a high school student, but literally a "person-of-society" (*shakaijin*). The *hikikomori* subject is not considered a "person-of-society," on the contrary: being out of work, studying or training, and remaining a recluse in his room, he is considered "out of society." It would seem that those who are themselves in a minority or marginal position "in society" assume the burden of understanding, explaining, and treating those who do not enter society. Anthropologists (Japanese and foreign) and foreign psychologists can understand and explain, but they cannot treat the people concerned, nor help their families. The difference between social scientists (Japanese and foreign) and foreign clinical psychologists is that the latter have clinical knowledge, so they can look in detail at the practice of their Japanese colleagues in order to know the strengths and weaknesses.

Although Japanese Studies specialists often have a scholarly knowledge of their area of specialty, they sometimes lack knowledge of the subtle nuances of clinical terms and "tricks," knowledge accumulated through years of clinical groups, supervisions, successes, and therapeutic failures. A recent example can be provided by Jeffrey Angles' translation of Saitō Tamaki's book. Angles makes translation errors related to specialty terms. For example, he sometimes translates *kyohaku shinkeishō* as obsessive-compulsive disorder. But the translation of *kyohaku shinkeishō* is obsessional neurosis, and the translation of obsessive-compulsive disorder is *kyohakusei shōgai*. This could be judged as a slight translation error, but it is actually a significant change of meaning that indicates a lack of knowledge about both source and target texts. First of all, the conceptual universe of the author Saitō Tamaki has its own specific history, and second, the target terms are subject to fierce conflicts between psychiatry and psychoanalysis with heavy consequences in the mental health field. While Jeffrey Angles might know the differences in translations above, he might have preferred to use the term obsessive-compulsive disorder, because the term obsessive neurosis is no longer used by American psychiatrists: it fell into disuse from 1980, with the disappearance of the term neurosis in DSM-III®. Saitō Tamaki claims the legacy of Jacques Lacan and opposes the DSM. Therefore, he uses *kyohaku shinkeishō* on purpose, and Jeffrey Angles underestimated the weight of the shortcut that his translation operates. Only specialists are likely to be aware of this, but the progress of research in the field that interests us cannot do without rigor and precision on the terms of specialty, behind which sits a whole world of conflicts and struggles.

At the turning point of clinical psychopathology and the anthropology of mental health, we can, therefore, expect an increase in knowledge: a contribution to anthropological inquiry; an improvement in the training of psychologists, and the treatment of those who consult them. In interviews with his Japanese counterparts, the foreign psychologist is condemned to stay liminal, but, exercising a similar job, he can do clinical investigations, as well as treatment and prevention proposals that are not the field of specialization of researchers in the social sciences and the sciences of education.

Transgenerational trauma

As we have seen in this chapter, Japanese associations (NGOs and NPOs) are diverse. They can use coercive methods (TYS), be affiliated with Buddhist schools, or be inserted into the city's welfare services. But they can also be initiated by Japanese citizens who have close relations with Korea (K2 International, Newstart, NPO M.). Obviously, this is only part of the support organized for these young people: it is necessary not to exaggerate the presence of the NPOs for *hikikomori-nīto* where a strong relationship with Korea exists. Nevertheless, this is one I have had access to. Or more exactly, it is the one that has interested me the most for a simple reason: they carry an ideal that is lacking in other NPOs. Newstart is by far the most visible and the most dynamic. Also, the National Association of Hikikomori Parents held one of its most important international symposia in South Korea. Is it only because these young people are also present in South Korea? I think that beyond a cultural proximity often invoked, lies a forgotten memory: that of the sufferings of World War II, the post-war period (US occupation, Korean War from 1950 to 1953) and the period of high growth (1955–1973). My terrain with *hikikomori* subjects led me, unintentionally, to touch an extremely sensitive point in Japanese history: its relations with Korea and *zainichi* Koreans.

It seems useful to recall a number of historical facts, especially at a time when Prime Minister Abe Shinzō (1954–) was photographed, posing on a plane marked with the number 731 (Spitzer 2013). The number evokes the 731 unit where Dr. Ishii Shirō (1892–1952) conducted large-scale medical experiments on human guinea pigs, comparable to those conducted by the Nazi doctor, Josef Mengele. Ishii Shirō concludes a pact with the Americans who exempted him from prosecution in the Tōkyō trial, by communicating the results of the experiments of his team (Harris 2002). At the same trial, another official escaped judgment: Abe Shinzō's maternal grandfather, Kishi Nobusuke (1896–1987). After joining the Ministry of Trade and Industry in 1920, he became a senior minister in Manchukuo in 1935, and Minister of Commerce and Industry in 1941. After the defeat, he was imprisoned and was one of the suspects of rank A war crimes. Released in 1948, he went back to politics in 1952 and became Prime Minister of Japan between 1957 and 1960. He was nicknamed the Shōwa Ghost (*Shōwa no yōkai*). Holding up the number 731, and considering his family's history, Prime Minister Abe's action insults the memory of the victims of these experiments.

I wanted to mention these facts in order to briefly indicate the complex coordinates of the type of work of remembrance in Japan: the continued strained relations between Japan and the two Koreas invite us to not assume a work of remembrance comparable to that which we know in Europe, and that we could summarize by the term "French-German friendship." There is present an implicit delimitation about which we can talk and about which we must remain silent in terms such as these. In order to maintain coherence in my remarks, I will not engage in the themes that regularly make the front page of the media of the issue of "comfort women"; territorial disputes related to the Tsushima Islands; Japanese anti-Korean nationalism of the far-right Zaitokutai; or Finance Minister Asō Tarō praising Adolf Hitler's "right motives" (McCurry 2017). All this raises eminently complex questions that can be seen through a brief review of the literature. The situation is so strained – for several decades – that any further elaboration requires infinite precautions and historical references that would separate us from the thread of an exploratory inquiry (Note: for more details on memory and trauma see: Hashimoto 2015, Lucken 2017).

Intergenerational transmission issues were already raised by the women interviewed by Margaret Lock in the 1980s. Lock (1995) was doing a survey about menopause but ended up collecting childhood memories of women traumatized by the experience of war and abuse during the catastrophic state of post-war Japan: either directly as a child or indirectly as a child whose parents experienced these hardships. The generation Lock studied is that of the mothers or grandmothers of shut-ins (*futōkō* and *hikikomori*); some in Lock's and Susan Holloway's investigations (2010) are actually socially withdrawn. It must be added that the American Occupation and the Korean War were a considerable upheaval, and their psychological consequences are still difficult to think about today. The upheaval of values following defeat was also stronger because a whole generation of men had died in combat. The Korean War and the consecutive period of high growth have accentuated this upheaval of values. According to Mr. Murata, parents of *hikikomori* subjects attribute a traumatic value to what they experienced during the period of high growth. What is this trauma? Is it a screen memory? Is it expected in Japan that a researcher and foreign clinical psychologist investigate such questions? Are these questions conceivable, and if so, under what conditions and in what context?

My exploratory research thus ends with a question: do *hikikomori* subjects embody what two generations – that of their parents and grandparents – would have tried to forget? If we make this assumption, *hikikomori* would then be the embodiment of a hidden memory in every Japanese household where he or she is present: the figurative "skeleton in the closet." However, this transgenerational hypothesis alone would be far too deterministic, and should only be a speculative first step. The *hikikomori* individual is also an "irreducible" subject. The necessary second step is to articulate family and transgenerational problems with individual and intrapsychic problems. Why in this particular family? And why he or she in particular? In the following chapter, I continue this questioning through the study of individual situations, and I analyze the accounts of *hikikomori* subjects I met, in Japan, between August 2010 and July 2013.

References

Borovoy, Amy. 2008. "Japan's Hidden Youths: Mainstreaming the Emotionally Distressed in Japan." *Culture, Medicine and Psychiatry* 32: 52–56.

Cave, Peter. 2007. *Primary School in Japan. Self, Individuality and Learning in Elementary Education*. London: Routledge.

Furlong, Andy. 2008. "The Japanese Hikikomori Phenomenon: Acute Social Withdrawal among Young People." *The Sociological Review* 56: 309–325.

Futagami, Nōki. 2012. *Nīto ga hiraku kōfuku shakai nippon - 'shinka-kei jinrui' ga hataraki kata · ikikata wo kaeru* ニートがひらく幸福社会ニッポン—「進化系人類」が働き方·生き方を変える (Happy Japan with NEETs). Tōkyō: Akashi shoten.

Futagami, Nōki, and Shirō Asano. 2006. "The 'Integrated Community': Toward the Transformation of the Hikikomori Archipelago Japan. A Dialogue between Asano Shirō and Futagami Nōki." Translated by John Junkerman. The Asia-Pacific Journal: Japan Focus. http://www.japanfocus.org/-Asano-Shirou/2239.

Guyotat, Jean. 2005. "Traumatisme et lien de filiation." *Dialogue* 168: 15–24.

Grabosky, Tomoko Kudo, Harue Ishii, and Shizuno Mase. 2012. "The Development of the Counseling Profession in Japan, Past Present and Future." *Journal of Counseling and Development* 90: 221–226.

Halfon, Olivier, François Ansermet, and Blaise Pierrehumbert. 2000. *Filiations psychiques*. Paris: Presses Universitaires de France.

Harris, Sheldon H. 2002. *Factories of Death. Japanese Biological Warfare, 1932–1945, and the American Cover-Up*. New York: Routledge.

Hashimoto, Akiko. 2015. *The Long Defeat. Cultural Trauma, Memory, and Identity in Japan*. New York: Oxford University Press.

Horiguchi, Sachiko 2011. "Coping with Hikikomori. Socially Withdrawn Youth and the Japanese Family." In *Home and Family in Japan. Continuity and Transformation*. Edited by Richard Ronald and Allison Alexy. Oxon, UK: Routledge.

———. 2012. "Hikikomori: How Private Isolation Caught the Public Eye." In *A Sociology of Japanese Youth, From Returnees to Neet*. Edited by Roger Goodman, Yuki Imoto, and Tuukka Toivonen. Oxon: Routledge.

Holloway, Susan D. 2010. *Women and Family in Contemporary Japan*. Cambridge University Press.

Inui, Akio. 2005. "Why Freeter and NEET Are Misunderstood: Recognizing the New Precarious Conditions of Japanese Youth." *Social Work and Society* 3 (2): 244–251.

Ishikawa, Ryōko, Tatsushi Ogino, Minoru Kawakita, Kōji Kudo, Rūtaro Takayama, Yoshitaka Nakamura, Akihiko Higuchi, and Sachiko Horiguchi. 2008. *"Hikikomori" e no shakaigakuteki apurōchi – media, tōjisha, shienkatsudō* 「ひきこもり」への社会学的アプローチ—メディア・当事者・支援活動 (Sociological Approach to *Hikikomori* – Media, Person Concerned, Support Activities). Tōkyō: Mineruva shobō.

Kaneko, Sachiko. 2006. "Japan's 'Socially Withdrawn Youths' and Time Constraints in Japanese Society: Management and Conceptualization of Time in a Support Group for Hikikomori." *Time & Society* 15 (2/3): 233–249.

Kitanaka, Junko. 2003. "Jungians and the Rise of Psychotherapy in Japan: A Brief Historical Note." *Transcultural Psychiatry* 40: 239–247.

———. 2012. *Depression in Japan, Psychiatric Cures for a Society in Distress*. Princeton, NJ: Princeton University Press.

Kondo, Naoji, Motohiro Sakai, Yasukazu Kuroda, Yoshikazu Kiyota, Yuji Kitabata, and Mie Kurosawa. 2013. "General Condition of Hikikomori (prolonged Social Withdrawal) in Japan: Psychiatric Diagnosis and Outcome in Mental Health Welfare Centres." *International Journal of Social Psychiatry*." 67: 193–202.

Kondo, Naoji. 2001. *Hikikomori kēsu no kazoku enjo - sōdan ・ chiryō ・ yobō* ひきこもりケースの家族援助 - 相談・治療・予防 (Support to Families in case of Hikikomori). Tōkyō: Kongōshuppan.

Kyodo. 2006. "Nagoya NPO Head Held over Captive's Death." *The Japan Times*, January 12, 2006.

———. 2012. "Suicide leap at disciplinary school." *The Japan Times*, January 12, 2012.

Lee, Young Sik, Jae Young Lee, Tae Young Choi and Jin Tae Choi. 2013. "Home Visitation Program for Detecting, Evaluating and Treating Socially Withdrawn Youth in Korea." *Psychiatry and Clinical Neurosciences* 67 (4): 193–202.

Letendre, Gerald K. 1995. "Disruption and Reconnection: Counseling Young Adolescents in Japanese Schools." *Educational Policy* 9 (2): 169–184.

Lévi-Alvarès, Claude. 2007. "L'adhésivité d'un monde professionnel." In *Enseignants et écoles au Japon – Acteurs, système et contexte*, edited by Claude Lévi-Alvarès and Manabu Satō, 157–190. Paris: Maisonneuve et Larose.

Lock, Margaret. 1986. "Plea for Acceptance: School Refusal Syndrome in Japan." *Social Science & Medicine* 23: 99–112.

———. 1995. *Encounters with Aging. Mythologies of Menopause in Japan and North America*. Berkeley, CA: University of California Press.

Lucken, Michael. 2017. *The Japanese and the War. Expectation, Perception, and the Shaping of Memory*. Translated by Karen Grimwade. Columbia University Press.

Maisterra, Pauline. 2013. "Treize gifles en 16 secondes : la vidéo qui choque le Japon." *Le Figaro*. September 18, 2013.

McCurry, Justin. 2017. "Japanese minister Taro Aso praises Hitler, saying he had right motives." *The Guardian*, August 20, 2017.

McLelland, Mark J. 2009. The role of the 'tojisha' in current debates about sexual minority rights in Japan, *Japanese Studies*, 29 (2): 193–207. Taylor & Francis.

Miller, Aaron L. 2012. "Taibatsu. From Educational Solution to Social Problem to Marginalized Non-Issue." In *A Sociology of Japanese Youth, From Returnees to Neet*. Edited by Roger Goodman, Yuki Imoto, and Tuukka Toivonen. Oxon: Routledge.

Miller, Aaron L., and Tuukka Toivonen. 2010. "To Discipline or Accommodate? On the Rehabilitation of Japanese 'Problem Youth.'" *The Asia-Pacific Journal: Japan Focus*. http://www.japanfocus.org/-aaron-miller/3368.

Ministry of Health Labour and Welfare (MHLW) 厚生労働省. 2003. *Jūdai/nijūdai wo chūshin toshita shakaiteki hikikomori wo meguru chiiki-seishin hoken katsudō no gaidorain* 十代二十代を中心とした社会的ひきこもりをめぐるちいき精神保健活動のガイドライン (Guidelines for Mental Health Support and Evaluation of Hikikomori in their 10's and 20's – Full version). Edited by Jun.Ichirō Itō et al. Tōkyō: Kokuritsu Seishin/shinkei Centre.

Nakamura, Karen. 2013. *A Disability of the Soul: An Ethnography of Schizophrenia and Mental Illness in Contemporary Japan*. Ithaca: Cornell University Press.

Ogino, Tatsushi. 2004. "Managing Categorization and Social Withdrawal in Japan: Rehabilitation Process in a Private Support Group for Hikikomorians." *International Journal of Japanese Sociology* 13: 120–133.

———. 2006. "Interaction Rituals and Self Identities: A Short Ethnography of a Private Support Institution of Social Withdrawal." *Shakaigaku hyōron (Sociologie critique)* 58 (1): 19–20.

Rohlen, Thomas. 1983. *Japan's High Schools*. Berkeley: University of California Press.

Saitō, Tamaki 1998. *Shakaiteki hikikomori — owaranai shishunki* 社会的ひきこもり―終わらない思春期 (Social Hikikomori – Adolescence without End). Tōkyō: PHP Shinsho.

———. 2013. *Hikikomori: Adolescence without End*. Translated by Jeffrey Angles. Minnesota University Press.

Sakai, Motohiro, Shin.ichi Ishikawa, Hiroshi Sato, and Yuji Sakano. 2004. "Development of Hikikomori Behavior Checklist (HBCL) and Examination of Its Reliability and Validity." *Japanese Journal of Counseling Science* 37: 210–220.

Sakai, Motohiro, Shin.Ichi Ishikawa, Mizue Takizawa, Hiroshi Sato, and Yuji Sakano. 2004. "The State of Hikikomori from a Family's Point of View: Statistical Survey and the Role of Psychological Intervention." *Japanese Journal of Counseling Science* 37: 168–179.

Sartorius, Norman. 2010. "WPA Guidance on How to Combat Stigmatization of Psychiatry and Psychiatrists." *World Psychiatry* 9: 131–144.

Satō, Tatsuya. 2007. "Rises and Falls of Clinical Psychology in Japan: A Perspective on the Status of Japanese Clinical Psychology." *Ritsumeikan ningen kagaku kenkyū* 13: 133–144.

Spitzer, Kirk. 2013. "Sorry, But Japan Still Can't Get the War Right." *Time Magazine*, May 20, 2013.

Suzuki, Kunifumi. 2009. "A propos du phénomène de Hikikomori." *Abstract psychiatrie* 41: 4–5.

Sungwon, Roh. 2012. "Hikikomori and Internet Addiction in Korea" presented at the 1st International Workshop on Internet Addiction, March 16, 2012, Yokohama.

Toivonen, Tuukka. 2008. "Introducing the Youth Independence Camp. How a New Social Policy Is Reconfiguring the Public-Private Boundaries of Social Provision in Japan." *Sociologos* 32: 42–57.

———. 2011."Don't let your child become a NEET!' The strategic foundations of a Japanese youth scare." *Japan Forum* 23 (3): 407–429.

———. 2012. "NEETs. The Strategy within the Category." In *A Sociology of Japanese Youth, From Returnees to Neet*. Edited by Roger Goodman, Yuki Imoto, and Tuukka Toivonen. Oxon: Routledge.

Toivonen, Tuukka, Vinai Norasakkunkit, and Yukiko Uchida. 2011. "Unable to Conform, Unwilling to Rebel? Youth, Culture, and Motivation in Globalizing Japan." *Frontiers in Psychology* 2: 207.

6   *Hikikomori* subjects' narratives

Introductory cases

The first dropout?

When I was conducting my investigations at Kyoto University, a colleague told me he knew a Japanese researcher who pretended to be "the first *futōkō*". I had an interview with him on December 21, 2011 between 7 and 9 pm in a Kyoto Cafe. Here is his story. Born in 1948, Mr. Nomura is the youngest son of four. He has an elder brother, born in 1939, who also went through a period where he refused to go to school. Mr. Nomura starts his narrative before his birth and talks about the family's departure from Tōkyō to Nagano, during WW2: People in the village did not appreciate people from Tōkyō, and his brother's school refusal started in this context. Back to Tōkyō, the family welcomes my interlocutor's birth. His father is a university professor of science and his mother is from a wealthy family. She is described as very protective and did not want him to mix with other children in a public school. In fact, in the 50s, there were up to 60 students per class. Mr. Nomura says he always had troubled relationships with schools. Like his mother, he did not have a good opinion of public schools and attended several private schools. He changed his primary school 3 times. After a random draw in his family, he had to go to a school which was one-and-a-half hours from home. At one point while attending this school, he developed a serious illness and had to be hospitalized. A closer school was found, but he had to repeat a year, which was, according to him, very rare at the time. He described himself as someone who stayed in bed, often reading books, and was full of anguish. Childhood and adolescence were nightmares for Mr. Nomura, very difficult periods, especially during junior high school. Because his father was a university professor, he was able to contact a famous psychologist, Mr. Hirai, to treat his son. In fact, he was the first patient to experience Mr. Hirai's method, a method created for children who refused to go to school. In agreement with his parents, this psychologist came to Mr. Nomura's room one evening to take him to another family for 2 weeks. It was the family of one of his roommates. According to Mr. Nomura, transferring him to his classmate's family was not really a good idea, but it worked. Others after him "suffered" Mr. Hirai's method.

Mr. Nomura had bad memories of his experiences in Japan and decided to leave when he was young. In the schools, during the 1950s, there was strong discipline where the one who had a fever was blamed... "this discipline was the opposite of me... by the way, I guess I've never graduated from junior high school." At 16, a colleague of Mr. Nomura's father was going abroad for a certain time, and he took this opportunity to leave Japan with him. His parents were surprised but accepted it. Abroad, he was registered in high school. However, when he started the second year, Mr. Nomura asked the director to tell the school he could not attend classes any longer. It was not possible. After a dropout period, he became the assistant of a famous religious studies scholar. This encounter "determined the life I had after," he says. Mr. Nomura is from a Christian family on his mother's side and was not really interested in Buddhism and Shintoism before. At the end of the 1960s, students' and workers' uprisings were at their climax. While in Japan, he participated in students' movements but "after 1970, there were nothing to do anymore." I did not learn much concerning the period between 1970 and 2010: He was an independent researcher while taking care of his parents. Today, he is a specialist in Buddhist studies and got his first position at 60, the age of retirement!

In foreign media

Newspapers in English such as *The Lancet* (Watts 2002: 359), the *New York Times* (Jones 2006), and *BBC News Magazine* (Kremmer and Hammond 2013) have discussed the *hikikomori* phenomenon, and the *Japan Times* has given detailed accounts about the experience of social withdrawal. Here, I sum up three accounts.

Kikuchi Tatehiko, 52, is the author of a book published in 2011 entitled "The English Monster" (Kikuchi 2011). He is the creator of the "*hikikomori ryūgaku* method", allowing students to study English while being socially withdrawn (Ōtake 2011b). For him, it is not necessary to travel to develop English language skills. Although he never went abroad by lack of "administrative skills," he succeeded 27 times to get the maximum grade (990) on the *Test of English for International Communication* (TOEIC). Let us have a look at his life story. After entering high school, his family moved from Aomori (the extreme north of Honshū) to Kyūshū (an island located at the extreme south of Honshū), while Mr. Kikuchi decided to stay back. At one point, he did not take a shower for 3 months and also did not change his underwear for 1 month. It was a personal record, according to Mr. Kikuchi. At Sapporo University, he discovered a passion for the Russian language. After graduating, he worked 12 years selling books and pedagogical material for the study of English. He could not sell enough, so he felt guilty, worked more, and became exhausted. At 34, he decided to quit everything to live in a

10-sq-m studio in Sendai. He only watched television. After 1 year, when the situation became unbearable, he found an English conversation book. He read it in 3 days. Then he read *Newsweek* and *Time Magazine* but noticed he did not know half of the words written. Then he studied English intensively, alone, encyclopedically, for 7 years. Jobless, without friends, and after consuming all his savings, he went back to his parents' home, who by that time had moved back to Tōkyō. It was 2011 when he started TOEIC. From the beginning, he found it too easy because, without preparing, he obtained a score of 970 out of 990: He was surprised and wondered if the test operator did it on purpose, just for him.

Iwai Hideto, 35, owns a theater company (Hi-Bye) based in Tōkyō. During adolescence, he experienced *hikikomori* for 4 years and made several plays on the topic: *Hikky Cancun Tornado* in 2010 and an autobiographical one based on family conflicts entitled *"Te"* (Hand). He describes his father, a medical doctor in a university hospital, as

> the absolute ruler. He used violence to keep everyone, especially my elder brother, under control. My brother was also violent towards me, so there was an absolute power hierarchy at home that formed the basic social code in my childhood. At school, I would bash other children to get something I wanted, and I never even noticed that that was abnormal behavior. In fact, I didn't care what others felt about me because they were only in the background in my world. But eventually, a friend hit me back, and from that moment my self-righteous world collapsed with a bang and I started to worry about people looking at me—and that took over my world. I couldn't go to school and so stayed at home for four years between the age of 16 and 20. I stayed in my room and played computer games and watched movies every day. Eventually, I developed a desire to be a film actor and so I went to a preparatory school to get university entrance qualifications. All sorts of people went to that school—genius young students jumping ahead of their grade, retired people, delinquents and people on welfare. It was a chaotic situation, but the teachers treated everyone as individuals — unlike normal school teachers, who I hated because they would scold students illogically and one-sidedly. So that prep school suited me well and I was able to return naturally to society and get on a drama course at Toho Gakuen College...That four-year experience is now brilliant material for my plays. I was terrified to see real people and the real world then, but now I understand that the real world is not so scary and that it is much more terrifying to live in a room with your delusions, because there the delusions are limitless and you can fall into a kind of fantasy forever.
>
> *(as cited by Tanaka 2010)*

Theater director Miyamoto Amon, 53, was marginalized by his classmates when he was at school. During adolescence, he experienced *hikikomori* for

1 year, alone in his room, questioning himself about the meaning of life. Since his early childhood, he was influenced by traditional dance *Nichibu*, loved theater, and discovered the composer Stephen Sondheim while socially withdrawn. It was when he was *hikikomori* that he first dreamt of becoming a theater director, which he finally became after being a dancer and chore-ographer. His path was not so easy, though. After becoming a house cleaner for a Singaporean family living in London, he spent all his money going to the theater every evening:

> I saw about 700 plays and shows in two years, and I made notes about each performance along with my own direction ideas and detailed com-ments. One day, at a party, I was asked by a friend, "What do you want to do?" — so I said, "I want to be a theater director." Then my friend said, "I know that — but what do you want to do as a director?" At that moment, I was thunderstruck and woke up to a fundamental flaw in my thinking, because I'd always just dreamed about being a director — without ever really considering what it was that I wanted to deliver to audiences.
>
> *(Tanaka 2011)*

After returning to Japan, Mr. Miyamoto changed his first name Ryoji for Amon, whose *kanji* means "Asian gate."

Shut-ins' crimes

On July 23, 1999, a 28-year-old man, unemployed and *hikikomori* for 10 months, took a plane departing from Tōkyō. Soon after the departure, he threatened the crew with a knife and entered the cabin where he forced the pilot to divert the flight, killed him with the knife, and piloted the plane himself for a few minutes. Let us sum up, a description of his mental his-tory made by a Japanese psychiatrist (Kobayashi 2008). He had problems during his teenage years, university and in the workplace. The psychiatrist mentions his fear of a classmate penetrating his thoughts, depressive feel-ings, and several suicide attempts. After a period of 6 months' vagrancy in Japan, he returned to his parents' home, locked himself in his room without speaking, and then consulted a psychiatrist with his parents a few days later. During the first consultation at the end of March 1997, he responded to ques-tions nodding his head and denied having auditory hallucinations, despite feeling like someone was constantly speaking about him. He showed a fear of others and wanted to commit suicide. The psychiatrist observed a perse-cutory delusion, a state of stupor, and diagnosed him with schizophrenia, prescribing medication. His condition improved a bit. He started to speak, but was transferred to another clinic after complaining of medication side effects. In the new clinic, the psychiatrist diagnosed depression, prescribed tranquilizers and psychotherapy. One month after, he integrated back into society, trained in accounting, and graduated with excellent grades in 1997.

In March 1998, he searched for a job and found one in the countryside, but quit 5 days later. In September 1998, he was forcibly hospitalized with a diagnosis of catatonic schizophrenia. After leaving the hospital in October 1998, until the plane's hijack in 1999, he was socially withdrawn and planned different ways to commit suicide. The expert of the Nagoya Court of Justice diagnosed him with an autism spectrum disorder, described as Asperger's syndrome at the time. In this case, social withdrawal was clearly the symptom of a mental disorder: schizophrenia, catatonic schizophrenia, depression, or Asperger's syndrome.

In January 2000, another crime attributed to a *hikikomori* person was reported. Newspapers revealed that in the city of Kashiwazaki (Niigata prefecture), a *hikikomori* man aged 37 captured a woman, aged 19, and kept her 9 years in his room. The mother, aged 73, had not noticed anything and was not allowed to enter his room (Horiguchi 2012). In May of the same year, a man aged 17 hijacked a bus in Saga prefecture. Cases such as these ensured that the media started to talk about *hikikomori* individuals as potential criminals (Rees 2002, Ueyama, Tsuiki and Tajan 2010, Saitō 2013). Saitō (2013: 4) Tamaki has written that "since those two events, there were no major events related to *hikikomori*". However, on December 8, 2011, newspapers inform that a *hikikomori* individual, Iwase Takayuki, was condemned to 30 years' jail for the murder of two members of his family. He also wounded three other family members. The Nagoya Court of Justice found him guilty of murdering his father, 58, and his niece, aged 1. With a knife, he wounded his mother, aged 60, and two other family members: his brother aged 22 and his brother's girlfriend aged 27. Only his 24-year-old brother, absent from home during the incident, was spared. Then he tried to set their house on fire by burning a *futon*. The alert was given by a neighbor, and the police found the five corpses while the house was on fire. These acts were committed after his father denied him access to the internet. During the trial, learning difficulties and autism were hypothesized. Iwase Takayuki, who was aged 30 when the incident occurred, had been socially withdrawn (*hikikomori*) for 15 years.

My encounter with Ueyama Kazuki

Before starting my investigations as a Kyoto University researcher, I went to Japan during the summer of 2009: I met Professor Tsuiki Kosuke who had begun to support my project. He also spoke about a former *hikikomori* – Ueyama Kazuki – with whom he had the opportunity to meet. Because they already knew each other and had a trusting relationship, it was possible for Professor Tsuiki to introduce me to Mr. Ueyama during my second trip in August 2010. Mr. Ueyama is the second person who wrote about their *hikikomori* experience in a *best-seller* autobiography entitled *Hikikomori datta boku kara* (From me, who was *hikikomori*) published in December 2001 (Note: the first person who gave a detailed account about *hikikomori* experience is Katsuyama Minoru, in January the same year. See: Katsuyama 2001). Ueyama was interviewed by journalist Michael Zielenziger in his 2007 book, entitled *Shutting Out the Sun: How Japan Created Its Own Lost Generation* which contributed to the popularization of *hikikomori* at the international level. Ueyama Kazuki is the author of a hatena blog, "Freezing Point," where he not only writes about *hikikomori* but also his reflections on philosophy and the social sciences. During the first trimester 2013, he was involved in translating portions of Felix Guattari's book *L'inconscient machinique* (English title: Semiotic Subjection, Semiotic Enslavement). On July 13, 2013, he did a presentation at the symposium about social withdrawal that he and I organized with Professor Tsuiki at Kyoto University. In August 2013, he was preparing a diploma to become a social worker in the field of mental health services. I first met him in August of 2010, as a person who experienced *hikikomori*, and one of the first to have written an autobiography. I wanted to read portions of his book before our meeting, and Tsuiki Kosuke suggested a chapter (starting on page 40 and ending on page 48), which I will now summarize and comment upon.

Autobiographical fragments

At the heart of his book, Ueyama Kazuki evokes the trigger moment of his hardships: "The strangeness (*ihen*) started when I prepared for the entrance exam, in October, second year of junior high school" (Ueyama 2001: 40). Mr. Ueyama's *ihen* started with difficulties controlling his body: He would often go to the toilet (several times a day during class and break) to defecate and urinate, without managing to do so. In closed spaces, he would feel suffocated, with sweats, vertigo, and panics. For these reasons, he was bullied (*ijime*) and humiliated by his classmates. He could not concentrate on his studies and became absorbed by the anguish of dropping out, becoming homeless, and dying. While he noticed his father coming home from work at 1:30 am and leaving the house before he woke up, he questioned himself on the meaning of adults' society: "In the morning, my belly hurts and I have diarrhea. I beg my mother not to send me to school. As soon as she says, 'okay, you can stay at home today', it slows down. Before noon, the homeroom teacher phones to inform us that there will be a 'special home-visit'. Immediately, my stomach aches and diarrhea restarts." (Ueyama 2001: 41). Let us stop at this point and make some remarks. We observe a typical onset during adolescence where puberty modifications trigger bodily phenomena and preoccupations related to the body. It seems there is great difficulty in containing drives and elaborating personal experience. He feels lost and cannot find external support: His father is absent, the medical doctor's diagnosis is rejected, teachers distance themselves from him, and he is bullied by classmates. Only his mother seems to care and count. At the time, she alleviates his pain, and does her best for him to enter a first, and then a second high school.

He felt anxious and had somatic symptoms. He was more and more absent, and even when going to the *juku*, his grades collapsed. Professors and classmates made fun of him. Some of them did home visits and he liked it. However, when he compared himself to others, he felt miserable and isolated himself to the point of not attending school and *juku* activities at a critical moment for every Japanese junior high school student: high school entrance exams. He always compared himself to others who applied to a higher ranked high school. He started feeling despair and oscillated between pride and panic. Although he entered a good high school, he felt guilty because his mother cried, and he simultaneously blamed himself for not entering the high school he deserved. When he wrote, he felt disgust for the mindset he had at the time. Entering high school was a turning point in his life, followed by a second period of withdrawal stronger than the previous, as he attests with this event in his autobiography: "High-school, the first day, orientation. We put on our sports clothes, we get in line in the schoolyard. 'Order!' He hits, angry. I don't understand anything. 'What should the angle of my arms be?' Arms should have been a little bit lower. As my face showed confusion, he told me: 'What is this behavior?' and slapped me." (Ueyama 2001: 42–43).

At this moment, Mr. Ueyama said he became *hikikomori*. This teacher's attitude was not unusual for the time. In the past, corporal punishment (*taibatsu*) was widely reported in Japanese schools (Letendre 1995), but today it would be considered a scandal. In the context of bodily and mental changes related to adolescence, the brutal and incomprehensible behavior of a teacher precipitated Mr. Ueyama's social withdrawal. During the period when he did not attend school, he felt bad. He spent his time watching *anime*, reading informatics and pornographic magazines, masturbating, drawing *manga*, and listening to radio at night. The day–night cycle reversed. He wrote, "I was outside of the machinery of the 'world'. As an 'excluded boy', I spent my time doing nothing, masturbating, every day. Just restlessness, remorse, sexual drive. A piece of abandoned flesh. Just the sexual desire and the anguish for the future." (*Shōsō to, jiseki to, seiteki shōdō dake no ōchisareta nitsukai. Seiyoku to mirai he no fuan dake.*) He continues, "At the time, going to the toilets disgusted me. I was disgusted (*ken'o*) that 'I had a body'. I ate and evacuated stinky feces. It is because of this body that I could not go to school. This body I could not control. The only benefit was sexual pleasure. Only when I was absorbed in it, I could forget time and my situation (Ueyama 2001: 43–44)."

His diary "holds him", through a process which looks like what the surrealists call automatic writing. He started to write it after stopping high school, and it was his only reason to live:

> In the beginning, I recorded my everyday life, second per second, in a monomaniac fashion. Only what was written here was the evidence of my existence. Soon, it transformed into recording internal conflict. I wrote

> rarely 'what happened', but continued to write only 'what I thought' and
> my feelings. I could only write the anguish for my future, 'I want to have
> a girlfriend', and my dark sexual feelings (Ueyama 2001: 44).

Only the mail he received – which he cared for a lot – connected him to
the world. His isolation (broken by some outings at the pool or the library)
lasted a whole year. His mother found him a highly ranked boarding school.
He did not really want to stay in this situation. He succeeded on the entrance
exam and would even be exempted from paying the school fees. When writing, he was still moved by sexual frustration and reflection upon the future.
He felt strange: "I feel a part of me is like a fraud (Ueyama 2001: 46)."

The year after that, he flirted with a woman older than him. But in the
end, he sent her a letter that would rapidly make her flee: As he imagined,
she just could not understand anything about what he thought. He read a
lot, and noticed, after a while, it was only authors who committed suicide.
He came back to the bench where he kissed her. A man came, they talked,
the man touched his zipper and proposed to go to the hotel. Mr. Ueyama
ran away, felt dirty, and washed compulsively his body and genitals. He did
not understand why he felt dirty, while the man only touched his zipper, and
not his body. What appears, after reading Mr. Ueyama's (2001: 45) account,
is the portrait of an extremely fragile young man, who has great difficulty
in containing his affects and thoughts. He can connect to others but alternates between anger, panic, hopelessness, and extreme self-depreciation.
His relationship to his body and bodily fluids (sperm, urine, feces) seems
problematic, notably in terms of smell (sperm stinks) invading interpersonal
relationships: "Human relations stink of sperm," he wrote. With the feeling
of strangeness, and the feeling that a part of him was "like a fraud", a clinician might think that he could have committed suicide. Let us add that the
tonality of this fragment is rather crude, and the use of time is unusual. The
mix of present and past in his writing is not simply related to the autobiographical style. Indeed, in his book and when I met him, he speaks about the
junior high school period and the *hikikomori* experience as if it was now: He
wrote and spoke of events which occurred 20 or 30 years before, as if it were
yesterday, a distortion of time often seen in trauma survivors.

Our interview (2010)

I met Mr. Ueyama for the first time in the office of a university located in
the Kansai area during the summer of 2010, that is, 9 years after he published his autobiography. The interview was video-recorded and subtitled in
French for research purposes and investigations of a Parisian research team
(Ōtake 2011a). The questions I selected for this interview have been inspired
by many sources. First, the *Hikikomori Behavior Check List* (HBCL) developed by psychologist Sakai Motohiro (Sakai et al. 2004), in partnership with
the association of parents of *hikikomori* individuals. I also relied on items

from DSM-IV-TR® for the diagnosis of social phobia. My ten questions were developed in collaboration with my Ph.D. supervisors Pierre-Henri Castel and Marie-Jean Sauret. Tsuiki Kosuke played the role of the Japanese interpreter during the interview (Ueyama, Tsuiki, and Tajan 2010).

In response to my first pair of questions – when did you become *hikikomori*? When did you get out of the *hikikomori* situation? – Mr. Ueyama spoke about elements of his autobiography. With regard to the first question, he insisted on the medical diagnosis he was given at age 14. Before entering high school, he developed symptoms which included heart palpitations, diarrhea, and the anxious conviction he would become homeless if he dropped out. However, he gave more precise details related to dates, insisted on his difficulties in joining a society where the seniority principle is so strong, and showed a strong feeling of hopelessness:

> The diarrhea started in October 1982. I tried to stay at school. I put in a lot of effort until July 1993, the end of the first semester of the second year of junior high school. At the time, I didn't know how to 'administrate myself', how I could hold myself well. [...] When I tried to adapt to society, I could not stand it anymore. But when I tried to enter society, I was in that state ... so the question to ask when I entered and when I got out ... I repeated these efforts, and failures like that ... efforts to integrate [into] society, the failures of these efforts ... I don't know what happens in France, but in Japan, the value of people is determined by age. People who are in their twenties are quite aware of that. But me, when I was thirty, I was desperate, because I thought I could not live while working. At [the] age [of] thirty, I was hopeless.

The computer offered by his brother in 1998 allowed him to escape hopelessness. Thanks to the Internet, he created relationships with others, became friends with a woman, and was invited to university seminars. Moreover, he felt guilty and wanted to escape a condition he judged as "shameful." During the spring of 2000, he started to live with another person, house sharing.

My second question – why does one enter the *hikikomori* condition? – is not crucial for him. Rather, he asks himself "why is it lasting like that? Why is it lasting so long? Because once you enter this condition, and you withdraw so strongly, you can hardly escape the situation ... there are only a limited number of people who can go out." Here, we can hear the sketch of what he will say later. According to him, *hikikomori* individuals are survivors. Compared to the terrible suffering he experienced when he was 14, he is actually in a much healthier state. He warns us to carefully keep that in mind. Accepting to be video-recorded puts him into a legitimacy conflict, a "dilemma", toward pure *hikikomori* individuals that nobody can represent.

My third question – are there some moments where one feels good while in a *hikikomori* condition? If yes, when? – allows him to insist that for a decade, he met a lot of socially withdrawn individuals. A largely debated question is whether one is "mandatorily entering" or "willingly entering" the *hikikomori* situation. Some people leave the *hikikomori* condition through conformism, others while completely forgetting this period of their life, refusing to speak about it. His way of answering my question was to claim that there is a political dimension to *hikikomori* testimonies. Those who went through this hardship could better elaborate what they experienced instead of denying it, and then they would contribute to social change.

My fourth series of questions – what could help them? What shall we do to try to get *hikikomori* individuals out of their withdrawal? Is there a specific way to speak to them? – allowed him to tell us that former *hikikomori* individuals are forced to hide their experience in job interviews. It is partly true, but let us underline that Mr. Ueyama places importance on others' gaze and the shame of being outside of society: "It is shameful, being *hikikomori* is the most shameful thing, it wounds people, it is a stigma." He sees a solution in professional integration through employment in cleaning occupations, but this perspective aborts as soon as mentioned. In fact, *hikikomori* people are 80% men. Yet, men doing cleaning jobs in Japan are poorly regarded. In addition, he argues, "In Japan, if there was a system similar to PACS, it would help a lot of *hikikomori* people". Indeed, before marriage was made legal for same-sex couples (September 2013 in France), the French civil solidarity pact (PACS) offered legal status to same-sex couples. Should we see here an implicit reference to homosexuality? Or would his remark be more widely related to the norm of "compulsory wedding" (Tajan 2014)?

My fifth question deals with the "typically Japanese" characteristics of *hikikomori* and provokes a response where he refers to symposia that took place in South Korea, Italian *hikikomori* cases, and the representation of psychiatrists internationally. One might observe that Mr. Ueyama's fears of becoming homeless, 10 years after writing his autobiography, have not been dispelled. And he continues to have suicidal thoughts: "To me, *hikikomori* people, if their parents do not take care of them, would be homeless or would commit suicide. That's my opinion." This worrisome observation is immediately followed by a well-known mechanism, intellectualization: "An English sociologist, Anthony Giddens, proposes the notion of reflexivity. To him, this notion is related to addiction, and I think it is important because of the question of addictions and *hikikomori*."

The three following questions were based on criteria of social phobia in DSM-IV-TR®. At question nine, I explained to Mr. Ueyama how social phobia might be applied to *hikikomori* and asked for his response to this approach. My sixth question – when you were *hikikomori*, did you feel a discomfort in doing certain things or speaking to specific persons? To whom, and according to you, why? – also provoked the aforementioned coping mechanism, though the theme is now more psychological. The resort to a theory of human relationships allows him to answer in a more personal manner. It is always a position made from guilt and shame in relation to the gaze of others: "There's another problem, it's the family members, because these are the people toward whom I feel the most guilty, because I involve them. It is difficult to stand in front of them, and talk to them. Sometimes it's very hard ..."

The seventh question – being *hikikomori*, is it a situation where one avoids being at the center of the attention? – provokes a need for supplementary information on the situation where one is observed. According to him, the response is clear: "People who could answer this question without any problem would not fall into a severe state of *hikikomori*." He recounts that, in 2001, he was one of the first to expose himself, and that *hikikomori* individuals were considered as people who could commit crimes, they were considered as "potential delinquents." Then, he insists on the difficulties he had of communicating inside his family and the possibility of joining support groups in several associations: "In these associations, parents do not want to hear about politics, for instance. Rather, they want to hear the voice of their children who are pitiful subjects. They want to hear voices telling their suffering ... I have many things to say, but I will tell them on other occasions, little by little."

My eighth series of questions – when you were *hikikomori*, were you afraid of appearing stupid? Or being caught out in what you were doing? Did you have other, more important, fears? – Mr. Ueyama still tries to objectivize elements related to social phobia. His response could seem surprising at first hearing and concerns phobic and obsessive–compulsive dimensions. It was difficult to understand, first of all, and second, to translate. It deals with what he calls "the bath metaphor" and he explains it as follows:

> There are people who don't want to take a bath for months. They love cleanliness. They want to take a bath, but as soon as they want to take it, they start to clean up the whole bathroom. You need to get rid of dirtiness and mold. These people, as soon as they want to take a bath, they need to start by cleaning up the whole bathroom, the bathtub, etc. For instance, they enter the bathroom at 8 pm, and they go out of it the next morning. There are people like that. In this metaphor, the bath corresponds with society for *hikikomori*. *Hikikomori* people, they would like to enter society, but in order to do so, you should start by cleaning. To them, people who are not *hikikomori*, those who live in society, including me today, those people who are living normal life are dirty because they're taking a bath in a quite dirty bathroom. That's how *hikikomori* people think.

Oppositional pairs of inside-clean and outside-dirty, or self-clean and others-dirty, are explicit and refer to an attempt to distinguish pure and impure, where reclusive life (those of *hikikomori*) would be located on the side of purity, and social life (those of *shakaijin*) on the side of dirtiness. However, we should also mention an important clinical aspect: Is it really a metaphor? In fact, Saitō Tamaki himself wrote about obsessional symptoms related to cleaning the bath among a *hikikomori* population in similar terms as those used by Mr. Ueyama (Saitō 1998: 45). Added to the difficulties of understanding during the interview, these elements suggest that what Mr. Ueyama speaks about is something "real" (*un réel*). The way he speaks about this "*un réel*" is not completely metaphoric.

With my ninth question – the last of three questions that deals with social phobia – I asked the following: According to you, what is the difference between *hikikomori* and social phobia? I also encouraged him to associate the question of medicalized diagnosis with the potential for social and financial assistance toward *hikikomori* subjects. He himself refuses medicalization, but he confirmed that it is a relevant debate, mirroring the accounts I have come across between psychiatrists' and parents' associations. The major concern seems to be the recognition of a necessity to support struggling individuals without them being considered mentally ill or disabled.

In the last question, I explained my hypothesis, as it was formulated during the early moments of my research with my Ph.D. supervisors and taking into account the Japanese translation. Our idea was as follows: "We think *hikikomori* begins during childhood and appears later. In other words, people who become *hikikomori* at university, already have predispositions. What do you think?" Mr. Ueyama insisted that the shift from "school refusal" to "school non-attendance" during the 1990s was very important, which I could confirm in Shimizu Katsunobu's article published in 2011 in the journal *Social Science Japan Journal* (Shimizu 2011). Researchers and persons concerned (*tōjisha*) agree that, through the change of a name, the Ministry of Education erased the dimension of illness – as it had appeared in school refusal syndrome (*tōkō kyohi shō*) – in order to promote the category of school nonattendance (*futōkō*), which was seen as much more neutral.

In his response, Mr. Ueyama says Saitō Tamaki, as well as his master in psychiatry, Inamura Hiroshi, thought about *hikikomori* as a sequence of problems triggered during adolescence. Mr. Ueyama believes, however, that a certain number of people today start being *hikikomori* after their first job. Mr. Ueyama tries to find a new way of considering *hikikomori* and to propose solutions which do not make parents feel guilty and which do not "search for the criminal", which is often the case in Japan, according to him. Speaking about a "mother complex" (*mazakon*) does not bring any concrete solution: "When one attributes the responsibility or the cause of the problem, to the problems of childhood or the ways children have been raised by parents, then it comes back to *hikikomori* themselves." Finally, he quotes the debate on medicalization and, for instance, the psychiatric diagnosis of developmental disorder (*hattatsu shōgai*): "It's always the question of social assistance and medical insurance. But when there's a diagnosis, parents are not blamed, parents don't feel guilty anymore."

Correspondence (2010–2013)

Following this interview, Mr. Ueyama and I had several correspondences, met individually 3 times, and in group 4 times. He invited me to a seminar about "Institution" which I attended once and introduced me to NPO *leaders*, Mr. Wada and Murata, during meetings lasting sometimes 4 hours. Mr. Ueyama positions himself as having experienced *hikikomori* and having met hundreds of people who have had this experience. He is not a spokesperson but conveys accounts of those he has met. His reflections gravitate around the experience of social withdrawal.

Since the beginning of our correspondence, he has refuted the idea that *hikikomori* did not exist before the Internet (he himself got out of reclusion thanks to the Internet) and the idea that *hikikomori* would be more connected, compared to others, to the Internet. According to him, medical doctors and sociologists consider social withdrawal situations to have always existed, with *hikikomori* simply a recent manifestation. Also, socially withdrawn individuals say themselves that they are not especially avid users of the Internet. In an interview with the founder of the website *nichaneru,* Nishimura Hiroyuki, Saitō Tamaki argues that the number of heavy users of Internet – *netoge haijin* – would be less than 20%, with the 80% remaining reading books, watching DVDs or television, or just not doing anything. Mr. Ueyama gives the example of a tentative idea 7 years ago by several groups of former *hikikomori* to create social networks, but failed, however: "We do not know how to institute social networks. It's rather the style of social bond which is the crucial problem," he claims. As for the use of the Internet, he distinguishes the Japanese situation from the South Korean one, where intensive Internet users (those involved in MMORPG) represent a great portion of *hikikomori* (Sungwon 2012, Choi and Lee 2012, Lee et al. 2013).

Mr. Ueyama was gratified when he learned of the existence of the French neologism, *"retirant social,"* built by the Parisian research team; he believes the term *hikikomori* in Japanese is too pejorative and discriminatory, which is altogether avoided by the term *"retirant social."* The term *otaku* is also a problem:

> Many times I was assimilated to *otaku* culture, but I don't subscribe to it myself. I don't like *manga*, or *anime*, or characters (before I liked them but now I hate them). When Saitō Tamaki says '*hikikomori* should be *otaku*', he wants to say that if people really like the *otaku* culture, they could engage in social actions. As a Lacanian, Saitō wants *hikikomori* people to desire. He always quotes the Lacanian statement 'The only thing of which one can be guilty is having given ground relative to one's desire'. In fact, I tried to be *otaku*, to be a socialized and desiring person. Yet I failed.

The above was an important moment in our correspondence, because it signaled the way Mr. Ueyama connects his interest in Felix Guattari in opposition to that of Jacques Lacan, via Saitō Tamaki's personal interpretation which spread in Japan – and his theory of desire and signifier. Mr. Ueyama is first interested by questions of socialization and dependency (in terms of addiction) and quotes Felix Guattari, *"Les défoncés machiniques"* (Machinic Junkies) in *"Les Années d'hiver"* (Soft Subversions). The comment of this extract by Mr. Ueyama invites us to think about the *hikikomori* phenomenon in perspective with *"l'échappatoire improductive"* (the unproductive loophole), *"à la limite de l'effondrement"* (the point of collapse), evoked by Felix Guattari. It allows him to intellectualize something like a bond that has been broken across generations, and on the other hand, his relationship to death (suicidal ideation). In other words, Felix Guattari's thoughts afford him a coping mechanism, by operating a *bricolage* contributing to nurturing him intellectually and holding him into existence. In the logic of fostering this *"échafaudage sémiotique"* (semiotic scaffolding), a notion from Guattari which also interests Mr. Ueyama, I responded to his request to bring Guattari's book *L'inconscient machinique*, difficult to find in today's Japan in French. Mr. Ueyama started to translate some portions in Japanese in 2013.

Our correspondence reflected our interest in varied approaches to subject formation, *subjectivation* for me in a Lacanian fashion, and the "production of subjectivity" in the Guattarian sense for Mr. Ueyama. Several times he used the term "survivor" to describe *hikikomori* subjects. He also distinguished five types of theories developed by those who are investigating *hikikomori* phenomenon: sociological and anthropological, psychoanalytical and psychological, medical (DSM-IV, ICD-10), philosophical (e.g., notion of "ontological security"), and ideological (e.g., "victims of capitalism or deregulated society"). During the symposium Professor Tsuiki and I organized on June 30, 2012, he asked a question during the debate after my conference to underline there was *tōjisha* discourse that I had forgotten to mention, to which I replied: "If there is something like *tōjisha* discourse which could be separable from other discourses, could we locate it using the Lacanian theory of discourse, – university discourse, master discourse, hysteric discourse, psychoanalytical discourse?" Because he could not fully develop his point of view, Mr. Ueyama was invited as a speaker in the symposium we organized a year later (July 13, 2013) at Kyoto University, entitled "Past Present and future of *hikikomori*." He used this opportunity to explain to us what he meant by *"tōjisha* discourse," as opposed to academic discourse. However, his definition of discourse was not the same as the one used in the Lacanian theory of discourse.

Finally, let us underline the fact that Mr. Ueyama made other collective meetings possible. For instance, he introduced me to several associations. He introduced the Parisian interdisciplinary research team to the new reflection group on social withdrawal (*Shin hikikomori nitsuite kangaerukai*), where we could meet the first generation of *hikikomori*, today in their 40s or even 50s. Let us have a look at the narratives of two members of this group: Maruyama Yasuhiko and Hayashi Kyōko. Along with Mr. Ueyama and Katsuyama, they are the first generation of *hikikomori* survivors and were the first to create a support group reflecting on the issue at the very beginning of the 2000s.

Hikikomori generations

First generation: age 50

I met Maruyama Yasuhiko and Hayashi Kyōko during a meeting organized by Ueyama Kazuki in a Tōkyō support group dedicated to current and ex-*hikikomori* individuals. They both have an experience of school nonattendance (*futōkō*), social withdrawal (*hikikomori)* and are known as *hikikomori keikensha* (individuals who have experienced social withdrawal) from the first generation (mid-1990s). They are also considered as *tōjisha* (person concerned).

Maruyama Yasuhiko, born in 1964, is in his 50s and works as a school social worker, holding his own private counseling practice called "Human studio." When Mr. Maruyama speaks about his experience, he starts by saying that he dropped out (*taigaku*) from school just after the first semester of the first year of high school. More precisely, he repeated the first year of high school 4 times and graduated after 7 years. How could he come back to school? One day, when he was at home, he became aggressive with his parents, broke a lot of things in the house, and felt completely relieved. Then he had to "confront himself alone in his room" (*heya de jibun jishin to muki aimashita*) and was not afraid of being expelled anymore; after 4 years, he could finally come back to school. Because he had repeated his first year of high school 4 times, he had to go to counseling sessions where caregivers did not understand anything about school dropouts. The counselor took him to the hospital where he had to accept "brain waves" examination. It was an "inhuman treatment" (*hi ningenteki na atsukai*), and according to him, a lot of dropout students of his age had to suffer this treatment. Neither the interviews with the parents, the counselors nor the teachers had any effect on the decision he made to repeat the school year. Also, he was profoundly shocked when he noticed the whole education was based exclusively on the teachers' points of view, not caring about the students' opinions.

Concerning his adult-*hikikomori* period, he says that he wanted to be a teacher since junior high school and went to a highly ranked university until he obtained a 1-year part-time teaching position. However, an incident occurred where he completely lost his trust in human relationships, and at this point his *hikikomori* period began, lasting for a few years, he says. When he was *hikikomori*, he was over 30 years of age and despite wanting to come back to society, found it very difficult. An inner voice would say, "now you want to come back to society? But what are your qualifications to go back to society?" After complaining about the parents and society, when the *hikikomori* wants to come back, he says to himself he is lacking expertise and complains about himself: This is, in his opinion, a form of self-denial (*jikohitei*). Finally, Mr. Maruyama mentions his low self-esteem during the reclusion, a feeling related to being of a low rank in Japanese society. He describes a "way of living like a wild animal" (*yasei dōbutsu no yō na ikikata*), struggling between life and death, not knowing if someone will care if he dies. These worries are echoed by the contemporary theme of the aging of *hikikomori* individuals (*hikikomori no kōreika*).

Ms. Hayashi experienced a period of school dropout during the second year of high school. When she was approximately 25 years old, she lived a *hikikomori* life for two full years. In her narrative, she looks back to her *hikikomori* and *futōkō* experience and speaks about parent–child relationships (*oyako kankei*). After withdrawing from the second year of high school, her health progressively declined. Her family had to move for professional reasons and after 1 day in the new high school, she dropped out again. Then she entered a distance education system to pass an equivalence degree enabling her to take the university entrance exam. But at university, she also dropped out: At the time, she thought, "I guess I am the only one to become *futōkō* at university." From this moment, her "fight with her difficulties to survive" (*ikizurasa tono tatakai*) started. She had irregular contact with the hospital for a long time before being hospitalized for 2 weeks in a medical facility and had an awkward feeling that something was wrong in her. As her mother told her "if you don't go to school, work," she started part-time jobs at the age of 20 years old, but by 26, it became impossible to continue. She just could not go out. The 2 years of her withdrawn existence were marked by feelings of insecurity. The only thing that could alleviate these feelings was listening to the music that she liked and the prospect of going to a live concert, which required money. But the more she worked, the more she burned herself out, and for that reason, her health deteriorated to the point of hospitalization.

Her days were punctuated by inner conflict and foggy-mindedness, related to issues that she could not catch the meaning of. In her 20s, she also had daily disputes with her mother, a relationship that continued as such for 10 years, prompting Ms. Hayashi to seek an apology for a lot of what she said (*oya ni ayamatte hoshii*). She encountered personal and familial problems but found relief in learning she had friends who shared these experiences. They had the same feeling as her: As the whole society blames the parents, it prevents children from getting angry with them. She adds that when she realized they could not understand each other, and that it would never disappear, their conflicts diminished. A meeting with a certain doctor was another turning point in her life: This person became someone who she could trust. At 33 years old, she decided to attend a support group for ex-*hikikomori*. In this group, it was possible to have regular discussions with other group members. "After seventeen years 'my *futōkō*' finally ended," she says.

Mr. Onishi: age 39

In the first NPO I visited in X. city, there is a space open to the public where one can construct a sense of self (*ibasho*). The NPO is quite small with only one permanent employee and a few volunteers. Mr. Wada, the leader of this NPO experienced a 10-year period of social withdrawal between 19 and 29 years old. He said he used to go out every month with his mother to the doctor in order to renew his prescription (anxiolytic, antidepressant). During this period of his life, he had a lot of anxiety and it was very difficult to overcome these hardships. According to him, a lot of *hikikomori* individuals go to the doctor once a month for the same reasons. Now Mr. Wada is a caregiver and a leader of an NPO related to X. city welfare services. He told me it was a huge step for Mr. Onishi, a 39-year-old ex-*hikikomori* who attended the NPO, to explain his own experience in writing. His narrative is entitled "Looking back to my history" (*furikaeri jibun shi*). The confession starts in the September 2011s edition of the NPO magazine, with the subtitle "The Monotonous Age of School" (*monotōn gakkō jidai*) and continues in the October edition. The section titles for the first part of his testimony, translated into English, are as follows:

> The "bluff" of living alone (*kodoku wo ikiru to iu kyosei*)
> The tension (nervousness) that you cannot find your place (*mi no okiba no nai kinchō*)
> The joy of the honors and the mask of the literary youth (*homerareta ureshisa to bungaku seinen to iu kamen*)
> The principle of the independence from parents and the true Self (*oyabanare to iu tatemae to jissai no jibun*)
> Clutched by the mother (*haha kara no shigamitsuki*)
> Methods to cope with my lonely way (*jibun nari no sabishisa no taisho hō*)

The first paragraph of his testimony starts as follows. "I am looking back to the high school period. The high school period, if I had to give it a color, [it] would be grey and I think it was sad and hard. I succeeded in entering the S. high school and I went there; the reason why I chose this high school was because at the time of junior high school I was bullied and I didn't want to go to the neighboring high school selected by a lot of my schoolmates. This year the catchment area was extended, and we could choose several high schools. As the high school S. was an hour away, I had the feeling to escape from reality and search for a place that is not here. I wanted to reset my 'miserable ego' which endured the bullying and had been excluded by the schoolmates and I didn't want to be with those who bullied me. They were 'vulgar people' and I wanted to live as a 'noble' with the friend of 'solitude', even if I couldn't find someone to understand me."

This former *hikikomori* also experienced bullying (*ijime*) and encountered difficulties in his relationships with others, to the extent he had to choose a high school located 1 hour from his house to avoid his classmates. After three events, his social reclusion progressively started. First, he attended the high school rugby team for an experimental period. However, he felt scared and weak and another student noticed it while they were in the changing room: At this precise moment, Mr. Onishi really felt ashamed. Second, he was congratulated by his professor for an essay he wrote and then was rewarded for the same essay in the local library. After the professor had read some parts of the essay to the classmates, he could not stand the feeling of being under the spotlights, exposed in front of everybody. The third event was related to his family, which owned a local business (a small restaurant), and which included an older brother and a younger sister. One day, he was supposed to go to high school but decided to stay at home in the company of old friends from junior high school, and his mother was spying them. She was angry and spoke about this to his father, who scolded him: "we all work hard, but you... what are you doing!" They were naturally asking why he was not attending high school. Mr. Onishi did not say anything and kept his feelings inside, but "the most shocking thing" was the feeling that his mother was "clutching" him, he says. Then he went to the mountain alone and felt lonely.

In the following edition, he starts by summing up the first part and writes about the Swedish movie "Pelle the Conqueror" which tells the story of a young boy called Pelle and his father Lassefar, moving from Sweden to Denmark to improve their living conditions. At their arrival, they are prevented from working at the farm by the local people who shun them, but they somehow manage to survive. Mr. Onishi writes about the young boy's situation in terms of "awful bullying" (*hidoku ijimerare*) and enhances the last scene of the movie, in which the father, dying, tells his son to escape alone. The last image shows the young boy walking alone, next to the sea, under the snow, at dawn: "I couldn't understand what to do with myself, why couldn't I stand up with strength like Pelle." In addition, he reports another event. After the end of the school year, there was a party where the students went to Karaoke together. He did not know how to communicate with others and drank whisky until he was completely drunk. In this pitiful state, he was apologizing all the time to his schoolmates and could not understand why they were so kind, taking care of him to the extent of bringing him back to his home by car.

In his testimony, Mr. Onishi makes it clear that there were severe problems with his self-esteem, and that alcohol only worsened the situation. He has a lot of difficulties communicating with others and understanding them, and particularly the motives of their action. What could be easily understandable (the parents scolding him because he does not go to school, the kindness of some schoolmates toward him while he is ill) is to him completely senseless: In these situations, he does not understand the meaning of actions directed at him. These scenes – the changing room, the mother's spying and the reaction to his essay's success – underline his feelings of self-intrusion. It would be too long to continue developing in detail the case of Mr. Onishi, but it is important to show here the section headings for the second part of his testimony:

I thought about school dropout (*gakkō chūtai wo kangaemashita*)
Low altitude flight *versus* fake pride (*teikū hikō VS itsuwari no puraido*)
Remaining of the first love (*hatsukoi no nagori*)
X. was the support of my heart (*kokoro no sasaedatta* X.)
The beginning of alcoholism (*arukōru ison no hajimari*)

These section headings show the likelihood that Mr. Onishi suffered from at least one mental disorder and could be considered a case of "secondary *hikikomori*." In terms of some Japanese psychiatrists (Suwa et al. 2003), "primary *hikikomori*" is a situation characterized by a pathological social withdrawal without any other mental disorders, unlike "secondary *hikikomori*" which qualifies a comorbidity, or a situation where social withdrawal is only a symptom of a broader mental disorder (alcohol-related disorder, schizophrenia, depression, social anxiety disorder).

Mr. Arai: age 33

In an NPO located in a *jōdō shinshū* (Pure Land Buddhism) temple, I met a former *hikikomori* and spoke with him. After sleeping in the temple, I awoke at 6 am to attend the *nenbutsu* session (morning recitation of *namu amida butsu*) at 6:30 and then rang the bell at 7. At 8 am, my informer came with Mr. Arai, who is actually employed in a cram school (*juku*). He works from 11 in the morning to 11 at night. Children are there from four to nine in the afternoon. He works 6 days a week and rests on Sunday and two Saturdays per month. He lived in this city until he was 18 years old and studied at one of the most prestigious Japanese universities. Until 18, everything was "apparently OK," he says. After his bachelor's, he went to study abroad, which is, according to him, quite uncommon. He obtained a master's degree and attended a doctoral course. But after three-and-a-half years, he had to come back to Japan because his visa was ending and because his parents could no longer afford his studies (They had to pay for the studies of his younger two sisters). He started working in a *juku* only 2 days after he came back to his hometown but stopped after 6 months. He wanted to finish his Ph.D. dissertation, so he stayed in his room in the family house in order to achieve this goal. For him, the first year was different from the following two years. The first year was like a vacation and at the same time, coming back to his hometown after such a long period, was a "cultural shock," compounded by the fact that he no longer had any friends in the area. He confesses that during these 3 years of withdrawal, he stayed, in his mind, abroad. He continued to communicate with his friends abroad and still does. After 3 years of withdrawal, he felt a heavy social pressure because he had no professional experiences and did not finish university. He remained in seclusion until one day a *jōdō shinshū* monk he liked and knew for a long time came to visit him at home and told him it was enough, that now he had to come out from his isolation. After this experience, he went every day for 2 months to the temple. He decided to go as often as it was allowed, which meant almost every day (6 days a week). Like everybody else there, he was involved in farming; these 2 months were pretty long, he recounts.

Afterward, Mr. Arai rapidly found a job in another *juku,* which he holds to this day. It is a tenure contract, poorly paid – 210,000 yens – with no chance of increase: With such a salary, he complains he cannot have a good social status. In order to have a girlfriend, he says he first needs to have a better job. Between the ages of twenty-nine-and-a-half and thirty-three, he has now been working there – three-and-a-half years. During the first-and-a-half years of the new job, he was able to move from his parents' house to an apartment provided by the *juku* company, but after financial difficulties arose in the company, they had to get rid of this apartment at which time he decided to go back and live at his parents' house. Now he thinks this withdrawal period could be called *hikikomori*, but at the time, he did not realize it. During the first year, he "was really studying every day to finish the PhD," he says, but at a certain point, it changed. During the following 2 years, he could spend 6 hours a day playing chess online (which he learned abroad), which means 40–60 games. He thinks he was not a standard *hikikomori* because he was never afraid of others and had a lot of friends.

In a conversation that took place among him, my informer and me, Mr. Arai said that when he was younger, people told him he seemed older, but now he feels like he is 10 years younger: Specifically, he feels as if he is 23. This is the approximate age when he went abroad: He suggests that when one goes abroad for work or studies, upon his return, it is as if time stood still. It is as if the time spent abroad did not count according to the workplace system and Japanese society in general. Following this logic, as he started working 10 years after those from the same generation, it is as if today, he was 10 years younger. Obviously, there are examples of Japanese students who go abroad without experiencing such a feeling. This argument concerning the perception of time was previously advanced by Kaneko Sachiko in her article published in *Time and Society* (2006) and could also correspond with the concrete and wide problems of returnees (*kikokushijo*) that scholars such as Goodman (2012) have described. Another way of understanding the complex relations between time and society can also be found in a collective article published in French. Researchers from Japan and France working on the topic of young adults' social withdrawal (Furuhashi et al. 2013) introduced the difference between *seken* (world or imaginary community) and *shakai* (society). This difference was not immediately understandable from a foreigner's point of view. When I was in Japan in 2010 and when the psychiatrists of Nagoya University explained *hikikomori* individuals as "out of society," it was hard for me to consider it this way, but after my years of research, this description started to make more sense. For instance, Mr. Arai spent three-and-a-half years abroad and stayed three years in a social withdrawal situation. From the point of view of Japanese society, he is six-and-a-half years late, and from the point of view of *seken*, his situation is shameful for him and his family (*seken ni taishite hazukashii to omō*). When Mr. Arai and my informer talk together, they seem to completely agree on this point.

This interview leads us down various paths and does not fit into the ideal type of *hikikomori*. Notably, we cannot diagnose a mental disorder, but instead, many questions arise. First, there are some aspects of this story that are unclear: Why did Mr. Arai leave Japan after his bachelor's (quite uncommon as he says)? Why did he come back to Japan before finishing the doctoral course and submitting the Ph.D.? Why not engage in a part-time job abroad, which could have allowed him to graduate one-and-a-half years later? In other words, why not stay abroad while working (if he did not want to come back) instead of withdrawing during the next 3 years? Apart from these questions, another element is particularly interesting: When I ask, "Do you have a girlfriend?" he answers negatively arguing that with his salary, he cannot afford to propose to a woman. According to Mr. Arai, his income is preventing him from getting married; thus, he does not have a girlfriend, which might seem quite surprising to some: It is not because you are not rich enough that you have to forbid yourself any date, sexual affair, or love story with a man or a woman. But Mr. Arai seems to think this way. We have to underline that from a Japanese point of view, being 33 years old and earning 210,000 yens a month without any chance of an increase is not a good situation (it is not the worst, but it is below the average salary). Nevertheless, Mr. Arai chooses to accept a conformist point of view instead of dating a partner without marrying. Of course, if we consider the powerful conformist discourses in Japan, it is difficult, but it does not mean that Mr. Arai is not responsible for his situation. These events partly testify to what Lacanian psychoanalysis calls *"position subjective."* For instance, going out of this withdrawal situation thanks to a *jōdō shinshū* monk, being located in an apartment of his company, going back to his parents' house, and not engaging with a partner testify of his *"position subjective."* On this last point, a fact is obvious: Mr. Arai could find a partner even if his social status is not the one he, his family, and his potential partner hoped for; he could find a partner even if he cannot propose the ideal marriage he wanted to, or had expected to.

Furthermore, Mr. Arai escaped Japanese society at the very moment of his transition to work, where the vast majority of students seek employment through activities and forums organized between universities and employers (Brinton 2011). He was expected to find a job after completing his bachelor's degree, but he decided to go abroad rather than enter the Japanese society. Later, his decision to interrupt his doctoral course could have been related to his family's financial problems. He returned to Japan to fulfill his parents' wishes, and then he resigned from his job after 6 months and remained withdrawn for 3 years. These elements suggest a potential repetition of failure and a masochistic position. Although many unknown socially constructed possibilities could explain his withdrawal, some elements indicate repetitive failure: failing to enter the Japanese society after completing his bachelor's program, failing to continue his doctoral course, resigning from his first job, and then failing to write his Ph.D. thesis. The symptom of repetitive failure hides the position of Mr. Arai as a subject and could be a window to his mode of enjoyment (*jouissance*). Although the complexity of the motivations behind Mr. Arai's actions and his desires merits further investigation, his case clearly refutes the supposed "absence of subjectivity" of the Japanese, which has long been the rhetoric of essentialist discourses (Befu 2001). It is also congruent with Lacan's ideas of the Japanese as mentioned in *Autres Écrits* ("*Le sujet est divisé comme partout par le langage,*" Lacan 2001: 19). Mr. Arai's case is even more interesting because it shows the intersection of money, partnership, and identity, which are three key notions in psychoanalysis, from Lacan's return to Freud to graphs of desire and Borromean topology.

Supplementary interviews would be necessary but we might already notice these emerging questions are not related to *hikikomori* in itself. They are more widely connected to subjectivity in contemporary Japan, a topic I will now discuss in detail.

Discussion

> One of the main difficulties for those of us who do recognize the effects of the social is how to account for the effects of the social without succumbing to the reductionism of social determinism, and how to account for the idiosyncrasies of human subjectivity without removing subjectivity from its social and historical context.
>
> *(Layton 2008: 66)*

Will hikikomori people survive?

Let us go back to Ueyama Kazuki's point of view because he was one of the first members of the *tōjisha* group with Mr. Maruyama and Katsuyama, and Ms. Hayashi. Ueyama Kazuki knows Mr. Yamamoto and his parents' associations but they do not share the same point of view. According to Mr. Ueyama, social movements developed at the end of the 1980s, where parents claimed that school refusal is not an illness and that one should not force a child to go to school. According to him, those parents of the 1980s and the 1990s who, with their children, "refused school," are not those of the 2000s and the 2010s. Among those of *KHJ*, as we saw with Mr. Yamamoto, to consider *hikikomori* as an illness is popular. That is opposed to citizen movements where the motto was "school refusal is not an illness." Consequently, it is one of two things: whether the parents who had school refusal in the 1980s and 1990s are different from contemporary *hikikomori* individuals' parents, as Mr. Ueyama would tend to think, or we are dealing with the same parents, but they changed their mind. In this sense, many parents of students in school withdrawal who were fighting for values would have become parents of children older than age 30 in the 2000s, and older than age 40 in the 2010s: In their situation, framing *hikikomori* as an illness would make them receive compensation from social welfare, or social insurance. Struggles to make *hikikomori* recognized as an illness and a disability is consistent with social movements which claimed that school refusal was not an illness.

In fact, the promotion of *hikikomori* as a social anxiety disorder is well summed up by Mr. Ueyama: If selective serotonin reuptake inhibitors (SSRI) are efficient for social anxiety disorder, and if they are efficient for *hikikomori*, then *hikikomori* could be considered as an illness, and we should consider the people concerned as disabled (with associated compensations). A major problem exists with this reasoning: If SSRI were efficient with *hikikomori*, would not they stop being *hikikomori*? This aporia might also be identified in the case of depression and provokes a supplementary question: If antidepressants are really effective, how can we explain that, since they have appeared on the market, the number of depressed people has not stopped growing?

What preoccupies *hikikomori* individuals' parents in Japan is, above all, a reality: What will become of my child when I am dead? Will he be able to get by without me? This reality is quite concrete, it is material, it is economic, and concerns the financial situation of precarious individuals. But this is not the only concern. Even if parents are wealthy, discrimination ensures that they often have difficulties in finding a care facility for their child, even while they are alive. Considering this, they are rightfully preoccupied with their child's future after their death. The parent's association is not very popular among *hikikomori* individuals who do not want to be considered as ill or disabled. However, confronted by economic precariousness and aging, there is also a movement toward resignation among many *hikikomori*. Fundamentally, questions arising among parents of a *hikikomori* child are shared by many parents whose child is not autonomous. Even though they would be recognized as disabled and would receive sufficient compensation, their life expectancy is lower (Thomas and Barnes 2010), and we do not know clearly what the future holds for disabled and nonautonomous people after their parents' deaths. Is financial assistance enough? For *hikikomori* people, a basic demand would be to receive the minimum they need to have a home and eat. In other words: survive. Yet for that, they are pushed to make their hardships recognized in terms of illness or disability. They are trapped in a situation where they cannot work nor escape isolation through a life outside of work.

Postmodern social renouncers and social change

Recently, *hikikomori* has been interpreted as a modern social renouncer, or a Japanese version of the "Bartleby syndrome," (Fansten 2013), which raises an important question: Does this modern social renouncer called Bartleby fit with a concrete sample of Japanese subjects who have experienced *hikikomori*? In light of my investigations and the existing literature, I would rather define *hikikomori* as a postmodern social renouncer trapped in both the neoliberal matrix – the invasion of references to money in every sphere of individuals' lives (for an example of this, consider the account of Mr. Arai) – and the dominant Japanese identity discourse. As I have shown, according to Japanese normative fictions, such an individual is out of society (*shakai*) but cannot escape the world (*seken*). In a different area, Indian social renouncers were conceived by Dumont (1966, 1983) as individuals "out of the world" (in French, *individu-hors-du-monde*). Japanese postmodern social renouncers are in the world (*seken*), but out of society (*shakai*). The "traditional" social renouncers in India that Louis Dumont described should be clearly distinguished from the postmodern social renouncers known as *hikikomori* in Japan. This distinction also suggests that modern forms of social renouncing could be found during the Japanese modern period (namely, Meiji, Taishō, and Shōwa), or that social renouncers have never been modern. Here, a brief contextualization is necessary.

Shortly after the fall of the Berlin Wall (1989) and while Russia, India, and China were adopting a capitalist market economy, Japan was hit by what has become a widely discussed phenomenon: an economic bubble collapse (1991). Ever since, Japan has experienced increased rates of unemployment in the context of a persistently declining birthrate, dropping marriage rates, and aging population. In addition to these subjects of preoccupation, the number of shut-ins has also increased (696,000 *hikikomori* by 2010). Records also show a growth in the number of part-time workers (*furītā*); depressed people, including those with overwork depression (Kitanaka 2012); and individuals without employment, education, or training (known as "NEET" or "*nīto*").

Rather than reducing these statistics to aspects of the rhetoric of Japanese identity discourse (Befu 2001), these symptoms of major historical and socio-anthropological changes can be understood as elements at the end of metanarratives – an important characteristic of our postmodern condition (Lyotard 1979) – or be conceived as features of paradigm shifts in autonomy (Ehrenberg 2010, Castel 2012). The bursting of the bubble and the beginning of the Heisei period (1989–2019) ushered in the postmodern era in Japan. The dramatic increase of *hikikomori* could be viewed as a symptom of postmodern Japan, and the persons concerned, who experienced social withdrawal, could be considered as postmodern social renouncers. Should *hikikomori* be considered a post-humanist form of subjectivity, or what comes after the subject? Further, is *hikikomori* illustrative of a subjectivity that comes after the subject? These questions align with the recurrent inquiry into subjectivity (Balibar 1989, Callus and Herbrechter 2012), and the answers remain open. However, the answer to another question might already exist: Does *hikikomori* subjectivity promote social and political change?

In my opinion, *hikikomori* holds strong potential for producing social change. This potential may not necessarily reside with the person concerned but may reside with parents, family, friends, caregivers, teachers, researchers, and journalists, all of whom can contribute to address an issue that cannot be reduced to individual failures. The shut-in becomes a "person concerned" (*tōjisha*), whose distress and social identity fits into a wider arena of concern for grassroots activism and social movements. A way for postmodern social renouncers to politicize their distress is to transform into a "person concerned." In this sense, the Japanese advocacy for the "sovereignty of the person concerned" (Nakanishi and Ueno 2003) could be thought of as an equivalent of the French Lacanian claim of the "sovereignty of the singular subject." It is a similarity worthy of further investigation because it could foster reflections in the intersection of Japanese social movements, Lacanian inquiry, and interdisciplinary research into subjectivity (Berman and Rizzo 2019). However, those who choose the aforementioned paths of activism and reflexivity (i.e., attend support groups such as *kangaerukai*) are a minority. The majority of those who experience or have experienced social withdrawal have not used youth culture as a way of resisting the dominant identity discourse. Rather, their condition might be understood as a form of passive resistance to social pressure that fails to become politicized or subjectivized. Only those who participate in certain NPO activities can contribute to social change; those who are hospitalized in psychiatric clinics become trapped in medicalization.

Idioms of distress and subjectivity

Despite the social expectation of uniformity among individuals experiencing *hikikomori*, there is a great diversity in the contemporary situations of these individuals. That is, the diversity of *hikikomori* subjectivities has greatly surprised me while also making it difficult to establish the typical features of *hikikomori*. This is not only because this is a hidden population that is difficult to meet, but also because psychiatrists create fictive cases that are supposed to describe *hikikomori* cases, but that can describe non-*hikikomori* individuals with the same typical features as well (Kato et al. 2012). Should *hikikomori* subjects be seen as never-ending adolescents? As Internet addicts? As old sons? As shy? Many non-*hikikomori* cases do share similar characteristics, and until now, a significant difference from the control population has not been proved. *Hikikomori* is a significant social problem in Japan, and there is a wide diversity of individuals who experience withdrawal at some point in their lives. Being out of society may be thought of as a choice or a rejection by many individuals from many different social classes in many different situations. However, when I questioned *hikikomori* individuals during my fieldwork, many of them did not recognize it as a choice and responded that they had found themselves in this situation without actually choosing it.

From an anthropological perspective, *hikikomori* should not be reduced to a mental disorder; rather, it should be seen as an idiom of distress (Nichter 1981, Tajan 2015b). What exactly is an idiom of distress? How does it differ from a mental disorder or a syndrome? In short, when I have an acute difficulty, I express my distress through idioms that signal it to others and make them recognize my distress. The number of idioms is limited: I can present myself as addicted, depressed, traumatized, or socially withdrawn, or I can somatize. Using these idioms is the first step that I can take to gain recognition for my suffering. After I receive treatment from a caregiver or a doctor, it may be discovered that beyond social withdrawal (an idiom of distress), I have schizophrenia (a mental disorder): In this case, social withdrawal is not only an idiom of distress but also a symptom of a mental disorder. In other cases, social withdrawal is the idiom of distress that hides severe personal issues and a problematic mode of enjoyment (the subject suffers from it) without a mental disorder. Although the APA cultural psychiatrists and I differ in our approaches, the recent advances of the former also clearly differentiate "idiom" from "syndrome" (APA 2016).

Also, *hikikomori* could possibly be thought of as, like French sociologist Alain Ehrenberg would say, "a socially regulated expression of complaint" (2010). As we see in their narratives, these subjects have encountered personal difficulties, anxieties, and distress during their period of social withdrawal, but one should be very careful before pathologizing and essentializing the complexity of their hardships. They share the same idiom of distress (social withdrawal) and experiences (school absenteeism, being bullied, dropping out), but they report multiple ways of positioning as a subject. In order to investigate the subtle ways one uses to position as a subject, a Lacanian approach is an interesting tool. In academic research, the Lacanian theory of subjectivity remains underutilized (Hook and Neill 2008: 247), and when it comes to studies taking Japan as an object of investigation, notable exceptions such as studies by Miller et al. (1988), Parker (2008), and Tsuiki (2006, 2013) strongly confirm this view. From a Lacanian psychoanalytical perspective, *hikikomori* could possibly be thought of as a "position subjective de l'être," which blends "knowledge," being, and sex (*le savoir, l'être, le sexe*), as described in Lacan's 12th seminar, entitled "Crucial problems for psychoanalysis." Some consider social withdrawal as an empowerment (Yoneyama 2000: 77), or a reflexive process (Murasawa 2012), and I prefer to see it as a modality where one can recognize him/herself as a subject (*subjectivation*, that is, the process of becoming a subject). In other words, *hikikomori* can be seen as a step toward subjectivity, which cannot be experienced in the educational or social setting. It goes without saying that there are also cases where social withdrawal is coupled with major mental disorders:

These individuals need community support and medical help, and *hikikomori* might not be, in these cases, a process or experience where these individuals recognize themselves as subjects.

Abandonment, enjoyment, and conspicuous absence

Overall, there seems to be no desire for social withdrawal, but an idiom shared by many individuals whose mode of enjoyment needs to be investigated on a case by case basis. This enjoyment of withdrawal is probably related to different kinds of abandonment occurring during adolescence and young adulthood. In fact, although great support is made available to Japanese junior high school absentees, recent research shows that high school dropouts are abandoned by society (Tajan 2015a). Also, it is during the ages of high school attendance that student dropouts start becoming shut-ins or develop major psychopathologies. (In Japan, there is a poor continuity of counseling services between junior high school and high school, and counseling services are weak at the high school level because it is beyond the compulsory level of education.)

This societal abandonment of dropouts challenges the popular perception of Japanese society by showing that social pressure is low for certain portions of the population (e.g., high school dropouts), and this could also apply to individuals who become social renouncers. In other words, not only is there withdrawal from society because of tremendous social pressure, the opposite might also be true: At some point in their life, *hikikomori* subjects have been abandoned from the outside (e.g., high school teachers) and from the inside (e.g., their parents). In this case, becoming a shut-in is a child's reaction to a concrete feeling of abandonment from others (i.e., parents, friends, teachers).

For instance, artist Watanabe Atsushi, who has a 3-year *hikikomori* experience, describes his physical isolation as a mental suicide, a social death, and the loss of his place in society. "It was due to my feeling as if I had lost my place in the world, along with the many wounds left by ten years of depression, my fiancée's betrayal, worries about my future as a young artist, and my rejection by social movements I had been a part of (...) My mother did not intervene, and my father saw me as a nuisance to be removed, and to that end began planning to have me committed to a mental hospital." (Watanabe 2020: 6). He was living with his parents who rarely knocked at his door and, at some point, he broke the door of his room. "I got angry with my mother who stopped intervening, I went out of my room in which I had been housebound for a few months, and kicked the door. I shouted to my mother: This is the way to open the door!," he wrote (atsushi-watanabe.jp). More precisely, he explains in his book: "Once, I think around three months into my time as a *hikikomori*, my mother told me from the other side of the door that she wanted to help. But after that, several months passed without so much as a knock. I quickly grew enraged, less at the reasons that had made me a *hikikomori* to begin with, and more towards the circumstances that had left me feeling as if my mother had abandoned me." (Watanabe 2020: 51). Then he realized his mother had been paralyzed with constant concern about how to approach him, and he wanted to "protect" her (Watanabe 2020: 6). In other words, Watanabe Atsushi had conflicts with his father and felt "abandoned" by his mother, about which he reacted violently, leading to a creative outcome: The readers can see the door in the frontispiece of this book.

When doing field interviews, one of those who survived the *hikikomori* experience (Mr. Ueyama) told me: "At that time, if I had not had a home, I would have committed suicide or become homeless." The image that arises of a person being "homeless at home" illustrates the severity of the subjective abandonment. Mr. Ueyama is not alone in this case because "being homeless" is also a concern raised by Itoh Kohki and the father of Misaki as we will see in the next chapter. Also, it is important here to distinguish *hikikomori* from hoarding disorder (popularly known in Japan as *gomi yashiki*): The two do not necessarily overlap.

Simultaneously, the *hikikomori* phenomenon is also a passive resistance to the intense pressure that exists when one transitions from school to the workforce and wage labor. During young adulthood (after several years of withdrawal), supporters of NPO activities and parents' associations do their best, but that has not yet been enough to significantly decrease the number of shut-ins. Many of them still cannot find the support they need; most do not consult psychiatrists, and only some of them attend NPO activities dedicated to occupational integration. However, finding a job is not a major preoccupation for many *hikikomori* individuals. Many do not directly refuse to enter work and society. Rather, they find themselves in a specific moment of their life in which, while they are not disabled or mentally ill, they nonetheless simply cannot enter the workforce. I maintain that a "desire" for long-term social withdrawal is rare. Although a "desire" would represent significant progress for most *hikikomori*, what leads an individual to become a social renouncer might not reach the status of a desire or a decision. For some of these individuals, their situation might be so sad that they cannot recognize their social withdrawal as a desire or a decision they made. In other words, the withdrawal is not subjectivized at all. For others, I maintain that withdrawal would be a step toward subjectivity.

In all cases, social withdrawal feeds a particular type of *jouissance* that has been increasingly displayed over the past decades. In this respect, Horiguchi Sachiko is right when she describes "how *hikikomori* caught the public eye" (2012). I would add that during my fieldwork investigations, I noticed that distressed individuals who make themselves "visible" (i.e., those who are involved in social assistance and welfare) are located in districts where there is a large proportion of poor citizens and ethnic minorities. While one can, of course, find *hikikomori* individuals in the middle and upper classes, the social status of their families and the lack of community support make them "invisible." This phenomenon is even worse in the case of a "double *hikikomori*": a shut-in that is hidden by his or her family. Members of middle-class families – belonging to the most visible social class in Japan – sometimes make invisible those among them who are distressed, especially when distressed individuals exclude themselves from a value that unites all others: labor.

Qualitative and transcultural investigations about socially withdrawn emerging adults

All researchers have made an important observation: The majority of *hikikomori* subjects drop out of or stop attending school. Of course, this does not mean that all individuals who skip school and/or drop out become *hikikomori*. The important question is as follows: Among the population who skip school or drop out, why do only some become *hikikomori*, while others do not? One of the limits of this study is that it cannot answer this question. This is a fundamental question for providing solutions for Japanese *hikikomori* youth and their families. All previous studies, despite their quality, have not answered this fundamental question. In my opinion, it is necessary to make a radical shift into qualitative research in order to focus on the experiences of the socially withdrawn, using a rigorous methodology that can take into account their subjectivities. In other words, I suggest that a qualitative approach focusing on narratives is implemented, using a validated methodological tool, such as the McGill Illness Narrative Interview (Groleau, Young, and Kirmayer 2006). This questionnaire has been recently translated into Japanese and is suitable for an investigation of illnesses, mental disorders, and idioms of distress such as *hikikomori*. I suggest that this investigation compares two populations in Japan: those who experienced school nonattendance and did not become *hikikomori* and those who experienced school nonattendance and did become *hikikomori*. An urgent need exists for qualitative investigations, and I feel that the relationship between school nonattendance (*futōkō*) and *hikikomori* should be given further attention in future research. Using the MINI would allow us to improve our knowledge about the initial narrative, the prototype narrative, the explanatory model narrative, the services and response to treatment, and the impact on life.

Despite the criticisms I made about the DSM-5®, the Cultural Formulation Interview (CFI) could be implemented with socially withdrawn individuals and their parents (CFI – *informant version*) in order to better understand the cultural definition of the problem; the cultural perception of cause, context, and support; cultural factors affecting self-coping and past help-seeking; and cultural factors affecting current help-seeking (APA 2013: 884–891; APA 2016). These two questionnaires are great achievements in the field of transcultural psychiatry and they are underused in qualitative research.

In Japan, the two distinctive features of mental health problems in emerging adults are suicide and acute social withdrawal (Arnett, Žukauskienė, and Sugimura 2014: 574). It is striking to see that the preoccupations about social withdrawal in Japan started at the same time (Saitō 1998, 2013) when Arnett published his first articles on emerging adulthood. It is now recognized that *hikikomori* affects between 541,000 and 696,000 individuals between 15 and 39 years old (Cabinet Office 2010, 2016). In Japan, those described as *hikikomori* are not "withdrawn adolescents" (Fansten et al. 2014). Although the first signs are detected during high school or junior high school, *hikikomori* phenomenon concerns mainly adults. In fact, according to an epidemiological survey (MHLW, 2010), 99% are older than 20, and 38% mark the onset of their *hikikomori* between 16 and 20 years of age. More recent estimations (Cabinet Office 2016) confirm that *hikikomori* people are not mainly adolescents because only 10.2% of them are less than 20. And yet, over the life course, childhood and adolescence appear to be an important stage for *hikikomori*. A quarter of them are school or university dropouts, and 30.6% report the onset of their withdrawal between 15 and 19. These results (MHLW, 2010, Cabinet Office 2016) should be put in perspective with the abandonment of high school dropouts described in Chapter 2.

Reflections should consider the concept of emerging adulthood, which is another aspect I will now introduce. In fact, another aim of this book is to show that emerging adults, who are neither adolescents nor adults, do exist. We face a hidden population that is quite difficult to investigate and support. Emerging adults who are not in employment, education, or training (NEET) are observed in East Asian countries and throughout the West. However, a widely held belief is that those between 18 and 25 years of age are making their way into existence, and that this period of moratorium does not need support by the state. In this sense, the Japanese situation might be quite similar to what is observed in the United States: It is actually difficult to distinguish between those "who are having normal identity struggles that will eventually be resolved by around 30 years of age and those who have more serious difficulties that are likely to hamper their functioning well into adult life" (Arnett, Žukauskienė, and Sugimura 2014: 570–571).

Behind the increasing number of Japanese distressed emerging adults is a lack of recognition for emerging adulthood as a specific life stage. However, counterarguments, such as those of Arnett (2015), are highly convincing and still need to be spread internationally. Industrialized countries have shifted from a manufacturer-based economy to a knowledge economy: worldwide, scientific, and technological discoveries constantly erupt, and it takes longer for individuals to integrate them. It takes longer for individuals to prepare themselves for the workplace, to commit themselves to a love partner, to have their first child and to marry, to get a long-term job, etc. In other words, the transition to adulthood has shifted from age 20 to 30, and Arnett proposes five features for emerging adulthood in the

United States: identity exploration, instability, self-focus, feeling in between, possibilities, and optimism (Arnett, Žukauskienė, and Sugimura 2014: 571–572). Moreover, this new life stage also has mental health implications in Europe where "unemployment has been associated with increased risk of depression, especially for emerging adults who do not have strong parental support" (Arnett, Žukauskienė, and Sugimura 2014: 572).

Other aspects of the phenomenon could also be investigated. An interesting focus could be on the peculiarities of consultations with medical doctors, psychiatrists, and their representations in Japanese society (Lock 1995, Kitanaka 2012). In fact, as I have shown, these narratives have been gathered in NPOs, which play an important role in supporting the *hikikomori* population and their families, who only consult psychiatrists when there is a major mental disorder.

An important issue that should also be addressed is the aging of the *hikikomori* population and their difficulties in finding a place in society (and a job) after their *hikikomori* experience. This theme, of the aging of the *hikikomori* population, could be connected to the issue of the aging of the general population. A focus on the role of education and the changing society in Japan could also help us deepen our perspectives; they could be summed up as follows: What does *hikikomori* say about the evolution of Japanese society? What does *hikikomori* say about "being a subject" in contemporary globalized societies? Does the Japanese epidemic of social withdrawal perfectly fit the neoliberal matrix, or does it nurture new alternative forms of living together? Like every society, Japanese society, through its educational system and social pressures, produces wounded subjectivities. But the notable specific here is that the condition of social withdrawal affects more than half a million individuals, a huge population compared to other countries.

Conclusions

Japanese postmodern social renouncers are in the world (*seken*), but out of society (*shakai*). From an anthropological perspective, *hikikomori* should not be reduced to a mental disorder but should be seen as an idiom of distress. From a sociological perspective, it is a socially regulated expression of complaint. From a psychoanalytical perspective, it could be considered as a modality where one can recognize him/herself as a subject, a position subjective, or a mode of *jouissance*. Although the behavior (social withdrawal) is the same, the causes of this behavior cannot be generalized, making it difficult to treat. Overall, *hikikomori* phenomenon is not a socially acceptable situation, but it is socially validated as an expression of distress. Simultaneously, it could be seen as a child's reaction to a concrete feeling of abandonment from others and as a form of passive resistance when confronted with the high pressures of the school-to-work transition. If *hikikomori* is coupled and understood within the context of other issues related to the "aging society" (e.g., declining birthrate, sexless couples, and NEET), the fact of not participating in society and reproductive behaviors could be considered as a passive and very "successful" way of disrupting social order in the long term.

The research intends to significantly contribute toward suggesting directions for further investigations by shedding new light on the mass production of social renouncers in postmodern Japan. *Hikikomori* phenomenon, far from being homogeneous, begins to appear as it really is: the history of a myriad of singular subjects who, despite themselves, draw attention to their absence while making social renunciation an idiom that is deeply subjective and eminently social.

References

American Psychiatric Association. 2013. *Diagnostic and Statistical Manual of Mental Disorders, 5th Edition: DSM-5 [Paperback].* Washington DC: American Psychiatric Publishing.
———. 2016. *DSM-5 Handbook on the Cultural Formulation Interview*, edited by Roberto Lewis-Fernandez et al. [Paperback]. Washington, DC: American Psychiatric Publishing.
Arnett, Jeffrey, Rita Žukauskienė, and Kazumi Sugimura. 2014. "The New Life Stage of Emerging Adulthood at Ages 18–29 Years: Implications for Mental Health." *Lancet Psychiatry* 2014 (1): 569–576
Arnett, Jeffrey. 2015. *Emerging Adulthood: The Winding Road from the Late Teens Through the Twenties* (2nd ed.). New York: Oxford University Press.
Borovoy, Amy. 2008. "Japan's Hidden Youths: Mainstreaming the Emotionally Distressed in Japan." *Culture, Medicine and Psychiatry* 32: 52–56.
Balibar, Etienne. 1989. "Citoyen Sujet. Réponse à la question de Jean-Luc Nancy: Qui vient après le sujet ?" *Cahiers Confrontation* 20: 23–47.
Befu, Harumi. 2001. *Hegemony of Homogeneity: An Anthropological Analysis of Nihonjinron.* Melbourne: Trans Pacific Press.
Berman, Naomi and Flavio Rizzo. 2019. "Unlocking *Hikikomori*: An Interdisciplinary Approach." *Journal of Youth Studies* 22 (6): 791–806.
Brinton, Mary C. 2011. *Lost in Transition: Youth, Work, and Instability in Postindustrial Japan.* New York: Cambridge University Press.
Cabinet Office of the Government of Japan (Director-General for Policy on Cohesive Society) 内閣府政策統括官 (共生社会政策担当). 2010. *Wakamono no ishiki ni kansuru chōsa – Hikikomori ni kansuru jittai chōsa* 若者の意識に関する調査・ひきこもりに関する実態調査 (Survey on Youth Consciousness – Survey on *Hikikomori*). https://www8.cao.go.jp/youth/kenkyu/hikikomori/pdf_gaiyo_index.html
———. 2016. *Wakamono no seikatsu ni kansuru chōsa hōkokusho* 若者の生活に関する調査 報告書 (Research Survey on Youth's life). https://www8.cao.go.jp/youth/kenkyu/hikikomori/h27/pdf-index.html
Callus, Ivan, and Stefan Herbrechter. 2012. "Introduction: Posthumanist Subjectivities, or, Coming after the Subject". *Subjectivity* (Special issue: Posthumanist subjectivities) 5: 241–264.
Castel, Pierre-Henri. 2012. *La Fin des coupables, suivi de Le Cas Paramord. vol. II: Obsessions et contrainte intérieure, de la psychanalyse aux neurosciences.* Paris: Ithaque (Collection Philosophie, Anthropologie, Psychologie).

Choi, Tae Young, and Young Sik Lee. 2012. "Home Visitation Program for Managing Korean Hikikomori." In The 108th Annual Meeting of the Japanese Society of Psychiatry and Neurology.

Dumont, Louis. 1966. *Homo hierarchicus. Essai sur le système des castes*. Paris: Gallimard.

———. 1983. *Essai sur l'individualisme*. Paris: Le Seuil.

Ehrenberg, Alain. 2010. *La Société du malaise. Le mental et le social*. Paris: Odile Jacob.

Fansten, Maia. 2013. "Se retirer dans une société de communication – l'exemple du hikikomori." In *L'incommunication*, edited by S. Lepastier, 71–88. Paris: CNRS éditions, Essentiel Hermès.

Fansten Maia, Cristina Figueiredo, Natacha Vellut, Nancy Pionnié-Dax, et al. 2014. *Hikikomori, ces adolescents en retrait*. Paris: Armand Colin.

Furuhashi, Tadaaki, Hitoshi Tsuda, and Toyoaki Ogawa. 2013. "État des lieux, points communs et différences entre des jeunes adultes retirants sociaux en France et au Japon (Hikikomori)." *L'Évolution Psychiatrique* 78 (2): 249–266.

Goodman, Roger. 2012. "From Pitiful to Privileged? The Fifty-Year Story of the Changing Perception and Status of Japan's Returnee Children (kikokushijo)" In A Sociology of Japanese Youth, From Returnees to Neet. Edited by Roger Goodman, Yuki Imoto, and Tuukka Toivonen. Oxon: Routledge.

Groleau, Danielle, Allan Young, and Laurence J. Kirmayer. 2006. "The McGill Illness Narrative Interview (MINI): An Interview Schedule to Elicit Meanings and Modes of Reasoning Related to Illness Experience." *Transcultural Psychiatry* 43 (4): 671–691.

Hook, Derek, and Calum Neill. 2008. "Perspectives on 'Lacanian Subjectivities'." *Subjectivity* 24: 247–255.

Horiguchi, Sachiko. 2012. "Hikikomori: How Private Isolation Caught the Public Eye." In *A Sociology of Japanese Youth, From Returnees to Neet*. Edited by Roger Goodman, Yuki Imoto, and Tuukka Toivonen. Oxon: Routledge.

Jones, Maggie. 2006. "Shutting Themselves in." *New York Times*. January 15, 2006.

Kaneko, Sachiko. 2006. "Japan's 'Socially Withdrawn Youths' and Time Constraints in Japanese Society: Management and Conceptualization of Time in a Support Group for Hikikomori." *Time & Society* 15 (2/3): 233–249.

Kato, Takahiro, Masaru Tateno, Takaoka Shinfuku, Daisuke Fujisawa, Alan R. Teo, Norman Sartorius, Tsuyoshi Akiyama, and Ishida Tetsuya. 2012. "Does the Hikikomori Syndrome of Social Withdrawal Exist Outside Japan? A Preliminary International Investigation." *Social Psychiatry and Psychiatric Epidemiology* 47 (7): 1061–1075.

Katsuyama, Minoru 勝山実. 2001. *Hikikomori karendā* ひきこもりカレンダー (Hikikomori Calendar). Bunshun nesuko.

———. 2011. *Anshin hikikomori raifu* 安心ひきこもりライフ (Living hikikomori in peace). Oota shuppan.

Kikuchi, Tatehiko 菊池健彦. 2011. *Ingurisshu monsutā no saikyō eigo jutsu* イングリッシュ・モンスターの最強英語術 (The English Monster). Tōkyō: 集英社 Shueisha.

Kitanaka, Junko. 2012. *Depression in Japan, Psychiatric Cures for a Society in Distress*. Princeton, NJ: Princeton University Press.

Kobayashi, Yoshiki. 2008. "La psychanalyse appliquée aux Japonais". *Mémoire de master en psychanalyse*. Paris: Université Paris VIII.

Kremer, William, and Claudia Hammond. 2013. "Hikikomori: Why Are so Many Japanese Men Refusing to Leave Their Rooms?" *BBC News Magazine.* http://www.bbc.co.uk/news/magazine-23182523.

Lacan, Jacques. 2001. *Autres Écrits,* 497–499. Paris: Seuil.

Lee, Young Sik, Jae Young Lee, Tae Young Choi, and Jin Tae Choi. 2013. "Home Visitation Program for Detecting, Evaluating and Treating Socially Withdrawn Youth in Korea." *Psychiatry and Clinical Neurosciences* 67 (4): 193–202.

Letendre, Gerald K. 1995. "Disruption and Reconnection: Counseling Young Adolescents in Japanese Schools." *Educational Policy* 9 (2): 169–184.

Lock, Margaret. 1995. *Encounters with Aging. Mythologies of Menopause in Japan and North America.* Berkeley, CA: University of California Press.

Lyotard, Jean-François. 1979. *La Condition postmoderne. Rapport sur le savoir.* Paris: Éditions de Minuit.

Miller, Jacques-Alain, et al. 1988. *Lacan et la Chose japonaise.* Paris: Navarin éditeurs, diffusion Seuil.

Murasawa, Watari. 2012. "Saikiteki purosesu toshite no 'hikikomori'" 再帰的プロセスとしての「ひきこもり」 (Social withdrawal as a reflexive process). *Shinri kagaku* 33 (1): 61–74.

Nakanishi, Shōji 中西正司, and Chizuko Ueno 上野千鶴子. 2003. *Tōjisha shuken* 当事者主権 (Sovereignty of the Party Concerned). Tōkyō: Iwanami Shoten.

Nichter, Mark. 1981. "Idioms of Distress: Alternatives in the Expression of Psychosocial Distress. A Case Study from South India." *Culture, Medicine & Psychiatry* 5 (4): 379–408.

Ōtake, Tomoko. 2011a. "French Researchers Seek «Raison d'Être» of Hikikomori." *The Japan Times*, November 20, 2011.

———. 2011b. "Social Recluse Transforms Himself into 'English Monster.'" *The Japan Times*, August 21, 2011.

Parker, Ian. 2008. *Japan in Analysis. Cultures of the Unconscious.* New York: Palgrave Mac Millan.

Rees, Phil. 2002. "Hikikomori Violence." *BBC News World Edition.* October 18, 2002.

Saitō, Tamaki 斎藤環. 1998. *Shakaiteki hikikomori — owaranai shishunki* 社会的ひきこもり—終わらない思春期 (Social Hikikomori – Adolescence without End). Tōkyō: PHP Shinsho.

———. 2013. *Hikikomori: Adolescence without End.* Translated by Jeffrey Angles. Minnesota University Press.

Sakai, Motohiro, Shin.ichi Ishikawa, Hiroshi Sato, and Yuji Sakano. 2004. "Development of Hikikomori Behavior Checklist (HBCL) and Examination of Its Reliability and Validity." *Japanese Journal of Counseling Science* 37: 210–220.

Shimizu, Katsunobu. 2011. "Defining and Interpreting Absence from School: The Debate in Ministerial Discourses in Japan." *Social Science Japan Journal* 14 (2): 165–187.

Sungwon, Roh. 2012. "Hikikomori and Internet Addiction in Korea" presented at the 1st International Workshop on Internet Addiction, March 16, 2012, Yokohama.

Suwa, Mami, Kunifumi Suzuki, Koichi Hara, Hisashi Watanabe, and Toshihiko Takahashi. 2003. "Family Features in Primary Social Withdrawal among Young Adults." *Psychiatry and Clinical Neurosciences* (57): 586–594.

Tajan, Nicolas. 2014. "Le retrait social au Japon: Enquête sur le *hikikomori* et l'absentéisme scolaire (*futōkō*)." PhD diss., Toulouse University.

———2015a. "Adolescents' School Non-Attendance and the Spread of Psychological Counselling in Japan." *Asia Pacific Journal of Counselling and Psychotherapy* 6 (1/2): 58–69.

———. 2015b. "Social Withdrawal and Psychiatry: A Comprehensive Review of Hikikomori." *Neuropsychiatrie de l'Enfance et de l'Adolescence*, 63 (5): 324–331.

Tanaka, Nobuko. 2010. "Director-Actor Hideto Iwai Proves That Anything Is Possible When You Come out of Hiding." *The Japan Times*. April 16, 2010.

———. 2011. "Amon Miyamoto: Globe-Trotting Dramatist Seeks New Horizons." *The Japan Times*. June 5, 2011.

Thomas, Raji, and Michael Barnes. 2010. "Life Expectancy for People with Disabilities." *NeuroRehabilitation* 27 (2): 201–209.

Tsuiki, Kosuke 立木康介. 2006. "La psychanalyse au Japon." *Psychanalyse* 7: 69.

———. 2013. *Roshutsu seyo, to gendai bunmei wa iu :* 「 *kokoro no yami* 」 *no sōshitsu to seishin bunseki* 露出せよ、と現代文明は言う：「心の闇」の喪失と精神分析 (Expose yourself, says contemporary civilisation: absence of "darkness of the heart" and psychoanalysis). Tōkyō: Kawade shobō shinsha.

Ueyama, Kazuki 上山和樹. 2001. *"Hikikomori" datta boku kara* 「ひきこもり」だった僕から (From me, who was *hikikomori*). Tōkyō: Kōdansha.

Ueyama, Kazuki, Kosuke Tsuiki, and Nicolas Tajan. 2010. "Hikikomori nitsuite" ひきこもりについて (About *hikikomori*). Video-recorded interview.

Watanabe, Atsushi. 2020. *I'm here.* Yokohama: BankART1929

Watts, Jonathan. 2002. "Public Health Experts Concerned about 'hikikomori'." *The Lancet*: 359.

Yoneyama, Shoko. 2000. "Student Discourse on Tōkō Kyohi (School Phobia/Refusal) in Japan, Burnout or Empowerment?" *British Journal of Sociology of Education* 21 (1): 77–94.

Zielenziger, Michael. 2007. *Shutting out the Sun. How Japan Created Its Own Lost Generation*. New York: Vintage Books.

7   Beyond the *hikikomori* spectrum

How *hikikomori* phenomenon became global

Hikikomori is not limited to Japan

As seen in Chapter 3, Teo and Gaw (2010) proposed to include *hikikomori* as a Japanese culture-bound syndrome in the DSM-5 (2010). While their argument remains extremely interesting, the understanding of culture in the DSM-5 was amended; as a result, it could no longer include *hikikomori*. The ICD-11 does not include *hikikomori*, either. Indeed, the vast majority of the psychiatric community does not consider *hikikomori* as a mental disorder; they still regard it as a symptom of multiple diverse mental disorders (schizophrenia, depression, anxiety disorders, etc.). But what about the role of culture? After all, only one place in the world exists where more than one million *hikikomori* individuals live. Common sense would suggest that it cannot be unrelated to Japanese culture. This is partially true and partially false. In this section, I take into account the fact that "*hikikomori* is no longer culture bound" (Bommersbach and Millard 2019), but is "a global health problem" (Wu et al. 2019); I will examine arguments that prove how *hikikomori* is not solely related to Japanese culture.

The first argument is that we find *hikikomori* in many other countries; articles supporting this claim increased in the 2010s: these include ones from South Korea (Choi and Lee 2012, Lee et al. 2013), China (Liu, Li, and Wong 2020, Wong et al. 2019), the United States (Teo 2013), Canada (Stip et al. 2016), Australia (Kim et al. 2008), Oman (Sakamoto et al. 2005), Tunisia (Souilem et al. 2019), Spain (Garcia-Campayo et al. 2007, Ovejero et al. 2014), Brazil (Gondim et al. 2017), Nigeria (Bowker et al. 2019), Croatia (Silic et al. 2019), Finland (Husu 2016, Välimäki, Kivijärvi, and Aaltonen 2019, Haasio and Naka 2019), and city-states such as Hong Kong (Wong et al. 2015, Yuen et al. 2018) and Singapore (Bowker et al. 2019).

In Italy, a book edited by Giulia Sagliocco, a psychiatrist from Napoli, was published as early as 2011. This book was the combined effort of 14 specialists working on the topic in Japan and Italy (Sagliocco et al. 2011). In Milan, a nonprofit organization (NPO) called "*Minotauro*" supports these individuals.

In fact, the Italian *hikikomori* population was estimated to be 30,000 in 2016. More recently, Ranieri (2018) published an important contribution in the area of psychoanalytic psychotherapy for Italian *hikikomori* adults.

In Sweden, cases similar to *hikikomori*, called *hemmasittare*, are described, and *hikikomori* projects have been developed. For instance, in Uppsala, "*Hikikomori Uemå*" is a health project for young adults ages 16–25 who do not work or study, and spend most of their time at home. The organizers write in their website:

> The purpose of the project is to offer you an early support to interrupt isolation. We want to meet you in the environment that suits you best [:] at home, via social media or at our location at KFUM (YMCA). We meet every individual where they are at [,] and our work is based on your needs. Some of the things we offer are: visits at home, support when/if you need to contact government authorities, individual meetings, support in meetings, training in social activities, group activities, for example, visits at the cinema, board games, road trips. Does this sound interesting to you, or do you know a person who you think would be supported by this?

A brief overview of French hikikomori studies

While it is difficult to pronounce in French, the word "*hikikomori*" is still used. This phenomenon has been studied for a decade now, resulting in articles in major newspapers, television programs, symposia, and books.

The first article on the topic followed a symposium held in 2009, and was published in a renown psychiatric journal. The article was written by a Parisian-based psychiatrist, Marie-Jeanne Guedj-Bourdiau (2011), who saw predecessors to *hikikomori* in Europe when quoting early notions of "*claustration*" (Gayral 1953) and more recent notions of pathological withdrawal of teenagers (Jeammet 1985). Moreover, she studied 21 cases the participants of which were younger than 30 years of age, were withdrawn at home, and had received home visits from her unit. Among these 21 cases, 16 were diagnosed with a mental disorder, 4 were diagnosed as being "*hikikomori*," and 1 committed suicide before the home visit. The first interesting point here is that the author considers *hikikomori* as a diagnosis, which is consistent with the notion of primary *hikikomori* explained by one group of Japanese psychiatrists (Suwa et al. 2003). Also, the author found mental disorders among the *hikikomori* population: schizophrenia (7/16); major depression (3/16); social or school phobia (3/16); developmental disorders (1/16); OCD (1/16); persisting delusional disorder (1/16). These results have to be understood with more refined studies on the psychiatric background of *hikikomori* in Japan, such as the one conducted by Kondo et al. (2013). Among the *hikikomori* help-seeking group, they found the following diagnosis: schizophrenia (17/49); mood disorders (16/49); anxiety disorders (14/49); personality disorders (5/49); developmental disorders (3/49); and others (3/49). In 2019, symposia researchers were organized in Paris and Nagoya to commemorate the 10 years of research on *hikikomori*.

A team based in Lyon, led by psychiatrist Chauliac, published a paper in the *International Journal of Social Psychiatry* (2017). Their psychiatric outreach team, called "Psymobile," was able to reach *hikikomori* patients who were not seeking mental health care. The authors aimed to identify the clinical and socio-demographic characteristics of *hikikomori* patients referred to their unit. They carried out a retrospective study on the records of patients aged 18–34 who were referred to their unit for "withdrawal" between April 2012 and December 2015. In total, 66 patients were included in the study. They were predominantly male (80%) from large or single-parent families. About 42% had no prior contact with a mental health professional before being referred. The mean duration of withdrawal was 29 months. In total, 42% of the *hikikomori* youth used cannabis, and 73% presented disorders in their sleep–wake schedules. About 71% maintained relations with their families, and 73% went out occasionally. They were mostly diagnosed with schizophrenia (37%) or mood disorders (23%).

An important series of works on the topic comes from an interdisciplinary team of researchers: the core group was composed of Maia Fansten (sociology), Cristina Figueiredo (anthropology), Natacha Vellut (psychology), Nicolas Tajan, and others. The Japanese group members were Nagoya University professors Suzuki Kunifumi, Ogawa Toyoaki, Tsuda Hitoshi, and Furuhashi Tadaaaki along with sociologist Sachiko Horiguchi and others. Some members were interviewed by the Japan Times (Ōtake 2011), and several articles and books in Japanese and French were published (Fansten et al. 2014). Between 2009 and 2014, a series of symposia was organized in Paris and Nagoya. After 2014, some group members chose not to continue, while new members joined the effort. The main Japanese correspondent was Furuhashi Taddaaki. Later on, the French psychiatrist Guedj-Bourdiau, the French sociologists from IEHSP in Rennes, Céline Rothé and Claude Martin, the Italian colleagues Antonio Pioti and Giulia Saggliocco joined the group. The second volume of the team's work will be published as a book in French in 2021. The book will gather contributions from French and Italian social scientists and clinicians (psychiatrists, psychologists, psychotherapists) about the support of *hikikomori*. Book chapters' topics will include problems associated with transition to adulthood, the difficulty of psychiatric diagnosis, aging, school, family, social bonding, local support services, and international initiatives.

Interview with a mother and a male hikikomori in his 20s

The French first heard of the *hikikomori* phenomenon back in 2004 when France's 2nd TV channel made a short news report. There are now novels (Aubry 2010, Marcotte 2014), artistic performances (plays such as *le Grenier* or *le Refuge*), and short movies on this topic. In June 2016, a TV program was specifically dedicated to French *hikikomori*. The name of the program was *"Toute une histoire"* and the title was "Who are these young people who refuse to leave their homes?" It was the first time we could observe individuals saying they were *hikikomori* and giving accounts of it. Also, there was an account of a mother whose son was 25 years old and had been in a *hikikomori* situation for 5 years; she described a similar situation as *hikikomori* in Japan (Box 7.1). He ate alone, he was always on the computer, he did not go out, he had no friends, he slept during the day, etc. In addition, the mother described her son as a perfectionist who liked to have everything in order, like her. Describing his education, she added that he failed to graduate as a bachelor in engineering; he could not stand failure, and he did not like competition. She also mentioned another failure when he had to do an internship, along with general difficulties in confronting the adult world. The six family therapy sessions did not make much of an improvement.

A young man's account also deserves our attention:

> I started locking myself up two years ago when I left my preparatory classes. Then, I couldn't enroll in college, and beyond being unable to, I didn't want to. And I started to lock myself in. One of the hardest things to witness is 'see yourself frozen,' do nothing, and see all of your loved ones move on. (…) My days are pretty simple. I usually get up late, because sleeping also gains time on the day. So, one tries to get through daytime as quickly as possible. That's all that allows you to escape for a moment. (…) My family, they worried and after the worry it's mostly a kind of anger. Because they want one to move, to go out, then seeing that it is useless, it is detachment. And the fact that these interactions disappear with the family is because one isolated themselves, one wanted to be lonely, and in the end it went too far. One didn't become lonely but embraced loneliness.

BOX 7.1: Interview with a mother of a *hikikomori* subject

INTERVIEWER (I): How is your son doing today?
MOTHER (M): It's always the same, he's at home, and he doesn't go out.
I: How old is he today?
M: 25 years.
I: Does he not study?
M: No, he stopped.
I: Since when?
M: Since he was at home, that is to say, for 5 years.
I: And how does he spend his time?
M: He's on his computer almost all day

(Continued)

BOX 7.1: Interview with a mother of a *hikikomori* subject *(Continued)*

I: What is he doing?

M: He plays I guess. He's a grown up now, I'm no longer behind him. He plays, and he studies in his own way, because he likes to hear from the world, so he watches things.

I: How does he justify his situation?

M: Well, the outside world doesn't interest him.

I: He eats?

M: Yes (laughs).

I: Does he share meals with you?

M: No, he doesn't eat with us. He eats alone in his spare time, because he does not live at the same pace as us. Currently, I don't see him since he sleeps during the day and is on the computer at night.

I: How do you live this situation? I imagine it got on your nerves …

M: For the past two months, I have been a little calmer, because I realized that by trying to force him to do something it resulted in very bad relationships. So, I calmed down a bit, well I don't know if it will last or not, but now it is better between us.

I: You consulted specialists to try to get out of this situation.

M: Yes, exactly. Psychologists, psychiatrists, and it didn't work.

I: What is he saying?

M: He says he is happy. He says that he was not happy in life before, and that today we are leaving him alone. It is quiet …

I: How does he see his future?

M: He doesn't envision it.

I: How do you see it?

M: Now I live day by day, because otherwise it's too much suffering.

I: I imagine that you want him to take off, to be independent, to make a living …

M: Of course, like any mom. Of course.

I: Does he know you are here today?

M: I don't know, I haven't seen him for three days, we're not at the same time, but when he doesn't see me, I guess he will know that I went there. I don't know if he knew the specific day.

I: You have finally discovered the *hikikomori* phenomenon; how did you learn about this disorder?

M: I have a sister-in-law who is a pharmacist, who subscribes to a magazine, and one day she showed me where we were talking about it, and she said to me: it looks like your son.

I: I imagine there were a lot of conflicts between you; you must have been annoyed by this situation.

M: Of course, and then looking for solutions … today he tells me that he is happy, he states that he is happy. He did not say it before, he claims it is his choice.

I: Is he aware that someday he'll have to make a living?

M: He lives day by day. For him the future… he will see at the right time.

I: Do you ever plan to kick him out?

M: I thought about it. But it's not in the family tradition (laughs).

Case study of a binational *hikikomori*: Misaki and her parents

The aforementioned findings have not yet been applied to the *hikikomori* population in the context of a qualitative study with the most recent and stringent methodological tools of transcultural research. First, I used the Cultural Formulation Interview (CFI)-informant version (American Psychiatric Association, 2013, 2016, Lewis-Fernández et al. 2014), which has never been used with *hikikomori* individuals' parents. One of the objectives is to explore the suitability of this tool for this population, and assess the role played by culture. Second, I used the McGill Illness Narrative Interview (MINI) (Groleau, Young and Kirmayer 2006), with Misaki (case study). The present investigation is, above all, exploratory: it has been done as a qualitative trial, in preparation of future qualitative or mixed-methods investigations, to assess different positive and negative methodological aspects and identify problems that might occur when using MINI and CFI in a larger sample.

Themes I selected are the most salient features of *hikikomori* subjects' affective distress, including feeling depressed, anxious, and abandoned. They also include the experience of having been bullied, attention problems, communication problems, problems with friends, and risk factors such as a "freeter" (part-timer) lifestyle preference, a lack of self-competence, and unclear ambitions about the future. Those three risk factors have been identified by Uchida and Norasakkunkit (2015) who postulates a "NEET-*hikikomori* spectrum."

The case study is composed of material I gathered during three audio-recorded interviews in July and August (Box 7.2): the first with Misaki's mother (CFI: 40:00), and the second with Misaki's father (CFI: 34:00). We managed to arrange an appointment during the summer break. Misaki could not come, and I only met the parents (3:00:00 interview in total). When I came to the country they currently live in, 1 month later, I did a home visit at their daughter's apartment (2:30:00 interview in total and 1:51:00 with Misaki alone) and proceeded to the third recorded interview with Misaki

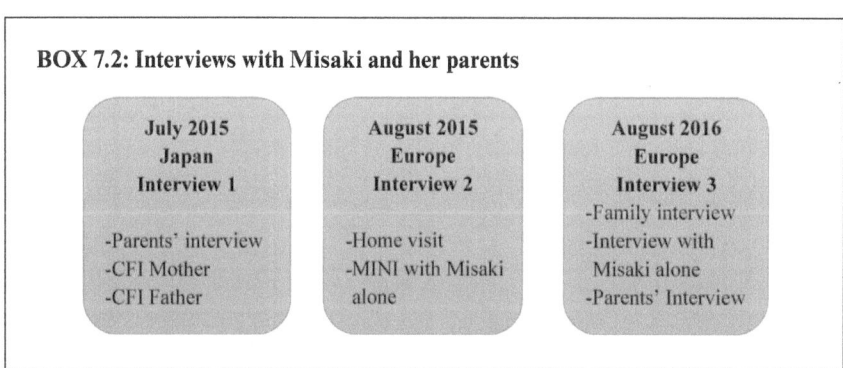

BOX 7.2: Interviews with Misaki and her parents

July 2015	August 2015	August 2016
Japan	Europe	Europe
Interview 1	Interview 2	Interview 3
		-Family interview
-Parents' interview	-Home visit	-Interview with
-CFI Mother	-MINI with Misaki	Misaki alone
-CFI Father	alone	-Parents' Interview

herself (MINI: 1:21:00). A fourth interview took place in 2016 and could not be recorded. The three of them signed a letter of consent, information about privacy and confidentiality were given, and any information that might reveal their identity has been changed to respect their privacy.

Parents' interview and cultural formulation

In February 2015, I received a message from Misaki's mother: she contacted me to ask for advice about her 18-year-old daughter who was experiencing affective distress. Misaki was 19 years old when I met her. Before being *hikikomori,* she dropped out of school (Box 7.3). At the moment of our interview, she had already met with a psychiatrist and had been hospitalized 1 year earlier in a day care hospital where she lived full time for one-and-a-half months. She was not diagnosed with a mental disorder, yet she was prescribed antidepressant medication. After the hospitalization, she went back to her parents' home, but they could not live with her, knowing that she would not do anything all day long. Consequently, they asked her to find an apartment, which she did. But after she moved, she entered into a *hikikomori* period, which lasted 9 months. That is when I met her. She has one younger brother and lives alone in her studio.

Before meeting her, I had corresponded with her mother and had met her parents. I first met the parents in Japan, and interviewed them using the CFI. When I asked Misaki's mother about the cultural formulation of the problem, it was very difficult for her to describe: she confessed she was "completely lost" and did not know "how to handle it": "It's something that started during her childhood because she had no friends, she did not contact others by phone, and never saw her friends at home," she recounted. According to

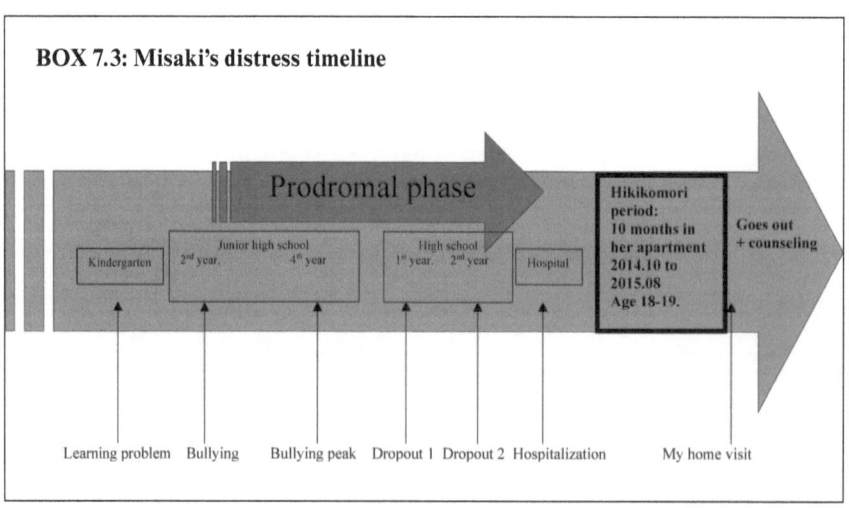

BOX 7.3: Misaki's distress timeline

Prodromal phase

Kindergarten Junior high school 2nd year. 4th year High school 1st year. 2nd year Hospital

Hikikomori period: 10 months in her apartment 2014.10 to 2015.08 Age 18-19.

Goes out + counseling

Learning problem Bullying Bullying peak Dropout 1 Dropout 2 Hospitalization My home visit

Misaki's mother, her daughter has a low self-image and thinks others think bad things about her, which is most often not the case. Misaki's mother felt she was "punishing herself" and was very worried by the fact that "she does not take care of herself" and she was "destroying herself." She described her daughter as someone who has a tendency not to be interested in others, and to not form social relationships.

When I asked about the cultural perceptions of the causes, her mother responded that she refuses to grow up, to take responsibility, and manage her life. The Japanese uncles know about the problem, yet the Japanese grandmother does not because she is old and they do not want to shock her. Misaki's father formulated that there could be a physical cause (her brain) or something that had happened during childhood or adolescence, but the psychiatrist and psychologist they saw did not diagnose any mental disorder or speak about that. He did not speak with others about the problem because he was afraid that she would lose the few social relationships she has.

Concerning the stressors and supports, both parents acknowledged that after the one-and-a-half months of hospitalization, she got better for a while. She found herself an apartment and did all the paperwork herself. Unfortunately, a new period of acute social withdrawal started, which lasted for 9 months; she was not ready to search for a job at this time.

According to Misaki's mother, cultural identity plays a role: she hoped that her daughter would have the good values of Japanese culture, such as respect for others. She noticed that Misaki was always described as shy and restrained by her teachers and she feels the same, as a Japanese, compared to non-Japanese. However, Misaki's mother did not think her culture could be a problem. On the contrary, it helps a great deal to make friends who are interested in Japanese culture and *manga*. Misaki's father thought somewhat differently because he felt culture plays a role in her daughter's problem. He recounted, for example, that she started school with linguistic problems in her second language (European language), and it was difficult to adapt to European kindergarten for her, also because it was in the countryside with few foreigners. For primary school, they moved to a big city, in a multicultural context, and it was no longer a problem.

As for the cultural factors affecting self-coping, Misaki's mother confessed that she could not analyze them, and simply did not know. She felt guilty about the situation because perhaps they pushed her too much to study, while simultaneously recounting they were not so strict. Misaki's father added that his daughter did not do anything to help herself. As for the past help-seeking, the mother tried to be positive and believe everything was useful, especially the hospital. Misaki's father shared her opinion, but he underlined that the positive effects only lasted 1 month. A major problem was quite evident for both: their daughter simply does not ask for support.

As for the cultural factors affecting help seeking, the mother would prefer home visits, while the father believed that activities through social welfare, or part-time work would be helpful. He added that work should be made of repetitive tasks and should not involve too much stress and social relationships. The father insisted that it is not only Misaki's problem, but also a family problem. Professionals should also know that it is no use waiting for the patient to ask for support since the very fact of asking is impossible for them, he insisted. He also said that his biggest trauma was to tell his daughter to leave home, and the possibility that she could become homeless.

I corresponded with her mother (July–August 2015) and was informed that Misaki agreed to a home visit. The second time I met the parents was when I did the home visit. They were here at the beginning and the end of the interview. Between, I was alone in Misaki's room with her, first simply talking with her, and then questioning her with the MINI.

Misaki: "I've always felt abandoned by my parents"

During the interview, she often cried and I had to give her a lot of tissues. She was quite distressed, and her mind seemed unclear because she often interrupted sentences. She looked fragile, weak, and obviously did not eat enough in the past month. Her handshake was quite floppy. When we look at the full interview, the most frequently reported affect is feeling abandoned: "I've always felt abandoned by my parents," she said. She expressed feeling abandoned 11 times. Then, we found communication problems, compulsive behavior, feeling depressed, problems with friends, feeling anxious (social anxiety), feeling guilty, a lack of self-confidence, being bullied, feeling bizarre, attention problems, and suicidal ideation.

When questioned about the initial narrative, she responded that, according to her, *hikikomori* started when she was in the second year of junior high school: "I felt I didn't want to belong to this world anymore." When she was in school, she was always thinking about something else like books or *manga*. She had friends, but they started to ask her why she was not saying anything: it made her uncomfortable, yet it was just that she did not have anything to say. She thought that she started to socially withdraw because she did not get along well with others. She insisted that she experienced humiliation at the end of junior high school and she reacted by escaping in books. The humiliation was caused by two boys who were always making fun of other students when going up to the whiteboard. These two boys made her a recurring target because she never answered back. Her coping strategy was to erase from her memory all the names of the people she could not stand.

She was also worried about her situation and not graduating from high school. *Hikikomori* is a problem for her because there are many things she would like to do, but she cannot because she cannot leave her apartment.

She reported feeling more secure inside. Outside, she sometimes had palpitations, difficulty breathing, or panicked – especially when someone was interrogating her. She stays at home to avoid panic, and books always helped to relieve her from these feelings of social anxiety. She added that she tried to commit suicide once when she felt she could not deal with life and her difficulties anymore. She took a knife in the kitchen, started to cut her belly, and stopped: "I was not brave enough (...) all is my fault," she said, while bursting into tears. Her parents requested hospitalization because she was not attending school anymore and because of psychological problems.

When questioned about the prototype narrative (analogical reasoning), she responded by saying that her brother is always on the computer (online games and social networks), whereas she stopped Facebook after being humiliated and bullied by other girls online.

As for the explanatory model narrative (causal reasoning), she believed that the cause of her *hikikomori* situation is that she was very sensitive, and she did not speak much. Her coping strategy was to always conceal her sensitivity by saying she did not care for others, or just put on a fake smile. Often, she did not agree, but still she did not say anything. She was afraid of speaking her own mind, and feared she might say evil things to others. She felt she had to remain friendly to others. However, at home she went "bananas," cried, and screamed, alone: it seems her parents never noticed anything, including what she reported as a suicidal attempt. She felt she was not normal, not like the others. She felt abandoned by her parents during kindergarten and at the beginning of primary school. She felt lost. This feeling has continued until the time of the interviews: "I don't know if it's me who is going away from other people, or if it's other people who are going away from me, but I have the impression that somehow it's my fault, and after that, it becomes people who go away." She felt she had always been like that, having problems expressing herself. And then she became fed up with school while simultaneously developing what she calls an "addiction for books" (reading books was a need, and she felt bad if she could not do it).

Regarding the services and response to treatment, because she spent 1 year eating alone at the canteen and felt humiliated (last year of junior high), she had counseling sessions at the end of junior high and the beginning of high school. She did not feel that the antidepressant prescribed during her hospitalization helped her at all.

As for the impact on her life, it obviously changed many things for her, including the way she perceived herself: she felt that she could not make it on her own in life, and that she would be homeless if her parents were not there.

The period after our interview and the situation's improvement

At the end of the interview with her, I was both feeling worried and at the same time optimistic: that is what I told her and her parents. I was worried because she was obviously distressed: "I'm really wound-up, and I don't know how to get by" she said. Simultaneously, she seemed conscious that she no longer wanted to remain in that situation anymore and was willing to change. She was also able to smile sometimes, which is important. I gave her the contact information of a psychologist. Spontaneously, she wrote down the name, address, and phone number and said she would contact her. After a few weeks, I asked the psychologist if she had been contacted by Misaki and, as it was not the case, I sent an email to her mother insisting that if her daughter was not able to contact the psychologist, then she might have to come with her to the consultations at the beginning. However, by the time I sent the email, Misaki had contacted the psychologist.

Misaki attended psychoanalytic counseling sessions for 4–5 months from October 2015 to March 2016. When she stopped, I was emailed by her mother. Following her email, I contacted the psychologist. For reasons of professional confidentiality, many aspects cannot be disclosed. However, the psychologist said that it was not depression, rather something that was related to her personality and her development. We shared similar hesitations about considering whether it could be the prodromal phase of a psychotic disorder, without obtaining sufficient evidence. We were both worried about what would happen to her. Replying back to her parents by email, I proposed an interview in Europe in August. I was expecting a catastrophic situation and had already contacted two psychiatrists and tried to find a therapy group. I also knew that her parents would expect a psychiatric diagnosis, and after careful elaboration, I found that avoidant personality disorder would be the most accurate diagnosis, although it is quite uncommon in the European tradition of psychiatry. During the August interview, they told me they met a Japanese psychiatrist in July, who gave the same diagnosis. Consequently, the European psychologist, the Japanese psychiatrist, and I excluded diagnoses such as schizophrenia, depression, social anxiety disorder, developmental disorder and converged on the diagnosis of avoidant personality disorder. The psychologist and I consider this diagnosis as a temporary working hypothesis. It should be noted that recent psychiatric research found that 41% of participants with a history of *hikikomori* have a co-occurring diagnosis of avoidant personality disorder (Teo et al. 2015).

Surprisingly, when I met them in August 2016, Misaki was much better, and the parents were very satisfied. I was astonished because there were many improvements. In fact, she stopped the counseling sessions because she had insight that she had to move forward and do something with her life. She feels better, and she is now involved in occupational integration in a local social center. She goes there every day at nine in the morning. She goes to the swimming pool and does athletics with her parents every week; she also went on vacation with them. The relationship with her parents might still be somewhat "too close" for an emerging adult, yet I found improvements: before it only involved rigidity, anger, and stress, and now they share something together. She still lives in her apartment and sometimes goes to dinner with them. She now has a friend she met at the social center, which might have played an important role as well. She told me that now, when someone attacks her or says something bad to her, she does not repress her feelings, but answers back, which is a significant change in her coping strategies. She also said that, before, she did not want to answer back because she was afraid of losing the relationship. With the same logic, I had to tell her that she could go back to counseling sessions when she feels the need. She did not know she could. She still relates her difficulties in communicating with others, but everybody notices it is much better. In addition, she no longer attributes her failures to others. She gained weight, which is good compared to her poor weight 1 year ago, and her handshake is far more energetic. Finally, she wants to obtain her bachelor's degree in Japan, so she is trying to find a program. That is not for now, but is a project for the future.

Discussion

The research tools I used proved to be very interesting and should be used in a larger sample. The MINI can be used by many health and mental health practitioners, social workers, and researchers during the first interview; it is very convenient when doing a home visit; it combines the collection of data and the inquiry on deep aspects of subjectivity. As for the CFI, it is useful to investigate how *hikikomori* might be related to culture. For instance, Misaki's mother hoped she had the good values of Japanese culture (respect for others), and also noted that Japanese culture helps in making friends. In this case, the relationship with culture was seen as positive and, simultaneously, difficult to gauge. Would the relationship to culture be difficult to gauge in a survey with Japanese *hikikomori* in Japan? And, further, would it make sense to interview Japanese parents, in Japan, about their distressed child, using the CFI? I believe so, due to the idea that *hikikomori*, as related to Japanese culture, is widespread: we need to assess more precisely the relationship between *hikikomori* and culture, considering that shut-ins are observed in diverse cultural areas. We also need to assess with a stringent methodology what is specific to Japan society and culture, outside of the spectrum of Japanese identity's essentialization, the old chestnut of Japanese studies.

This case cannot be reduced to avoidant personality disorder, but should be seen as avoidant personality disorder associated with *hikikomori*. We have to listen to parents' and patients' distress: they are recognizing the situation as "*hikikomori*," a word from the mother's and the daughter's culture.

In the case of Misaki, what did I do? What was efficient? I used illness narratives to foster subject formation. What I did for Misaki was to empower her and make her an agent of her own change. Also, subject formation was fostered through transference: that is, I influenced her in a way in which she would recognize herself as a subject. In Lacanian terms, I tried to temper (to help her regulate) her mode of *jouissance*, and also intervened in the network of significant others: namely, her parents. A concrete example of her mode of *jouissance* is elicited by the theme of "abandonment": "I've always felt abandoned by my parents," she said. She has been ruminating over this scenario since her childhood: She was abandoned by the others; that is part of her identity, the place she has in life, the story she tells herself. It is a commonly held belief that psychoanalysts work only from chairs behind the couch: I broke with this tradition, and, proceeding like the pioneers of psychoanalysis with the hysterics at the end of the 19th century (e.g., Breuer with Anna O.), I did a home visit, and, because we are in the 21st century, I used diverse research methods, social networks, and messaging to monitor the situation from Japan.

More generally, the theme of abandonment is important, as it is rarely reported in the literature on *hikikomori* still contaminated by the accepted idea that they are immature spoiled children hypnotized by their computers. This is clearly not the case for many of them who might experience subjective abandonment and a feeling of being homeless at home (Tajan 2015a,b,c, 2017a,b).

Recommendations

When there is a person in a *hikikomori* situation, it is crucial to consider the following. First, parents should consider acute social withdrawal as a problem. It may seem obvious, but in Japan, that is often not the case: some families hide or do not seek support; others who are searching for support are never satisfied with it. "Due to prejudice and lack of knowledge, in many cases family members cannot respond directly to individuals with this problem, are unable to intervene at all, and tend to turn a blind eye for many years without seeking help" (Kato, Kanba, and Teo 2018). Some parents are simply not looking for support for their child. They may complain, but there is a considerable amount of passivity because at the same time, they do not go to NPO activities, for instance. Money could be a problem as well for some families. That is the first thing, if it is not a problem for the parents, then caregivers and social workers cannot effectively support the patient and his or her family.

Outside Japan, parents' reaction might be to kick them out of the house (this is extremely rare in Japan). Of course, that is not the right thing to do, and would be considered by psychoanalysts as an "acting out": the risk of becoming homeless should not be underestimated. Also, one should carefully assess for the potential prodromal phase of a psychotic disorder (Stip et al. 2016).

Second, it should be a problem for the *hikikomori* person himself/herself. In the case of Misaki, she acknowledged that the situation could not last and she wanted her life to change. However, most of the time, this is not the typical response. The next thing to do would be to continue talking to the subject and try to discover what might be a problem for him or her.

Third, it is important, even for psychologists, to do home visits – in other words, to get inspiration from social work practice. You cannot help shut-ins without doing home visits in the first place. In the West, however, this is problematic since most psychologists cannot do home visits because it requires too much effort in terms of time and energy, and they have many other patients.

Fourth, it is very important to contact and respond to the parents when they need it, as I did in our correspondence. In this situation, I was not a therapist, but I monitored the situation by talking to the parents together, separately, responding to emails, talking with Misaki, introducing a psychologist, talking to the psychologist, etc., like a social worker would do. The combination of counseling sessions, my monitoring of the situation (the network built around her case), referring to some aspects of social work practice (such as home visit), and combining some tools of anthropological investigations on illness narratives proved efficient. And, of course, on Misaki and her parents' side, the will to change was essential.

Fifth, I would add that early intervention is crucial. This has already been said in many articles of Japanese scholars. The longer you wait, the more difficult it is to help. In this respect, I hope my contribution will benefit social workers and mental health practitioners who are at the forefront of these complex situations of distress.

Rethinking *hikikomori*

To come back to our initial statement, *hikikomori* is not a culture-bound syndrome or a cultural concept of distress. However, there should be a cultural component explaining the 1,154,000 *hikikomori* individuals aged 15–64 years in Japan. *Hikikomori* is partially related to culture, and explaining cultural components related to Japanese *hikikomori* is still extremely difficult. This issue should lead to further substantial research, but without taking the popular path of the essentialization of Japanese identity, which is a dead-end.

Psychiatrists are in consensus. In very simple terms, if you manage to reach *hikikomori tōjisha*, their psychiatric background is often composed of depression, anxiety, schizophrenia, and other developmental disorders. For those who are not diagnosed with a mental disorder, a minority of psychiatrists propose *hikikomori* as a mental disorder. In doing so, they transform a symptom into a pathology; we might say that the old notion of "*apragmatisme*" (found in schizophrenia, depression, and *psychasténie*) is transformed, refined, and adapted to our contemporary globalized era.

There are a myriad of singular subjects behind the *hikikomori* category. The question of whether it should be considered a spectrum must lead to some reservations. In fact, the trend of labeling mental disorders using the word "spectrum" started with schizophrenia and has more recently been extended to autism, becoming autism spectrum disorders (ASD) in 2013. However, a recently published meta-analysis showed that it has become impossible to distinguish individuals diagnosed with ASD from those who were not (Rødgaard et al. 2019). This should invite all of us to be extremely cautious when considering the reliability, validity, and overall scientific grounds of disorders or conditions described as spectrums. While the Cabinet Office reports consider *hikikomori* as a spectrum comprising the *hikikomori* group, quasi-*hikikomori* group, and *hikikomori* affinity group, it does not correspond to what I would call a "*Hikikomori* Spectrum Disorder (HSD)." In the case of *hikikomori*, it appears that with regard to the literature on the topic, it does meet cohesive and consistent criteria for being described as a spectrum in the psychiatric sense. However, *hikikomori* is a psychosocial condition, and resists medicalization.

Two exclusions

If we consider the Japanese situation, it is obvious that we face at least two extremely serious issues: (1) the exclusion of individuals with schizophrenia from the *hikikomori* group, and (2) the *hikikomori* population that does not present a mental disorder.

Although the Ministry of Health Labour and Welfare (MHLW) (2010) guideline and reports from the Cabinet Office of the Government of Japan (Director-General for Policy on Cohesive Society) (2010, 2016, 2019) should be seen as significant achievements (Tajan, Hamasaki, and Pionnié-Dax 2017), the definition of the *hikikomori* group always excludes schizophrenia. What contributes to the complexity of the phenomenon is that individuals describe themselves, and are described by others, using the term *hikikomori*; when they are met by psychiatrists, the latter can hypothesize the presence of schizophrenia. However, if you were to make a survey about homelessness, why would you exclude subjects with schizophrenia? And why are people with schizophrenia so often excluded? In my opinion, *hikikomori* is not a mental disorder: *hikikomori* is a social condition, or more precisely, a psychosocial condition. Therefore, one should not exclude individuals who have been hypothesized by psychiatrists as having mental disorders from the *hikikomori* category. I often say that *hikikomori tōjisha* are the "homeless at home." *Hikikomori*, like homelessness, is a social condition, a psychosocial condition if you prefer; in any case, it is a condition that needs psychosocial support (Tajan and Shiozawa 2020).

The fact that the *hikikomori* population is underestimated has been repeated for almost three decades by psychiatrist Saitō Tamaki. And he is right. Many *hikikomori* subjects are reluctant to see a psychiatrist. In other words, there is a hidden population that does not consult psychiatrists, and we do not know if they have a mental disorder or not. We have to recognize that there is a logical impossibility here. If you go out, you are not a representative of individuals who never go out. The very moment you enter the room of a *hikikomori tōjisha*, he stops being a representative of those whose rooms have never been entered. There are always individuals who do not allow you to enter their rooms, or go out – meaning you cannot accurately represent or identify them. This is the pure form of *hikikomori*. Perhaps it is a patient who has schizophrenia or depression, but you cannot say it definitively without meeting him or her. We have many examples of *hikikomori* subjects who do not present mental disorders. As a consequence, we should be very careful when it comes to studies conducted by psychiatrists; they might overestimate the prevalence of mental disorders among the *hikikomori* population or underestimate the *hikikomori* population that does not present a mental disorder.

Hikikomori studies are confronted with a structural impossibility: the character of "pure" *hikikomori* (*junsui hikikomori*). It embodies an inaccessible, an impossible, a real. "Pure" *hikikomori* is, by definition, one who cannot bear witness to his experience. In order for him to bear witness to this, he would still have to come out of his withdrawal: either spatially, when leaving his room, or by consenting that someone enters the room and/or by agreeing to communicate (i.e. interpersonal exchange). In either case, those who accept these conditions are no longer considered members of the category they used to represent. This is exactly what Mr. Ueyama evokes when he says: "*Hikikomori* people who really suffer cannot be filmed. So, as soon as I agree to be filmed, it is in a sense that I am no longer a *hikikomori*. It is even possible that if you look at me like that, being filmed by you, there will eventually be people who criticize me, saying 'you are no longer *hikikomori* because you are filmed like that'." (Ueyama, Tsuiki, and Tajan 2010). The category of "pure" *hikikomori* is, therefore, a logical impossibility around which possibilities organize. These possibilities are often thought of in terms of "joining society," most often via part-time professional integration, followed by full-time employment. For others, the link with the experience of social withdrawal will be maintained through recruitment in an association responsible for their assistance, or employment in a business dependent on this association. Very few, like Mr. Ueyama, are engaged in the practice of researching these questions.

I highlighted the dropout rates of high school students, but no one actually abandons young *hikikomori* adults. Some of them may feel a sense of abandonment, but their supporting networks are still present. Although shut-ins are the focal point of negative judgment from a society that values work enormously, many try to help them within the framework of the NPO. *Hikikomori* remains an often shameful situation, which reinforces the impossibility of testifying for some of them.

Overall, criticizing the exclusion of schizophrenia, and underlining the *hikikomori* population that does not present a mental disorder is underestimated, could seem awkward to some. If we include socially isolated subjects, such as people with schizophrenia or depression, women who describe themselves as doing housework help (*kaji tetsudai*) socially iso-lated individuals above 40 years, the *hikikomori* population might reach 10 million! The Ministry of Health Labor and Welfare did not implement successful policies, and the Cabinet office simply produces reports. In this respect, I wanted to mention an initiative by Kato Takahiro and Kanba Shigenobu who have established a *hikikomori* clinical research unit in a university hospital and collaborate with *hikikomori* support centers. The project is remarkable, especially when they established educational pro-grams for parents of *hikikomori* subjects taking into account that, in the vast majority of cases, parent counseling comes first. Moreover, 5-day programs for family members have been recently implemented (Kubo et al. 2020). A similar program was attempted at Nagoya University in the 2000s, but, unfortunately, could not be perpetuated. Also, some of the NPOs I have described are doing extremely valuable work, but some of them are struggling too, and hardly manage to make ends meet. They sometimes have to reduce their activities after a few years, or remain at a small scale.

> Currently there are more than 50 government-funded community support centers for *hikikomori* located throughout the prefectures of Japan, pro-viding services such as telephone consultations for family members, the creation of "meeting spaces" for affected people, and job placement sup-port. In addition, various private institutions provide treatment for *hikiko-mori* sufferers. However, there is yet to be a unified evidence-based method for these public/private interventions (Kato, Kanba, and Teo 2018).

Indeed, after more than two decades, measures implemented under the leadership and relying on the guidelines of the Japanese Ministry of Health Labor and Welfare have failed to solve issues related to *hikikomori*. Perhaps it is time to think about a Ministry of Loneliness (Pimlott 2018) that would not only provide the psychosocial support that the population desperately needs, but most of all, restore the dignity of the millions who are socially isolated.

Social class, poverty, and ethnic minorities

My inquiry into *hikikomori* unintentionally led me to address questions relating to social class, poverty, and ethnic minorities. In Japan, ethnic minorities are mainly made up of communities located in Hokkaidō (Ainu), and Okinawa, as well as *Zainichi* Koreans and discriminated communities (*burakumin*). However, Kansai, the region in which I mainly investigated, is also a place with high numbers of *burakumin* and *Zainichi* communities. The underlying reasons are historical; the presence of *burakumin* in the Kansai region is the heritage of the caste system of the feudal era, and the presence of Korean residents has its roots in the colonization of Korea. The figures provided by Sugimoto Yoshio are striking; in the Kansai region, there are 2,000,000 *burakumin* and 400,000 Korean residents (Sugimoto

2010: 192). Note that obtaining accurate data on these issues is difficult, and the previous figure is probably overestimated. Indeed, the research institute for human rights and the release of *buraku* provided data 5–6 times lower (Aoki 2009: 192). Obviously, many in a *hikikomori* situation do not belong to these discriminated or *Zainichi* communities. From this point of view, one could ask: What population is more likely to ask for support? In the H. prefecture, Dr. Matsuda's answer is clear, and is based on statistics from the guidance center: these are the populations located in places where the highest concentrations of poor, discriminated, and *Zainichi* communities are found.

However, a counterpoint to the preceding thoughts is that the request for psychological help is not only addressed through social assistance. The call for social assistance can convey the idea of stigmatization of people seeking help. According to this line of reasoning, one might think that the discriminated communities, already being stigmatized, would have less difficulty in seeking social assistance. This fact remains to be confirmed, but it seems clear, in the H. prefecture, that non-discriminated populations make less use of social assistance. *Hikikomori* and *futōkō* are obviously present in the middle and upper classes, but my investigation focused, without me having decided it beforehand, on NPOs who are in places where there is a high concentration of poor, discriminated communities, and *Zainichi*. The NPO A. is an example, and my participation in NPO M. illustrates this fact in the most significant way: to accompany them as they trace their "origins" in South Korea.

The NPO P. is located on the outskirts of a town in the G. prefecture, and its name refers to the culture of prefecture D.: the place of concentration of another ethnic minority. When I met Prof. Kubo, it was part of a university event on prefecture D.'s culture. In this conference, a speaker from an NPO presented her work, highlighting that 80% of the people in her community had at least one family member who had perished during World War II. All of this data invited us to think of testimonies and trauma as they manifest themselves in the Japanese archipelago. The accounts of *hikikomori* subjects collected in places with a high concentration of ethnic minorities and discriminated communities naturally brought to light the most salient and constitutive elements of the identity of these populations: ostracism from society (discrimination), survival situation in poverty, memory of the hardships of history, and experiences of anxiety (Aoki 2009: 191).

My investigation of the assistance systems, the testimonies of *hikikomori* subjects, and the system of assistance to youths in absenteeism from school highlights a fact: Individuals who are in distress and who become "visible" are those located in poor neighborhoods with a high concentration of ethnic minorities (discriminated communities or *Zainichi*). Socially withdrawn individuals from the Japanese middle and upper classes are, therefore, very present, but the social statuses of these families and the lack of integration into a community make them invisible. In other words, those who are socially withdrawn from the middle and upper classes are another hidden population. In my investigation, Dr. Matsuda affirms that the large traditional families of the middle and upper class of the city of H. did not reveal their family secrets (*ie no himitsu*). When there is a child with developmental disabilities, for example, they have family members who can take care of them. The hardships and secrets of middle and upper class families remain undisclosed, unlike poor nuclear families who can "open their secrets" to social assistance. Overcoming the tendency to keep problems within the family is precisely the intention of the leader of K2 International, and is the slogan of the NPO M., "open the family" (*kazoku wo hiraku*).

In other words, the upper and middle classes, that is to say, the most visible social classes to the point that it has long been considered the one and only (Satō 2000), make invisible those among them who are suffering … and all the more so, since they exclude themselves from a central value that unites all the others: work.

What work means to subjectivity and identity

When children refuse school or when adults refuse society, they refuse schoolwork and salaried work, respectively. From this point of view, do they not relay the dramatic changes experienced by previous generations? Or is it a form of resistance, a way of refusing Japanese society, as it is today? An answer to these questions is only satisfactory on a case-by-case basis. The fact that solutions for these individuals can only be found one by one is perfectly illustrated by the successive attitudes of psychiatrists whose common denominator is embarrassment. Basically, shut-ins resist them, and as some psychiatrists have told me, they do not understand why they do not want to work. At first, this was considered an exclusively Japanese phenomenon known as *taijin kyofushō*. Later, patients with retreat neurosis (*taikyaku shinkeishō*) (Kasahara 1978), or students with apathetic syndrome (*apashī shindorōmu*) (Kasahara 1984), shared with their mother the diagnosis of imbalance of the autonomic nervous system (*jiritsu shinkei shicchōshō*) (Rosenberger 1992, Lock 1986, 1995). Its contemporary figure is now the young adult experiencing social withdrawal (*shakaiteki hikikomori*). And it is the latter that most embarrasses psychiatrists: Either he has a mental disorder (*seishin shōgai*) that can be identified and he could obtain a job corresponding to his disability (*shōgai*), or he is not afflicted with any disorder and, not falling within the competence of psychiatrists, he can work. However, finding a job is not an immediate concern of an individual experiencing social withdrawal. Many do not voluntarily refuse society and work, but they find themselves at a time in their life when they are unable to do so without being disabled, handicapped, or mentally ill.

In other words, those labeled *hikikomori* are contemporary subjects confronted with intrapsychic conflicts and struggling in their subject formation – in the context of the current Japanese society. From this point of view, they find few interlocutors who can allow them to break out of their isolation. Here, I am not only targeting psychiatrists but also members of NPO: The latter, in fact, manage to rehabilitate only a third of the individuals who contact them. However, there are a large number of cases, currently unknown, who do not contact NPOs or psychiatrists. This embarrassment is, therefore, not only that of psychiatrists, but also that of the Japanese society as a whole. Given the continuing demographic decline, the Japanese need all of their youth to work. In a way, the fact that *hikikomori* individuals are not working is one more threat to the future of Japan. But on the other hand, the idea that "even if they worked, it wouldn't change the future of Japan" fuels their despair.

Another idea must be brought up: Japanese society should change to accommodate its weakest members. Policies for the professional integration of the disabled can already boast significant results (Dervelois 2011), but depressed and *hikikomori* individuals represent a new challenge. Depressed employees and *hikikomori* express distress in two ways: of exhaustion linked to either excess work or a lack of it. All the current difficulty resides in the resistance to conceive an identity where work would not occupy a central place. This is exactly what the depressed and the *hikikomori* expose. More particularly, concerning *hikikomori*, the persons concerned very often testify to the involuntary nature of their withdrawal, and at the same time, their conditions cannot be reduced to a handicap (*shōgai*). In my opinion, shut-ins represent a problem that is at the crossroads of transgenerational and subjective questions.

Beyond a central value placed on work as a constituent of identity, the testimonies I have gathered have brought to light the motive of "survival." Inspired by Michel Foucault, Giorgio Agamben proposes to grasp the specificity of biopower in the 20th century. According to him, it would be formulated as follows:

> ...no longer either *to make die* or *to make live*, but *to make survive*. The decisive activity of biopower in our time consists of the production not of life or death but rather of a mutable and virtually infinite survival [...] Biopower's supreme ambition is to produce, in a human body, the absolute separation of the living being and the speaking being, of *zoè* and *bios*, the inhuman and the human: survival (Agamben 1999: 155–156).

Ueyama (2001) mentions this type of "survival" in his autobiography and in our interview, when he talks about his fear of becoming homeless should his parents die. Then, in the context of our correspondence, he is gradually led to define *hikikomori* as a survivor: this experience of confinement at home, for him as for Iwai Hideto or Mr. Wada, is marked by significant anxieties and even suicidal ideation. Ueyama Kazuki says the longer you stay in this mindset, the harder it is to get out. In this sense, *hikikomori* and ex-*hikikomori* subjects can be considered "survivors." The motive for "survival" is also present in a quote by Maruyama Yasuhiko, who describes a "way of living like a wild animal" (*yasei dōbutsu no yō na ikikata*), fighting between life and death, not knowing if someone would take care of him if he were to die.

The motive for survival suits the theme of trauma. This is all the more visible since the concerned population has a low social status. A question then arises: How should one think of testimony, trauma, transmission, and subjectivation in East Asia and, more particularly, in Japan? To explain social withdrawal of the Japanese children, adolescents, and young adults, one should not resort to stereotypical explanations. Japanese *hikikomori* subjects are not spoiled children addicted to the internet. This representation is unsatisfactory if we wish to think of an experience lived by millions of people.

Confronting this phenomenon of social withdrawal leads the clinician to reconsider global history: the history of Japan and its social classes, but also that of Japanese–Korean relations. In this sense, I maintain that the expression "a skeleton in the closet" could be applied to *hikikomori*. Psychological theories will explain this in different ways. For systemicians, he is the "identified patient." For post-Freudian or post-Kleinian psycho-analysts, it crystallizes family secrets and unspoken family histories. For Lacanian psychoanalysts, "the child's symptom is in place to respond to what is symptomatic in the family structure." From this perspective, a *hikikomori* person embodies, like any child with regard to his parents, not only a phallus but also an object a (Note: object a is a Lacanian concept). But, like any child, he too is a subject with a desire in a position not to be the pure object of his parents' fantasy. In other words, I maintain that the *hikikomori* situation can be seen as a subjective position, the coordinates of which must be determined on a case-by-case basis that necessarily involves enjoyment (*jouissance*). In summary, social withdrawal can be explained from a transgenerational and family point of view on the one hand, and from the point of view of the *jouissance* of the person concerned (*tōjisha*), on the other hand. This must take into account historical, sociological, and anthropological determinisms (Lucken 2017, Hashimoto 2015).

To explain views held in psychoanalytic clinics in a Japanese context, one will face several difficulties. An example of resistance from the clinical and psychoanalytic points of view can be summarized by an expression: "seek the criminal" (*hannin sagashi*). Against the subtlety that I wish to point out, this thought pattern will guide the understanding of our interlocutor toward a conclusion: "it is the fault of the parent(s)," or "it is the fault of the child." In the West, this misrepresentation can also be noted, but, in Japan, it fits into a cultural particularity that the expression "seek the criminal" illustrates well.

My purpose here is to call for a different kind of assistance to the fam-ilies and the persons concerned and, more generally, for a renewal of the theory of subjectivity via the Japanese example. We must, therefore, take into account the dimension of trauma, not only by considering the Freudian discovery but also by considering the anthropological coordinates of Japan in East Asia. From this point of view, trauma is no longer only thinkable in the Viennese context of the end of the 19th century, or that of Paris in the second half of the 20th century: The insistence on an individual trauma as trauma lived by a group (ethnic minority) must be the subject of a thorough reflection. Does the reduction of individual trauma to that of the group prevent psychic elaboration? When individual trauma is not expanded to that of a community group, how do clinicians manage treatment? In other words, I raise the question of the subjectivation process and its assistance via psychiatrists, child psychiatrists, and clinical psychologists.

Twenty lessons on *hikikomori*

In this exploratory investigation, I interviewed a large number of actors who are in the field of assistance to *futōkō*, *hikikomori*, and *nīto*. I have also described the accounts of socially withdrawn subjects (Box 7.4 and Box 7.5).

Most *hikikomori* subjects have a history of absenteeism or dropping out of school either in junior high or high school **(1)**. In my investigation, I discovered an important, but little-known fact, namely, a vastly different level of assistance is offered between these two groups of distressed students – with

---

BOX 7.4: Fieldwork and field interviews

In this book, I described in great detail the accounts of seven subjects who experienced prolonged social withdrawal throughout their life:

1. Mr. Ueyama
2. Mr. Maruyama
3. Ms. Hayashi
4. Mr. Onishi
5. Mr. Arai
6. Mr. Nomura, for his account on school nonattendance (*futōkō*)
7. Misaki

I recorded eight field interviews with

1. Ms. Otsuka (school counselor)
2. Mr. Sakurai (coordinator of a guidance center)
3. Doctor Matsuda (child and adolescent psychiatrist)
4. Prof. Kubo (university professor)
5. Mr. Ueyama
6. Misaki's mother
7. Misaki's father
8. Misaki

(Continued)

BOX 7.4: Fieldwork and field interviews *(Continued)*

I interviewed six NPO coordinators

1 Mr. Wada
2 Mr. Sano
3 Mr. Taniguchi
4 Mr. Murata
5 NPO M.'s founder
6 Mr. Yamamoto (*hikikomori* parents' association)

I briefly introduced the situation of eleven individuals who recently got out of their *hikikomori*, and joined NPOs where I met them. In NPO P:

1 Mr. Ando
2 Ms. Kojima
3 Mr. Takagi
4 Mr. Endo
5 Mr. Chiba

In NPO C:

6 Mr. Goto
7 Mr. Hirano
8 Mr. Iwasaki

In NPO A:

9 Mr. Onishi

And in NPO M

10 Mr. Kinoshita
11 Mr. Matsui

I visited six associations and three centers:

1 NPO A.
2 NPO C.
3 NPO P.
4 *Newstart*
5 NPO M.
6 Reflection Group of ex-*hikikomori* (*Shin hikikomori nitsuite kangaerukai*)
7 Guidance center X. (H. city)
8 Guidance center J. (H. city)
9 Centre F.

BOX 7.5: Twenty lessons on *hikikomori*

1 Most *hikikomori* subjects have experienced school absenteeism or dropout.
2 High school dropouts are abandoned by Japanese society.
3 Psychiatrists and NPO members meet a non-representative part of the socially withdrawn population.
4 Psychiatrists are not the only ones to meet *hikikomori* subjects who are often met by NPO members.
5 NPO staff members rarely have master's degrees in psychology, social work, or nursing.
6 NPOs are not the place for psychiatrists.
7 NPOs receive around a third of people with psychiatric illnesses.
8 The Japanese *hikikomori* I met (19) do not present an online gaming disorder, or internet overuse. There is a specific *hikikomori* profile of decline of the internet use across the lifespan.
9 There are hidden populations among the Japanese *hikikomori* population.
10 The period of social withdrawal could be a moment of subject formation.
11 More than 90% of the Japanese *hikikomori* individuals are adults, not adolescents.
12 The *hikikomori* phenomenon is not exclusively male, and women are much more numerous than previously thought.
13 The socially withdrawn population is aging.
14 One is led to the *hikikomori* situation: it is not a conscious decision or a voluntary refusal.
15 Some *hikikomori* individuals have mental disorders, some not.
16 *Hikikomori* is not a spectrum (i.e., Hikikomori Spectrum Disorder, HSD) but a psychosocial condition.
17 *Hikikomori* subjects are the "homeless at home."
18 *Hikikomori* is not limited to Japan and is not solely related to Japanese culture.
19 The Japanese Ministry of Health, Labor and Welfare has failed to solve issues relating to *hikikomori*.
20 A ministry of loneliness could be successful in responding to the needs of the socially isolated.

---

an abandonment of high school dropouts **(2)**. While junior high school students are the subject of intensive assistance, distressed high school students, in some cases, are voluntarily abandoned and left by themselves. In a way, the end of compulsory education is taken quite literally; since high school is not compulsory, society is not obligated to help distressed senior high school students. Logically, this fosters the school dropout of distressed adolescents, who then become more involved in delinquent behaviors or in situations of social withdrawal and trigger various psychiatric pathologies. This consequence is supported by the following four professionals I interviewed. Ms. Otsuka, for example, recounted a difficult experience from her practice as a school counselor, and provided the example of a teenage girl who had attempted suicide. She had insisted that the teachers of the junior high school make a connection with the high school to plan counseling sessions, only to realize a few months later that this teenager had returned to the junior high school to ask for help. The teachers had not, in fact, planned for psychological counseling. Another professional, Mr. Sakurai, who is the coordinator of the X. guidance center, notes that high school students are not received for consultation. Also, on a table about truancy provided by Dr. Matsuda, we can observe a massive difference between the reception of junior high school students and high school students. High school students were not received by guidance centers. (Note: Regarding these two guidance centers, it is worth remembering that they are *allowed* to take charge of high school students. Further examination would be necessary to understand the factors involved with the low number of high school students. Are these situations of domestic violence or of a psychiatric nature? Or, is it a continuation of the follow-up of certain middle school students who were already supported? And if so, why them and not others?) Finally, when I asked Prof. Kubo to tell me the most difficult example of her clinical practice, her words again illustrate this fact. According to her, the situation of high school students dropping out of school is eminently problematic because "everyone gives up" on them. The clinical psychologist, on his own, fails to make others (parents, teachers, students) understand that the young person is experiencing a distress that he could overcome. Some students drop out of school when occasional help, awareness of those around them, and the teaching community could be enough for them to finish high school.

This slackening of assistance for distressed students is also visible in the discourse of former *hikikomori*: Messrs. Ueyama, Maruyama, Onishi, Ms. Hayashi, and Misaki, to name but a few, and all of whom experienced being a dropout during high school. We also observed in their remarks that social withdrawal begins with symptoms in junior high school, which are accentuated in high school and later crystallize in the expression of distress in the form of social withdrawal during adulthood. This observation is made *a posteriori*. At the present time, one cannot predict that a *hikikomori* situation will be experienced in adulthood based on symptoms present in junior high school. From this point of view, studies on the risk factors of *hikikomori* have just started (Uchida and Norasakkunkit 2015, Wong et al. 2019) and are consistent with my findings. For instance, Yong and Nomura (2019) have conducted a secondary analysis using the Cabinet Office of the Government of Japan (Director-General for Policy on Cohesive Society')s (2009) survey data to identify the factors associated with *hikikomori*. Interestingly, they found that "*hikikomori* is associated with interpersonal relationships, followed by suicide risks. *Hikikomori* people are more likely to be male, have a history of dropping out from education, and have a previous psychiatric treatment history" (Yong and Nomura 2019).

Psychiatrists and members of NPOs meet a non-representative part of the socially withdrawn population **(3)**. More specifically, psychiatrists meet those of who are most likely to have a psychiatric pathology, and association members meet a subcategory of *nīto* and *hikikomori* individuals. In my survey, I focused on these associations, because, contrary to widely held belief, psychiatrists are not the only ones to meet *hikikomori* subjects **(4)**. It is, above all, the members of the associations (NPOs) who weave a local, sometimes national (e.g. KHJ parents' association), and international network (e.g., Newstart, NPO M) to help socially withdrawn youths. Consequently, I focused on the NPOs in order to better describe their roles and the affected population. On many points, my results correspond with other researchers who have already investigated this phenomenon in these types of associations (Ogino 2004, Kaneko 2006, Furlong 2008, Ishikawa et al. 2008, Toivonen 2008, Miller and Toivonen 2010, Horiguchi 2011, 2012).

NPOs voluntarily employ staff members who, for the most part, do not have master's degrees in psychology, social work, or nursing **(5)**. Note that Mr. Sano is a retired teacher, and Mr. Murata holds a bachelor's degree. NPOs give a chance to people who are on the margins of society. The founder of Newstart (Futagami Nōki) has an atypical career path, and recruits others like him. The founder of NPO M. had a chaotic education, and Mr. Wada, while he manages Association A., was himself a *hikikomori* when he was 19–29 years old. From this point of view, the presence of former *hikikomori* in assisting *hikikomori* individuals is seen repeatedly; the Japan Times has echoed this by taking the example of a Nagoya cafe run by a former *hikikomori* individual employing former *hikikomori* individuals (Takeuchi 2013).

NPOs work within a network of partners in hospitals or psychiatric clinics. They will invite certain psychiatrists for a conference or a meeting under some circumstances, but psychiatrists are generally not welcome in NPOs **(6)**. I have observed this in NPOs I have attended, and has been confirmed to me many times by psychiatrists themselves.

According to my investigations, about one-third of the people NPOs receive have psychiatric illnesses **(7)**. However, these results should be taken with caution, and it would be necessary to conduct a survey of a larger sample. Indeed, out of the 17 individuals participating in the activities of associations surveyed, 6 of them presented a psychiatric pathology at least once in their life: Mr. Onishi (alcoholism), Mr. Wada (social anxiety disorder, depression), Mss. Kojima and Hayashi (depression), and Messrs. Ando and Takagi (schizophrenia). It has not been shown that the chess practice of Mr. Arai and the interest in Mr. Endo's for horse racing was addictive. It is difficult to assess how many of them have met a psychiatrist, but it seems that most have met with general practitioners.

None of the 19 people interviewed showed intensive and addictive internet activity **(8)**. This is consistent with what recent studies have shown. Those who use the internet longer are not *hikikomori* subjects but rather the at-risk group: "subjects with high risk for *hikikomori* (…) used the internet longer than subjects with low risk for *hikikomori*" (Tateno et al. 2019: 6). Note that the image of *hikikomori* addicted to the internet and online games is not representative of the majority of *hikikomori* people in Japan, which does not seem the case in the United States and Australia (Stavropoulos et al. 2019). On the other hand, in Japan, a subcategory of individuals addicted to the internet and online games does exist; first, there is the group at risk of *hikikomori* and, second, a hidden population within the *hikikomori* population. With *hikikomori* women and the *taijin kyōfushō* cases, these three populations are hidden among the *hikikomori* population and are the most difficult to access and meet.

As we have seen in Chapter 4 with the Cabinet Office of the Government of Japan (Director-General for Policy on Cohesive Society) (2010, 2016, 2019) surveys, it appears that *hikikomori* adults aged 40–64 use the internet less than those aged 15–39. Consequently, internet use among *hikikomori* varies depending on the age range: there is no significant difference between *hikikomori* individuals aged 15–39 and the general group, while those aged 40–64 use the internet less compared to the general group [Cabinet Office of the Government of Japan (Director-General for Policy on Cohesive Society) 2019: 43]. Recent research proves an overuse of the internet among the child and adolescent recluse population (Hamasaki et al. 2020). It sketches a specific *hikikomori* profile of decline of the internet use across the lifespan, i.e., from overuse to underuse.

Indeed, there are six hidden populations **(9)** among the Japanese *hikikomori* population that sometimes overlap: (1) Individuals with an internet gaming disorder, (2) women, (3) severe *taijin kyōfushō* cases, (4) individuals from lower social classes who do not access social welfare services and who cannot afford NPO or NGO services, (5) individuals from middle and upper classes who are too ashamed to search for support, and (6) "pure" *hikikomori* subjects.

In some cases, the period of social withdrawal is experienced as a moment in a process of *subjectivation*, subject formation **(10)**. Yoneyama's (2008) comments consider school refusal from this point of view. Certain accounts, such as those published in the Japan Times, and part of those of Mr. Ueyama, Mr. Maruyama, and Ms. Hayashi also go in this direction. The period of social withdrawal was a time when they could live as a subject, in a way that was impossible through the role that was prescribed for them in Japanese society. Parents are well aware that Japanese society, for some children, can make it difficult to express their subjectivity. Hence, an understandable attitude authorizing social withdrawal for a few months does not necessarily evoke particular concern. Some leave after a few months or a year and resume a social life; it was merely a moment in their life. In many accounts, anxiety, torment, remorse, despair, guilt, and shame are indeed present. The difficulty lies in the fact that one cannot know in advance whether the subject is taking a break or whether he is falling into a morbid process.

However, this difficulty is characteristic of a phase of development little known and seldom studied in Japan: emerging adulthood (Arnett, Žukauskienė, and Sugimura 2014, Arnett 2015). Although social withdrawal can be triggered in adolescence, those known as *hikikomori* in Japan are not adolescents. As of 2016, almost all of them are adults (between 89% and 99%), and a third of them are emerging adults **(11)**. Also, the fact that a *hikikomori* subject does not marry, in a nation where marriage is still considered as "the completion of transition to adulthood" (Hendry 2017: 121), means that they are not fully considered as "adults." It reinforces their perception as "never-ending adolescents," which can be explained by the lack of recognition of emerging adulthood as a life stage, and the still-pervasive idea that marriage is a marker of transition to adulthood.

The *hikikomori* phenomenon is not exclusively male: 36.7% of *hikikomori* individuals are women, and 59.3% women are in the affinity group. In other words, women are much more numerous than previously thought, especially in what some might be considered the population at risk **(12)**.

There is an aging of the socially withdrawn population: The people concerned may be over 40, and were not taken into account in epidemiological surveys until 2019 **(13)**.

There is a difference between school nonattendance (*futōkō*) and school refusal (*tōkō kyohi*). And just as it is true that children who do not go to school do not necessarily refuse school, so one can also enter the *hikikomori* situation without necessarily refusing society **(14)**. Acknowledging an agency would already mean an important step in subject formation that cannot be assumed for all cases.

Among the *hikikomori* population, there is a diversity of individuals who have been diagnosed with mental disorders and those who have not. **(15)**

Hikikomori resists its medicalization and does not meet clear and consistent criteria for being described as a spectrum in the psychiatric sense (i.e., HSD). Rather, it should be seen as a psychosocial condition. **(16)**

Hikikomori subjects are simultaneously pressured by society and their families, and at the same time abandoned in a situation that I would call "homeless at home." **(17)**

Hikikomori is not limited to Japan and is not solely related to Japanese culture. **(18)**

For more than two decades, the Japanese Ministry of Health, Labor and Welfare has taken measures to address *hikikomori*; however, these measures have not been able to get mass numbers of *hikikomori* individuals back to work and have not solved the issues raised by the parties concerned. On the contrary, more issues have emerged, such as "double *hikikomori*," and the aging of children and parents, leading to what is called the "80/50 issue." **(19)**

Every country struggles to respond to the needs of individuals in social isolation, whether they are with *hikikomori*, depression, schizophrenia, homelessness, etc. The failure of existing health ministries worldwide should give birth to a new kind of ministry or agency dedicated to loneliness. **(20)**

References

Agamben, Giorgio. (1999). *Remnants of Auschwitz. The Witness and the Archive.* New York: Zone Books.

Aoki, Hideo. 2009. "Buraku Culture." In *The Cambridge Companion to Modern Japanese Culture*. Edited by Yoshio Sugimoto, 182–198. Melbourne: Cambridge University Press.

American Psychiatric Association. 2013. *Diagnostic and Statistical Manual of Mental Disorders, 5th Edition: DSM-5 [Paperback].* Washington DC: American Psychiatric Publishing.

———. 2016. *DSM-5 Handbook on the Cultural Formulation Interview.* Edited by Roberto Lewis-Fernández et al. [Paperback]. Washington DC: American Psychiatric Publishing.

Arnett, Jeffrey. 2015. *Emerging Adulthood: The Winding Road from the Late Teens through the Twenties* (2nd ed.). New York: Oxford University Press.

Arnett, Jeffrey, Rita Žukauskienė, and Kazumi Sugimura. 2014. "The New Life Stage of Emerging Adulthood at Ages 18–29 Years: Implications for Mental Health." *Lancet Psychiatry* 2014 (1): 569–576.

Aubry, Florence. 2010. *Je suis un hikikomori.* Namur: Mijade.

Bommersbach, Tanner, and Hun Millard. 2019. "No Longer Culture-Bound: Hikikomori Outside of Japan." *International Journal of Social Psychiatry* 65 (6): 539–540.

Bowker, Julie C., Matthew H. Bowker, Jonathan B. Santo, Adesola Adebusola Ojo, Rebecca G. Etkin, and Radhi Raja. 2019. "Severe Social Withdrawal: Cultural Variation in Past Hikikomori Experiences of University Students in Nigeria, Singapore, and the United States." *The Journal of Genetic Psychology* 180 (4–5): 217–230.

Cabinet Office of the Government of Japan (Director-General for Policy on Cohesive Society) 内閣府政策統括官 (共生社会政策担当). 2010. *Wakamono no ishiki ni kansuru chōsa – Hikikomori ni kansuru jittai chōsa* 若者の意識に関する調査・ひきこもりに関する実態調査 (Survey on Youth Consciousness – Survey on *Hikikomori*). https://www8.cao.go.jp/youth/kenkyu/hikikomori/pdf_gaiyo_index.html.

———. 2016. *Wakamono no seikatsu ni kansuru chōsa hōkokusho* 若者の生活に関する調査 報告書 (Research Survey on Youth's life). https://www8.cao.go.jp/youth/kenkyu/hikikomori/h27/pdf-index.html.

———. 2019. *Seikatsu Jōkyō ni Kansuru Chōsa* 生活状況に関する調査 (Survey on Living Conditions). https://www8.cao.go.jp/youth/kenkyu/life/h30/pdf-index.html.

Chauliac, Nicolas, Audrey Couillet, Sophie Faivre, Nassima Brochard, and Jean-Louis Terra. 2017. "Characteristics of Socially Withdrawn Youth in France: A Retrospective Study." *International Journal of Social Psychiatry* 63 (4): 339–344.

Choi, Tae Young, and Young Sik Lee. 2012. "Home Visitation Program for Managing Korean Hikikomori." In *The 108th Annual Meeting of the Japanese Society of Psychiatry and Neurology.*

Dervelois, Michaël. 2011. "Le rôle de l'encadrement institutionnel et associatif pour l'insertion professionnelle des handicapés au Japon: Points communs et divergences avec le système français." PhD diss. Paris University.

Fansten, Maia et al. 2014. *Hikikomori, ces adolescents en retrait.* Paris: Armand Colin.

Furlong, Andy. 2008. "The Japanese Hikikomori Phenomenon: Acute Social Withdrawal among Young People." *The Sociological Review* 56: 309–325.

Gayral L., J. Carrie, and J. Bonnet. 1953. "La claustration." *Annales Médico-Psychologiques.* 111: TI, avril.

Garcia-Campayo, Javier, Marta Alda, Natalia Sobradiel, and Beatriz Sanz Abós. 2007. "A Case Report of Hikikomori in Spain." *Medicina Clinica (Barcelona)* 129 (8): 318–319.

Gondim, Francisco A. A., Adelmo P. Aragão, Joana G. Holanda Filha and Erick .L.M. Messias. 2017. "Hikikomori in Brazil: 29 years of Voluntary social Withdrawal." *Asian Journal of Psychiatry* 30: 163–164.

Groleau, Danielle, Allan Young, and Laurence J. Kirmayer. 2006. "The McGill Illness Narrative Interview (MINI): An Interview Schedule to Elicit Meanings and Modes of Reasoning Related to Illness Experience." *Transcultural Psychiatry* 43 (4): 671–691.

Guedj-Bourdiau, Marie-Jeanne. 2011. "Claustration à domicile de l'adolescent Hikikomori." *Annales Médico-Psychologiques* 169 (10): 668–673.

Haasio, Ari, and Hajime Naka. 2019. "Information Needs of the Finnish and Japanese Hikikomori: A Comparative Study." *Qualitative and Quantitative Methods in Libraries* 8 (4): 509–523.

Hamasaki Yukiko, Nancy Pionnié-Dax, Géraldine Dorard, Nicolas Tajan, and Takatoshi Hikida. 2020. "Identifying Social Withdrawal (Hikikomori) Factors in Adolescents: Understanding the Hikikomori Spectrum." *Child Psychiatry and Human Development.* Available from: https://doi.org/10.1007/s10578-020-01064-8

Hashimoto, Akiko. 2015. *The Long Defeat. Cultural Trauma, Memory, and Identity in Japan.* New York: Oxford University Press.

Hendry, Joy. 2017. *An Anthropological Lifetime in Japan.* Leiden, Boston: Brill.

Horiguchi, Sachiko 堀口佐知子. 2011. "Coping with Hikikomori. Socially Withdrawn Youth and the Japanese Family." In *Home and Family in Japan. Continuity and Transformation.* Edited by Richard Ronald and Allison Alexy. Oxon, UK: Routledge.

Horiguchi, Sachiko 堀口佐知子. 2012. "Hikikomori: How Private Isolation Caught the Public Eye." In *A Sociology of Japanese Youth, From Returnees to Neet.* Edited by Roger Goodman, Yuki Imoto, and Tuukka Toivonen. Oxon: Routledge.

Husu, Hanna-Mari, and Vesa Välimäki. 2017. "Staying inside: Social withdrawal of the young, Finnish Hikikomori." *Journal of Youth Studies* 20 (5): 605–621.

Ishikawa, Ryōko, Tatsushi Ogino, Minoru Kawakita, Kōji Kudo, Rūtaro Takayama, Yoshitaka Nakamura, Akihiko Higuchi, and Sachiko Horiguchi. 2008. *"Hikikomori" e no shakaigakuteki apurōchi – media, tōjisha, shienkatsudō* 「ひきこもり」への社会学的アプローチ—メディア・当事者・支援活動 (*Sociological Approach to Hikikomori – Media, Person Concerned, Support Activities*). Tōkyō: Mineruva shobō.

Jeammet, Philippe. 1985. "Actualité de l'agir," *Nouvelle Revue de Psychanalyse* 31: 201–222.

Kaneko, Sachiko. 2006. "Japan's 'Socially Withdrawn Youths' and Time Constraints in Japanese Society: Management and Conceptualization of Time in a Support Group for Hikikomori." *Time & Society* 15 (2/3): 233–249.

Kasahara, Yomishi 笠原嘉. 1978. "Taikyaku shinkeishō to iu shinkategorii no teishō" 退却神経症という新カテゴリーの提唱 (Proposition of a New Category Called Retreat Neurosis). In *Shishunki no Seishinbyōri to Chiryō* 思春期の精神病理と治療 *(Psychopathology and Treatment of Adolescence).* Edited by H. Nakai and Y. Yamanaka 中井久夫・山中康裕編, 287–319. Tōkyō: Iwasaki Gakujutsu Shuppan.

———. 1984. *Apashī shindorōmu — kōgakureki shakai no seinen shinri* アパシー・シンドローム—高学歴社会の青年心理 (Student Apathy Syndrome). Tōkyō: Iwanami Shoten.

Kato, Takahiro A., Shigenobu Kanba, and Alan R. Teo. 2018. "Hikikomori: Experience in Japan and International Relevance." *World Psychiatry* 17 (1): 105–106.

Kim, Jinkwan, Ronald M Rapee, Ja Oh Kyung, and Hye-Shin Moon. 2008. "Retrospective Report of Social Withdrawal during Adolescence and Current Maladjustment in Young Adulthood: Cross-Cultural Comparisons between Australian and South Korean Students." *Journal of Adolescence* 31 (5): 543–563.

Kondo, Naoji, Motohiro Sakai, Yasukazu Kuroda, Yoshikazu Kiyota, Yuji Kitabata, and Mie Kurosawa. 2013. "General Condition of Hikikomori (Prolonged Social Withdrawal) in Japan: Psychiatric Diagnosis and Outcome in Mental Healths Welfare Centres." *International Journal of Social Psychiatry* 67: 193–202.

Kubo, Hiroaki, et al. 2020. "Development of 5-Day Hikikomori Intervention Program for Family Members: A Single-Arm Pilot Trial." *Heliyon* 6: e03011.

Lee, Young Sik, Jae Young Lee, Tae Young Choi, and Jin Tae Choi. 2013. "Home Visitation Program for Detecting, Evaluating and Treating Socially Withdrawn Youth in Korea." *Psychiatry and Clinical Neurosciences* 67 (4): 193–202.

Lewis-Fernández et al. 2014. "Culture and Psychiatric Evaluation: Operationalizing Cultural Formulation for DSM-5." *Psychiatry: Interpersonal and Biological Processes* 77 (2): 130–154.

Liu, Lucia L., Tim MH Li, and Paul WC Wong. 2020. "Discovering Socially Withdrawn Youth in Shanghai through the Eyes of Social Workers: A Mixed-Methods Study." *Journal of Social Work*. doi: 10.1177/1468017320911509.

Lock, Margaret. 1986. "Plea for Acceptance: School Refusal Syndrome in Japan." *Social Science & Medicine* 23 (2): 99–112.

———. 1995. *Encounters with Aging. Mythologies of Menopause in Japan and North America*. Berkeley, CA: University of California Press.

Lucken, Michael. 2017. *The Japanese and the War. Expectation, Perception, and the Shaping of Memory*. Translated by Karen Grimwade. New York: Columbia University Press.

Marcotte, Josée. 2014. *Hikikomori*. Québec: L'instant même.

Ministry of Health Labour and Welfare (MHLW) 厚生労働省. 2010. *Hikikomori no hyōka/shien ni kansuru gaidorain* ひきこもりの評価ー支援に関するガイドラン (Guidelines for Support and Evaluation of Hikikomori). Edited by Kazuhiko Saitō et al. http://www.mhlw.go.jp/stf/houdou/2r98520000006i6f.html.

Miller, Aaron L., and Tuukka Toivonen. 2010. "To Discipline or Accommodate? On the Rehabilitation of Japanese 'Problem Youth.'" *The Asia-Pacific Journal: Japan Focus*. http://www.japanfocus.org/-aaron-miller/3368.

Ogino, Tatsushi. 2004. "Managing Categorization and Social Withdrawal in Japan: Rehabilitation Process in a Private Support Group for Hikikomorians." *International Journal of Japanese Sociology* 13: 120–133.

Ōtake, Tomoko. 2011. "French Researchers Seek «Raison d'Être» of Hikikomori." *The Japan Times*, November 20, 2011.

Ovejero, Santiago, Irene Caro-Cañizares, Victoria de León-Martínez, and Enrique Baca-Garcia. 2014. "Prolonged Social Withdrawal Disorder: A Hikikomori Case in Spain." *International Journal of Social Psychiatry* 60 (6): 562–565. https://doi.org/10.1177/0020764013504560.

Pimlott, Nicholas. 2018. "The Ministry of Loneliness." *Canadian Family Physician* 64 (3): 166.

Ranieri, Fiorenzo. 2018. "Psychoanalytic Psychotherapy for Hikikomori Young Adults and Adolescents: Psychoanalytic Psychotherapy for Hikikomori." *British Journal of Psychotherapy* 34: 623–642.

Rosenberger, Nancy R. 1992. "The Process of Discourse: Usages of a Japanese Medical Term." *Social Science & Medicine* 34 (3): 237–247.

Rødgaard, Eya-Mist, Kristian Jensen, Jean-Noël Vergnes, Isabelle Soulières, and Laurent Mottron. 2019. "Temporal Changes in Effect Sizes of Studies Comparing Individuals With and Without Autism: A Meta-analysis." *JAMA Psychiatry* 76 (11): 1124–1132.

Sagliocco, Giulia, et al. 2011. *Hikikomori e adolescenza. Fenomenologia dell'autore-clusione.* Milano: Mimesis.

Sakamoto, Noriyuki, Rodger R. Martin, Hiroaki Kumano, Kuboki Tomifusa, and Samir Al-Adawi. 2005. "Hikikomori, Is It A Culture-Reactive or Culture-Bound Syndrome? Nidotherapy And A Clinical Vignette from Oman." *International Journal of Psychiatry in Medicine* 35: 191–198.

Satō, Toshiki 佐藤佐藤. 2000. *Fubyōdō shakai nippon—sayonara sōchūryū* 不平等社会日本—さよなら総中流 (Unequal Society Japan—Farewell to the Mass Middle Class). Tōkyō: Chūkō shinsho.

Silić, Ante, Jakša Vukojević, Ilaria Čulo, and Hrvoje Falak. 2019. "Hikikomori Silent Epidemic: A Case Study." *Research in Psychotherapy: Psychopathology, Process and Outcome* 22 (2), 317–322.

Souilem, A, A. Mrad, Takoua Brahim, R. Hannachi, and Anwar Mechri. 2019. "Syndrome d'Hikikomori ou de claustration à domicile: À propos d'une observation Tunisienne" *Neuropsychiatrie de l'Enfance et de l'Adolescence* 67 (2): 106–108.

Stip, Emmanuel, Alexis Thibault, Alexis Beauchamp-Chatel, and Steve Kisely. 2016. "Internet Addiction, Hikikomori Syndrome, and the Prodromal Phase of Psychosis." *Frontiers in Psychiatry* 7: 6.

Stavropoulos, Vasileios, Emma Ela Anderson, Charlotte Beard, Mohammed Qasim Latifi, Daria Kuss, and Mark Griffiths. 2019. "A Preliminary Cross-Cultural Study of Hikikomori and Internet Gaming Disorder: The Moderating Effects of Game-Playing Time and Living with Parents." *Addictive Behaviors Reports* 9: 100137.

Sugimoto, Yoshio. 2010. *An Introduction to Japanese Society* (3rd ed.). Cambridge: Cambridge University Press.

Suwa, Mami, Kunifumi Suzuki, Koichi Hara, Hisashi Watanabe, and Toshihiko Takahashi. 2003. "Family Features in Primary Social Withdrawal among Young Adults." *Psychiatry and Clinical Neurosciences* 57: 586–594.

Tajan, Nicolas. 2015a. "Adolescents' School Non-Attendance and the Spread of Psychological Counselling in Japan." *Asia Pacific Journal of Counselling and Psychotherapy* 6 (1/2): 58–69.

———. 2015b. "Social Withdrawal and Psychiatry: A Comprehensive Review of Hikikomori." *Neuropsychiatrie de l'Enfance et de l'Adolescence* 63 (5): 324–331.

———. 2015c. "Japanese Post-Modern Social Renouncers: An Exploratory Study of the Narratives of Hikikomori Subjects." *Subjectivity* 8: 283–304.

———. 2017a. *Génération hikikomori.* Paris: L'Harmattan (Collection Japon).

———. 2017b. "Traumatic Dimensions of Hikikomori: A Foucauldian Note." *Asian Journal of Psychiatry* 27: 121–122.

Tajan Nicolas, and Meiko Shiozawa. 2020. "Hikikomori wo saikōsuru – kaigai, tokuni furansu no jirei 「ひきこもり」を再考する—海外、特にフランスの事例" (Rethinking Hikikomori – Examples from France and Abroad) *Kyōiku to Igaku* 教育と医学 3/4: 54–61.

Tajan, Nicolas, Yukiko Hamasaki, and Nancy Pionnié-Dax. 2017. "Hikikomori: The Japanese Cabinet Office's 2016 Survey of Acute Social Withdrawal." *The Asia-Pacific Journal* 15 (1): 1–11.

Takeuchi, Satoshi. 2013. "Former 'hikikomori' Helping Young Recluses Reintegrate into Society." *The Japan Times.* October 1, 2013.

Tateno Masaru, Alan R. Teo, Wataru Ukai, Junichiro Kanazawa, Ryoko Katsuki, Hiroaki Kubo, and Takahiro A. Kato. 2019. "Internet Addiction, Smartphone Addiction, and Hikikomori Trait in Japanese Young Adult: Social Isolation and Social Network." *Frontiers in Psychiatry* 10: 455.

Teo, Alan R. 2013. "Social Isolation Associated with Depression: A Case Report of Hikikomori." *International Journal of Social Psychiatry* 59 (4): 339–341.

Teo, Alan R., and Albert R. Gaw. 2010. "Hikikomori, A Japanese Culture-Bound Syndrome of Social Withdrawal? A Proposal for DSM-5." *The Journal of Nervous and Mental Disease* 198 (6): 444–449.

Teo, Alan R., Kyle Stufflebam, Somnath Saha, Michael D. Fetters, Masaru Tateno, Shigenobu Kanba, and Takahiro A. Kato. 2015. "Psychopathology Associated with Social Withdrawal: Idiopathic and Comorbid Presentations." *Psychiatry Research* 228 (1): 182–183.

Toivonen, Tuukka. 2008. "Introducing the Youth Independence Camp. How a New Social Policy Is Reconfiguring the Public-Private Boundaries of Social Provision in Japan." *Sociologos* 32: 42–57.

Uchida, Yukiko, and Vinai Norasakkunkit. 2015. "The NEET and Hikikomori Spectrum: Assessing the Risks and Consequences of Becoming Culturally Marginalized." *Frontiers in Psychology* 6: 1117.

Ueyama, Kazuki 上山和樹. 2001. *"Hikikomori" datta boku kara* 「ひきこもり」だっ た僕から (From Me, Who was *Hikikomori*). Tōkyō: Kōdansha.

Ueyama, Kazuki, Kosuke Tsuiki, and Nicolas Tajan. 2010. "Hikikomori nitsuite" ひきこもりについて (About *Hikikomori*). Video-recorded interview.

Välimäki Vesa, Antti Kivijärvi, and Sanna Aaltonen. 2019. "The Links Between Structural and Social Marginalisation – Social Relations of Young Finnish Adults not in Employment or Education." *Journal of Youth Studies* 0: 1–19.

Wong, Paul WC, Tim MH Li, Melissa Chan, Y Law, Michael Chau, Cecilia Cheng, KW Fu, John Bacon-Shone, and Paul SF Yip. 2015. "The Prevalence and Correlates of Severe Social Withdrawal (Hikikomori) in Hong Kong: A Cross-Sectional Telephone-Based Survey Study." *International Journal of Social Psychiatry* 61 (4): 330–342.

Wong, John Chee Meng, Michelle Jing Si Wan, Leoniek Kroneman, Takahiro A. Kato, T. Wing Lo, Paul WC Wong, and Gloria Hongyee Chan. 2019. "Hikikomori Phenomenon in East Asia: Regional Perspectives, Challenges, and Opportunities for Social Health Agencies." *Frontiers in Psychiatry* 10: 512.

Wu, Alison FW, Jinnie Ooi, Paul WC Wong, Caroline Catmur, and Jennifer YF Lau. 2019. "Evidence of Pathological Social Withdrawal in Non-Asian Countries: A Global Health Problem?" *The Lancet Psychiatry* 6 (3): 195–196.

Yoneyama, Shoko. 2008. "The Era of Bullying: Japan Under Neoliberalism." *The Asia-Pacific Journal: Japan Focus.* http://www.japanfocus.org/-Shoko-YONEYAMA/3001.

Yong, Roseline, and Kyoko Nomura. 2019. "Hikikomori Is Most Associated with Interpersonal Relationships, Followed by Suicide Risks: A Secondary Analysis of a National Cross-Sectional Study." *Frontiers in Psychiatry* 10:247.

Yuen, John, Yoyo K. Y. Yan, Victor C. W. Wong, Wilson W. S. Tam, Ka-Wing So, and Wai Tong Chien. 2018. "A Physical Health Profile of Youths Living with a Hikikomori Lifestyle." *International Journal of Environmental Research and Public Health* 15 (2): 315.

8   Conclusions

Social isolation, biopower, and the end of the clinic

Introduction

Hikikomori does not simply happen, and at no random point in history does it happen alone. The increase in the number of *hikikomori* individuals, including the fact that individuals self-identify as such and no longer rely on psychiatric categories, teaches us a great deal from the point of view of mental health anthropology, psychoanalysis, and the theory of subjectivity. To conclude this work and in order to open up new perspectives, I would like to invite you along with me to think about several issues that are in tension with certain aspects of Michel Foucault's work.

Psychiatry was to disciplinary power what mental health science is to biopower

We use the terms "psychiatry" and "mental disorder" as if they have always existed. However, they are very recent and have increasingly been emptied of their meaning to the extent that one can very easily imagine that they will fall into disuse by the end of the 21st century.

What has certainly existed throughout the ages is medicine. This was first a medicine to be subdivided into psychiatry and neurology during the second half of the 19th century. Psychiatry was not the brainchild of Philippe Pinel (1745–1826) and neither was it that of William Tuke (1732–1822) or Francis Willis (1718–1807), nor did it develop with the French alienists of the 19th century, nor even with Jean-Martin Charcot or Sigmund Freud, whose profession, needless to say, was that of a neurologist. It must be taken literally that none of the doctors of the 18th century and French alienists of the 19th century used the term psychiatry to describe their discipline, and they did not designate themselves by the term psychiatrist. Admittedly, we speak for ease of understanding rather than for the sake of accuracy of the history of psychiatry, but before Kraepelin, it was "proto-psychiatry," if I may quote the term used by Foucault. Psychiatry was the brainchild of Kraepelin, and to consider that the doctors who preceded him practiced psychiatry when they neither used the term nor designated themselves as psychiatrists is an intrinsic characteristic of a teleological approach (i.e., an approach where phenomena are explained through the intervention of a final cause – *telos* in ancient Greek).

Psychiatry, psychiatrists, and their disorders are recent, and there is no evidence that they will survive the 21st century. Indeed, since modern times, the object of medicine has been successive: unreason, madness, insanity, mental alienation, nervous disease, mental illness, and mental disorder. Unreason has been silent for a long time, but can the type of social withdrawal born in Japan – *hikikomori* – be considered one of the resurgences of unreason? What does unreason even mean? It is difficult for us to think about it today and understand what it is. In 1961, however, Michel Foucault gave a masterful explanation.

The great movement in the history of madness and unreason

Madness and Unreason. History of Madness in the Classical Age (Foucault 2015a: 1–669) is better known by its short title *History of Madness*, and it was not until 2006 that the full text was available in English. However, we cannot stress enough the need to remember that Michel Foucault's first major work was not only about madness; above all, it was also about unreason and the reason/unreason duality. Philippe Ariès, upon receiving Foucault's manuscript, spoke of a "philosophy thesis on the relationships between Madness and Unreason" (Artières and Bert 2011: 88). Louis Althusser insisted in his 1962–1963 seminar that "Foucault's book is therefore a book on Reason, as much as on Madness" (Artières and Bert 2011: 160).

Prior to the 17th century, there was not really madness or mental illness, which is difficult for us to imagine. There was unreason. One of its symbols is the ship of fools (*Stultifera Navis*), which appeared at the end of the 15th century, the best known representation of which is by Hieronymus Bosch. These boats, responsible for transporting madmen from one city to another, did exist, but it is difficult to understand the meaning of this custom. There have been places of detention for madmen since the Middle Ages: madmen were not systematically excluded, as they were entrusted to sailors. In the city of Nuremberg, for example, they were imprisoned in large numbers because madmen from other cities were sent there. Foucault's hypothesis is that foreigners were chased among the mad and that, in some cases, these ships were pilgrimages subsidized by a city or hospital (Foucault 2006a: 10). Unreason and madness were excluded from the city.

Thereafter, the 17th and 18th centuries were a period described by Foucault under the expression of the "great confinement," a period in which the classical age silenced madness, i.e., those whose voices had been released by the Renaissance. Madness leaves its boat, its exclusion, to maintain durability within establishments included in the cities: "embarkation has given way to confinement" (Foucault 2006a: 41). This time, there were no abstract types, like in the ship of fools, but concrete characters condemned by society.

They no longer displayed a visible evil, such as leprosy, but an invisible stigma, that of unreason, enclosed in houses of confinement and at the general hospital. Before being the object of psychiatric knowledge, unreason was the object of excommunication. Before being a coherent institution from a medical and psychological point of view, internment was a coherent institution from the point of view of a "police" and "perception." In Germany, they were in correctional houses (created in Hamburg in 1620). In England, they were in workhouses (created in 1697). In France, they were at the general hospital created in 1655 (Quétel 2012) and in houses of confinement (which disappeared at the end of the 18th century), then in private houses and boarding houses reserved for the insane (*les insensés*): the "Little Houses" that welcomed around 20 or 30 people (Foucault 2006a: 384). This dynamic was European.

Internment is simultaneously exclusion and organization: The 17th century banished and grouped, in a single gesture, a variety of figures and experiences that did not feature in the previous century, "thus forming a uniform world of Unreason" (Foucault 2006a: 82). Let there be no mistake: those who reproach Foucault for being against psychiatry or psychoanalysis, for standardizing unreason, or even for creating a myth of madness whose essence will cross the ages, or even, like Henry Amer, that his analyses rest on a "fixity of madness over time" (quoted by Artières and Bert 2011: 138), have not read until the end. I would highlight two essential contributions: (1) the general apprehension of unreason is simultaneous with the recognition of the diversity of internees and (2) the rejection of naturalist reductionism allows the development of ethical conscience and social sensitivity.

> A madman is not recognized as such because an illness has pushed him to the margins of normality, but because our culture situates him at the meeting point between the social decree of confinement and the juridical knowledge that evaluates the responsibility of individuals before the law. The "positive" science of mental illness and the humanitarian sentiments that brought the mad back into the realm of the human were only possible once that synthesis had been solidly established. They could be said to form the concrete *a priori* of any psychopathology with scientific pretensions (Foucault 2006a: 129–130).

First, Foucault insisted and continued to highlight the teeming and colorful multiplicity that has populated these establishments for 150 years: madmen, libertines, poors (Leblanc 2014), blasphemers, the insane, the debauched, dissipators, homosexuals, alchemists, idlers, vagrants, those who attempted suicide, followers of witchcraft and magic, etc. His thesis is that the Middle Ages gradually individualized the mad, while the 17th century undifferentiated them, dispelling them "in a general apprehension of unreason" (Foucault 2006a: 118). He highlighted a general apprehension of unreason and, simultaneously, the diversity of internees, "the multiple faces of madness" (Foucault 2006a: 131). According to him, there is no unity of madness but a plurality, a "constellation," a "torn presence." Although he never ceased to draw distinctions in this sense, they do not come under the differential diagnosis of psychiatrists. From this point of view, critics of Foucault have run up against what contributes to the philosophical significance of his work: the rejection of naturalist reductionism. Indeed, Foucault demonstrated that madness had never fully entered the garden of species. It resisted naturalization.

> Mental illness, in the classical age, does not exist, if what is understood by that is the natural homeland of the insane, the mediation between the madman who is perceived and the dementia that is analyzed, the link, in short, between the madman and his madness (Foucault 2006a: 206).
>
> Perhaps from one century to another, the same name does not refer to the *same sicknesses* – but this is because fundamentally it is not the *same* illness that is in question. To speak of madness in the 17th and 18th centuries is not, in the strict sense, to speak of "a sickness of the mind," but of something where both the body and the mind *together* are in question (Foucault 2006a: 214).

Second, it shows that classicism was opposed to madness through a refusal that was not so much a reaction to the transgressions of the moral rules in which it operated but, above all, the manifestation of an ethical conscience. In the 17th century, the internment decision was not a medical decision; it was a social one. This social sensitivity on which the medical conscience was formed made it possible to decide on internment and release.

The end of the 18th century also marked the end of the great confinement, and Foucault insisted on two medical figures of the time, Tuke and Pinel. This focus features in the last chapters of *Madness and Unreason*. These chapters do deserve a long overview here, but insofar as the lectures on *Psychiatric Power* will be devoted to asylum, I will provisionally conclude with two events that symbolize the passage of unreason from the classical age to mental alienation as an object of scientific knowledge: Sade being chased from Charenton and Pinel liberating the insane. Indeed, Doctor Royer-Collard no longer perceived unreason: for him, Sade was not insane, and his place was in prison. Gradually, an "asylum perception" of madness developed (Foucault 2006a: 390). The alienated (*l'aliéné*) and the insane (*l'insensé*) were initially confused, but this was no longer the case: The alienated became those who had completely lost the truth; they were absolutely blinded by their madness; they were foreign to others and to themselves. We can identify with the insane (we can understand them because they "imagine" this, they believe that ...), and the insane testify to the exchanges between reason and unreason. However, in alienation, there is a break between reason and unreason. With Pinel delivering the insane from their chains (men at Bicêtre in 1793, then women at

La Salpêtrière in 1795), unreason disappears almost completely, thanks to the creation of the concept of mental alienation. When the internees became alienated, i.e., becoming objects of scientific knowledge (Pinel), we excluded from internment those who were unreasonable (Sade), and we kept those who were mad: But madness has changed the name. It is now called mental alienation.

I suggest that the epidemic of contemporary social withdrawal must be understood in terms of the resurgence of unreason. In other words, the meaning of *hikikomori* is not to be sought in the context of a mental disorder or disability. Let us remember that we went from "free" unreason to a madness excluded in boats and interned on the outskirts of European cities. The hospitalization of patients was followed by confinement at home, bereft of all agency or link to the hospital environment. *Hikikomori* subjects are obviously not the abstract types found in the ship of fools; they do not exhibit a visible evil, such as a disease, but an invisible stigma, that of unreason, which can no longer be enclosed in psychiatric hospitals and clinics.

Hikikomori does not succeed in becoming the object of psychiatric knowledge; it is the sign of unreason. For this specific reason, it is not the object of an excommunication but of an abandonment at home. From a medical and psychological standpoint, hospitalization has lost all coherence. Hospitalization is exclusion and organization: The 17th century had banished and grouped, in a single gesture, a variety of figures and experiences that did not feature in the previous century, "thus forming a uniform world of unreason" (Foucault 2006a: 82). At the start of the 21st century, if we take the example of Japan, *hikikomori* has been misunderstood, excluded, a shameful situation, though not in the same way as individuals with disabilities or mental disorders. In the 17th century, the internment decision was not a medical decision; it was a social one. Today, abandonment in social withdrawal must also be thought of in terms of social sensitivity. Royer-Collard no longer perceived unreason: For him, Sade was not insane, and his place was in prison. An "asylum perception" of madness gradually developed (Foucault 2006a: 390). Today, a Japanese psychiatrist either identifies a psychiatric category as (comorbid) social withdrawal and orders hospitalization and medical treatment, or he finds himself without resources to think about the manifestation of unreason crystallized by the *hikikomori* subject. The shut-in is not crazy; he is not alienated because the alienated is the one who has completely lost the truth. The alienated is absolutely blinded by his madness, foreign to others and himself. We can identify with the insane (we can understand them because they "imagine" this, they believe that ...), and they testify to the exchanges between reason and unreason. In alienation and madness, there is a break between reason and unreason. While *hikikomori* can be thought of in the context of the insane (*l'insensé*), its idle situation is external to the central value of work, so precious to the Japanese who hope to bring the *hikikomori* back on the right path, that of work for all.

From psychiatric power to user biopower

January 1974 marked the start of the lectures on *Psychiatric Power*. It is not, strictly speaking, the second volume of *Madness and Unreason*. Indeed, since *Madness and Unreason*, there has been a book made up of his scraps, *The Birth of the Clinic*, then *Raymond Roussel, Me Pierre Rivière...*, and *Disorderly Families*. Let us therefore consider these lectures as a second step in which "there is a shift from the problematic of a history of representations towards the apparatuses of power producing *énoncés*" (Foucault 2015b: xx).

In *Madness and Unreason*, Foucault stopped at Pinel (late 18th century). In *Psychiatric Power*, he went as far as Charcot (late 19th century). If we had to highlight the most salient feature of these lectures, that which had not been detailed in *Madness and Unreason*, I would say that it is the central role attributed to the notion of power defined by the negative: It is not what someone holds or what emanates from someone: "Power does not belong to anyone or even to a group" (Foucault 2006b: 4). More specifically, Foucault attached great importance to the concept of disciplinary power. Indeed, disciplinary order is the condition of the therapeutic operation: Order and discipline are necessary for medical knowledge, and to ensure the conditions for healing. There are not really individuals but bodies, behaviors, and discourses distributed and regulated within the asylum: One can only heal within "this regulated distribution of power."

If the founding scene of the myth of the birth of psychiatry is that of Pinel liberating chained madmen, Foucault attached greater importance to another scene that took place in England in 1788: that of George III (1738–1820) being treated by Willis. According to Foucault, this scene illustrates the transition from sovereign power to disciplinary power. Disciplinary power has no particular target: silent, networked, it makes bodies docile and submissive. In this proto-psychiatry, we are dealing with "a tactic of the manipulation of madness" (Foucault 2006b: 31).

Disciplinary power, born in religious communities of the medieval period, was transmitted to secular communities. It became a generalized social form in 1791, with the Panopticon of Jeremy Bentham: "the most general political and technical formula of disciplinary power" (Foucault 2006b: 41). In disciplinary power, "the subject-function is fitted exactly on somatic singularity," i.e., it is "individualizing." It did this through writing and panoptic surveillance, where discipline constituted the individual. The Panopticon was designed as a model for all institutions: hospital, school, and workshop. It was a mechanism that gave strength to the institution that intensified power. One of its objectives was to make distractions disappear: copying in schools, strikes in factories, complicity in prisons. Surveillance must take place without the surveilled knowing whether or not they are being monitored. To be in the panoptic is the experience of being constantly "visible for a gaze" (Foucault 2006b: 76). In this apparatus, there are only individuals, and power is anonymous, completely deindividualized. Surveillance from the central tower can be ensured by anyone: the director, his wife, his children, a cleaner, or citizens who access it through an underground passage. For Bentham, this was democracy: Power was subject to the control of citizens who could verify how it is exercised.

During the first half of the 19th century, mental alienation was treated by a doctor: the alienist; in other words, not a psychiatrist, at least not until the very end of the 19th century. First, we talked about alienation and mental alienation, then disease, and then nervous disease. Pinel, for example, almost never spoke of "mental illness" (*maladie mentale*) for a simple reason: "in his intellectual universe, it makes no sense to make the distinction between mental illnesses in some cases and physical illness" (Dumouchel 2006: 21). This lack of usage of the term mental illness was visible up to Charcot. However, from Pinel to Charcot, if the terms alienation and disease were favored, some doctors were beginning to use the term "mental illness": Esquirol, Leuret, Falret, Voisin.

Jean-Etienne Dominique Esquirol (1772–1840) sometimes wrote about "*maladie mentale,*" a term featured in the title of his book with engravings by Ambroise Tardieu, and the expression was often used in *Des illusions chez les aliénés* and *Question médico-légale sur l'isolement des aliénés* (only a few times in *Examen du projet de loi sur les aliénés*). François Leuret (1797–1851) almost never used "*maladie mentale*" in *Fragmens psychologiques sur la folie* (1834); it was absent from the two tomes of the *Anatomie comparée du système nerveux considéré dans ses rapports avec l'intelligence* (1839), but it appeared more frequently in *Des indications à suivre dans le traitement de la folie: mémoire lu à l'Académie royale de médecine* (1845). "*Maladie mentale*" was frequently used by Jean-Pierre Falret (1794–1870) in *Des maladies mentales et des asiles d'aliénés: leçons cliniques et considérations générales* (1864), as well as by Félix Voisin (1794–1872) in "*Conférences cliniques sur les maladies mentales. Leçons sur l'idiotie*" (1881).

Therefore, there was first mental alienation and then the concept of mental illness, which spread gradually during the 19th century. It was from the second half of the 19th century that "neurologist" doctors appeared (Duchenne 1806–1875; Charcot 1825–1893), then psychiatrists (Kraepelin 1856–1926). Also, there was a historical sequence whereby certain notions stood out: unreason (until the 16th century), insanity (17th and 18th century), alienation (19th century), and mental illness (mid-19th and 20th century). I would add mental disorder (late 20th century and early 21st century), then spectrum, cluster, and biotype (21st century).

The period since the 1970s has witnessed a global transition from psychiatry to mental health. Psychiatry is included in the science of mental health, and psychiatrists have given up on curing mental disorders: Their goal is now to empower users. I emphasize this transformation: Disciplinary power (psychiatry) has been subordinated to biopower (mental health).

Self-diagnosis and hikikomori

In May 2017, I received an email with the title "Orientation of a long-term *hikikomori* schizoid in France." Mr. X. contacted me because he was in a state of distress consistent with the definition of *hikikomori*. He had also self-diagnosed. This is a situation that professionals are increasingly confronted with: self-diagnosed individuals. These are users who need support, though not in the same way as 20th-century patients. Very simply put, they are no longer patients. It is not only that the patient–psychiatrist relationship has changed from paternalistic to informative (Emanuel and Emanuel 1992); it is also that the doctor–patient relationship has collapsed. From this point of view, Alain Ehrenberg and Pierre-Henri Castel were correct in stating that we observe the transition from "autonomy as an aspiration" to "autonomy as a condition" (Ehrenberg 2010, Castel 2012). Autonomy is no longer what we aspire to in the future (i.e., an emancipation where heteronomy plays a role). From now on, autonomy is what we owe to users (e.g., an ordinary school for a nonverbal 9-year-old child who self-mutilates daily), and in medicine, treatment is subordinated to autonomy. One of the signs of this change is self-diagnosis. This has consequences from the viewpoint of the Foucauldian theory of psychiatric tests (*épreuves*).

According to Foucault, the first psychiatric test is to transcribe the motives of the request into symptoms of an illness. The second and very important test "involves making the power of intervention and the disciplinary power of the psychiatrist exist as medical knowledge" (Foucault 2006b: 268). Thereafter, disciplinary power begins to function as medical power: the request for internment turns into illness, and the doctor is the one who holds the power of internment. In other words, in medicine, there would be a "show me your symptoms, and I will tell you what patient you are." In the psychiatric test, there would be a "provide me with some symptoms (…) so that I can stand before you as a doctor" (Foucault 2006b: 268). As Foucault noted, the patient "enthrones" the doctor, either by sending him back to his purely disciplinary role or by making him play the role of a doctor: This is precisely what the hysteric has achieved with Charcot.

The whole problem with self-diagnosed users of the 21st century is that, even if they suffer, they do not really ask (*demande*) for anything, i.e., in the psychoanalytical sense. In addition, the doctor can only hospitalize them on very rare occasions. The patient is no longer available for questioning (assimilated to anamnesis and confession by Foucault), which holds a disciplinary dimension and has the function of "pinning the individual to his identity," forcing him to recognize himself in his past, in a number of events in his life. The user bypasses this because he has already questioned himself. Psychiatrists can no longer use disciplinary power to pin the individual to his identity. His identity already arrives ready-made "*hikikomori*-schizoid" and doctors are left with the role of providing guidance – an "orientation."

This dominance of biopower has not resulted in the disappearance of disciplinary power or sovereign power. They are simply subordinated to it; thus, the Foucauldian argument concerning the family still holds true in contemporary Japan, especially in the case of *hikikomori*. In fact, the family (sovereign power) has always played a central role because it pins individuals on the disciplinary apparatus. The family is the zero point, the exchanger: The individual is rejected from one system (e.g., school, work) to his family, who will pass him on to another system (e.g., special school, NPO, psychiatric hospital). Discipline did not dissolve the family: On the contrary, it intensified it. Bourgeois families always give rise to a "profit of abnormalities," as Foucault (2006b: 110) says. More precisely, when a disciplinary system is extremely tight, abnormalities and irregularities are numerous. For instance, the economic system of the 19th-century bourgeoisie made a profit from its abnormalities while reinforcing its power. Such disciplinary systems produce "the unclassifiable," "the unassimilable" (Foucault 2006b: 53): the delinquent, the mentally defective, the deserter. However, in the case of the current *hikikomori*, he is no longer watched by his family (e.g., his behavior, his sexuality) with a psychological gaze. The *hikikomori* user is abandoned, the "homeless at home," and is no longer the target of psychiatric intervention (Tajan 2017b).

According to Foucault, it was possible to make hysteria an illness because the hysteric first entered the medical field via the neurological apparatus (Charcot). It was only then that she was picked up by psychiatry: Hysterical neurosis had to go through the neurological clinic before it could become a psychiatric pathology. However, in the case of *hikikomori*, nothing similar can be observed. Also, the three great maneuvers in the struggle between the neurologist and the hysteric cannot really apply to *hikikomori*. First, the organization of the symptomatological scenario fails: *hikikomori* resists being a psychiatric category. The subjects falling into this condition are the bad patients who do not allow psychiatrists to self-recognize as good doctors (*hikikomori* individuals often do not want to see psychiatrists who struggle to treat them). Therefore, the maneuver of the "functional mannequin" fails because *hikikomori* is not an instrument that allows one to distinguish truth from simulation. Finally, I have shown elsewhere (Tajan 2017a) that the redistribution around trauma works only partially. *Hikikomori* is a form of passive aggression, unknown to the subject himself, hidden from the one who exposes his seclusion, despite himself. The *hikikomori* user, even if he excludes himself from work, meets the normative standards of capitalist societies and is one of their by-products. Yet, simultaneously, the *hikikomori* phenomenon can be seen as a struggle inside the home, outside social institutions, and against current mental health practices. While Foucault (2004) defined a group of abnormal individuals made of three elements – the human monster, the individual to be corrected, the onanist – my investigations contribute to the argument that the 21st-century shut-in might be a fourth element of Foucault's theory of the abnormal.

RDoC biopower

We know that the mission of agents in the mental health field is to achieve user autonomy. Indeed, according to the World Health Organization, "Health is a state of complete physical, mental and social well-being and not merely the absence of disease or infirmity," what Gori and Del Volgo have called "Totalitarian Health" (2005). This will to achieve total well-being and complete autonomy implies the destruction of human psychiatry.

DSM "is, at best, a dictionary, creating a set of labels and defining each"; "Patients with mental disorder deserve better"; "NIMH will be re-orienting its research away from DSM categories" (Insel 2013). These words were not uttered by Ronald Laing, David Cooper, Franco Basaglia, or any other anti-psychiatrist; they are the words of a scientist who was the director of the NIMH in 2013, Thomas Insel, known for popularizing the Research Domain Criteria (RDoC) project. This project testifies to the attempt to make psychiatric categories disappear. Indeed, psychiatry has failed to cure mental disorders. In truth, mental disorders are less and less precise (e.g., the notion of autism spectrum disorder), and their definition is sometimes criticized (e.g., depression). Moreover, the increased presence of comorbidities is seen as a problem: When a person is diagnosed with several mental disorders simultaneously (Barnhill et al. 2014), one can legitimately say that our categories are imprecise and that we might have missed an unknown and potentially distinct clinical category.

Considering that progress in psychiatry is much lower and slower than progress in other fields of medicine, some mental health researchers believe that biomedicine and big data can succeed where psychiatry has failed. Psychiatry has failed for a very simple reason: Its categories are based on symptoms. However, these categories must be based on data.

Data is provided through computational nosology, precision psychiatry, and many other biomedical disciplines. They are distributed in the RDoC matrix with units of analysis (gene, molecules, cells, circuits, physiology, behavior, self-reports, paradigms) and domains (negative valence systems, positive valence systems, cognitive systems, systems for social processes, and arousal and regulatory systems) divided into 23 constructs. We also know that biotypes (categories based on biomarkers) are more precise than traditional diagnoses (Clementz et al. 2016). We can even divide depression into four biotypes (Drysdale et al. 2016), and we have begun offering treatments (drugs, therapies, etc.) for each biotype (Williams 2016). Mental disorders considered as heterogeneous syndromes will be replaced by homogeneous clusters (Insel and Cuthbert 2015). For example, what we know as schizophrenia, depression, or bipolar disorder will become cluster x, y, z, etc.

Under the leadership of Thomas Insel, the RDoC project seemed to indicate the horizon of mental health without psychiatrists: Mental disorders are biological disorders. With the arrival of Joshua Gordon as the new director of NIMH in 2016, one has the feeling that a mental health science without psychiatric categories is still an objective, and yet that it is also necessary to cooperate with psychiatrists and the American Psychiatric Association. He wants to take into account DSM observation diagnostics along with behavioral constructs from the RDoC. According to Gordon, the categories of DSM (disciplinary power) are useful only if they are subordinate to those of the RDoC (biopower). Schizophrenia and depression, for example, are imprecise categories of symptoms because they reflect the observations of psychiatrists. These psychiatric categories are not the causes of the disease process that takes place in the brain (naturalistic reductionism): "Since we know the outcomes (DSM-based observations) but not the causes (underlying disease processes), we need a way of working backwards from outcomes to causes if we are to understand the neurobiology of mental illnesses" (Gordon 2017). Following is Gordon's definition of the ambition of the RDoC project:

> Imagine a world where your psychiatrist runs a panel of tests – behavioral and brain function tests – in addition to her clinical assessment. She gives you a diagnosis and realistic prognosis and helps you choose between treatments with the knowledge of your individualized chance of responding to each of them (Gordon 2017).

The evolution of biomedical research in mental health shows the relevance of biopower. Let us go back to the Foucauldian text. During his last lecture of *Society Must be Defended* (1975–1976), he questioned, "what does this new technology of power, this biopolitics, this biopower that is beginning to establish itself, involve" (Foucault 2003: 243)? He especially differentiated the mechanisms of disciplinary power from those of biopolitics. The mechanisms put in place by biopolitics are forecasts, statistics, and global measures: We do not intervene on the individual as such, but we lower morbidity, we lengthen life, we stimulate the birth rate.

> Unlike disciplines, they no longer train individuals by working at the level of the body itself. There is absolutely no question relating to an individual body, in the way that discipline does. It is therefore not a matter of taking the individual at the level of individuality, but on the contrary of using overall mechanisms and acting in such a way as to achieve overall states of equilibration, or regularity; it is, in a word, a matter of taking control of life and the biological processes of man-as-species, and of ensuring that they are not disciplined but regularized (Foucault 2003: 246–247).

This power of regularization consists in "make live" and "let die" (Foucault 2003: 247). Inspired by Foucault, Giorgio Agamben proposed an understanding of the specificity of biopower. According to him, it would be formulated as follows:

> No longer either *to make die* or *to make live*, but *to make survive*. The decisive activity of biopower in our time consists of the production not of life or death but rather of a mutable and virtually infinite survival [...] Biopower's supreme ambition is to produce, in a human body, the absolute separation of the living being and the speaking being, of *zoè* and *bios*, the inhuman and the human: survival.
>
> *(Agamben 1999: 155–156)*

Biomedicine has both disciplinary and regulatory effects. Norms apply to the body that we want to discipline and to the population (biological multiplicity) that we want to regularize. I would add that "make survive" is the point where disciplinary power (psychiatry) meets biopower (mental health science).

I will provisionally conclude this section with a Japanese word, *Bokuchikugyō*, meaning "stock farming." This is the term used by Takemi Tarō – a former director of the Japanese Medical Association – to refer to mental hospitals. Kitanaka (2012: 50) considered that it ridiculed psychiatrists, but it could also be seen as an insult to some stock farmers who treat their cattle in a humane manner. As a trained psychologist, I cannot help but think that "stock farming" is a projection; in truth, it applies to its speaker: a doctor. In the 21st century, it is not just psychiatry that falters; medicine also becomes uncertain. Reduced to a health science, contemporary biomedicine seems entirely doomed to a regularization, the objective of which is the tasteless horizon of biopower: make survive.

The end of the clinic

Foucault's famous *The Birth of the Clinic* relates exclusively to the medical clinic, and its scope did not go beyond the end of the 19th century. In other words, it contains nothing about the 20th century, nothing about medicine in the 20th century, nothing about psychiatry, nothing about psychopathology, and nothing about psychoanalysis. Thus, he did not explore the clinics of the medical subdisciplines, such as those developed in the 20th century – the psychiatric, psychopathological, psychological, psychoanalytic clinics – neither in *The Birth of the Clinic* nor in *Psychiatric Power*. These disciplines represent the development of the clinic, and all are rooted in clinical medicine.

If Foucault described the birth of clinical medicine and the 20th century saw the development of a diversity of clinics (medical, psychological, psychoanalytic, etc.), could the 21st century mark the end of the clinic? What, from the clinic, will survive the era of cost cutting and the promotion of artificial intelligence in healthcare? I suggest that we address these questions as follows. First, I will outline what Foucault's reading brings to the clinician. Second, I will return briefly to *The Birth of the Clinic*, which will, third, allow me to discuss the conditions of the clinic in the 21st century.

Read Foucault for the clinician

Beforehand, one must remember that *Madness and Unreason* and *Psychiatric Power*, despite the remarkable aspects highlighted previously, are satisfactory neither for the historian of medicine nor for the clinician. For clinicians, it suffices to compare his presentation of the case of Leuret, cited in *Psychiatric Power*, with the original source in *Fragmens psychologiques*. Foucault omits parts of the case written by Leuret. Why not? There is nothing wrong with cutting out parts of the original case study for reasons of length. This undoubtedly served Foucault's argument, even if Leuret's presentation of the original case was quite short. It is not the selection of parts of a doctor's case report that is problematic. What poses a problem for the clinician is that by reading Foucault's and Leuret's versions of the case, the diagnosis changes: Indeed, Foucault amputates certain parts of the text, of the dialogue, in fact, which are important for the diagnosis and, more fundamentally, for understanding the richness of the patient's lived experience.

Lectio pessima

Foucault's method in the area of scientific research consisted of amputating, erasing, cutting, and plugging holes, all of which are akin to data manipulation. In medicine and biology, data manipulation, if not detected and sanctioned, can have serious consequences on the lives of patients. Why should it be different in the humanities and social sciences? Why should erasing a stain on a DNA strip (Rossner and Yamada 2004) be different from the amputation of certain key words used by a patient, especially if these key words can influence the diagnosis? Foucault made believe that Leuret's patient never talked about her parents and never designated herself with the pronoun "I." However, in Leuret's text, she does speak of her parents and does designate herself by the pronoun "I." (Leuret 1834: 121–124). The patient described by Foucault is a much purer form (Castel 2009: 239), ideal in a sense, compared to that described by Leuret, which appears much more concrete, more contradictory, in a word: more alive.

Lectio optima

Importantly, Foucault was neither a professional historian nor a clinician. Yes, this should lead to criticism regarding aspects that can sometimes be of considerable importance. As Basso (2014) wrote, "the criticism about Foucault's 'romantic' view of madness is still topical today." However, the interest of *Madness and Unreason*, *The Birth of the Clinic*, and *Psychiatric Power* lies in the way in which Foucault thought of medicine – psychiatry, psychology, and psychoanalysis – on a longer time scale, within the framework of a history of systems of thought. Foucault necessarily cut, and by these gestures, if you allow me the expression "lost matter," which allowed him to identify categories that are useful to us, for example, sovereign power, disciplinary power, and biopower.

Foucault stopped at considerations of psychiatry as a form of disciplinary power. He did not know about the transition from psychiatry to mental health, i.e., the inclusion of psychiatry into the mental health field. However, his concept of biopower allowed us to think about this change. I stated earlier my argument that psychiatry was to disciplinary power what the science of mental health is to biopower. In other words, psychiatry is today subordinated to mental health: Disciplinary power has not disappeared, but it is subordinated to biopower. Could the advent of biopower have meant the death of the clinic, in other words, its end? To answer this question, let us return to *The Birth of the Clinic* by selecting elements that will be useful for the analysis of the contemporary period.

A glance at the birth of the clinic

The Birth of the Clinic is composed of scraps of *Madness and Unreason*. For Foucault, *The Birth of the Clinic* was a research, the project of which was historicocritical and the aim of which was to determine "the conditions of possibility of medical experience in modern times" (Foucault 1976: xxii). At that time, medicine was born as a clinical science, and Foucault supported the importance of the medical gaze in the constitution of medicine as a science:

> it was this constant gaze upon the patient, this age-old, yet ever renewed attention that enabled medicine not to disappear entirely with each new speculation, but to preserve itself, to assume little by little the figure of a truth that is definitive, if not completed, in short, to develop, below the level of the noisy episodes of its history, in a continuous historicity. In the non-variable of the clinic, medicine, it was thought, had bound truth and time together.
>
> *(Foucault 1976: 65)*

In other words, "the clinic gives medicine its true historical movement," and the advent of medical clinics was an essential moment in supporting its scientific consistency, where the medical gaze played a central role.

In another register, Foucault recalled that the simple fact of hospitalizing someone was criticized, even before the French Revolution, for moral and economic reasons: An illness treated in hospital would be a cost for society, the patient becoming chronic, he and his family losing money, which accentuated financial and moral distress. Foucault saw another moral problem here: that of the patient asking for help, finding himself obliged to be the object of a gaze – because it is through the clinic that we see the symptoms that are the telltale signs of an illness.

In his last chapter, he returned to the conditions of the possibility of medicine and especially the anatomo-clinical method.

> For clinical experience to become possible as a form of knowledge, a reorganization of the hospital field, a new definition of the status of the patient in society, and the establishment of a certain relationship between public assistance and medical experience, between help and knowledge, became necessary; the patient has to be enveloped in a collective, homogeneous space (Foucault 1976: 242).

It is, moreover, only at the end of the volume that Foucault mentioned the "Freudian man" and "the importance of Bichat, of Jackson, of Freud in European culture" (Foucault 1976: 245). No doubt, *The Birth of the Clinic*, which gives so much room to the gaze, could not integrate Freud, who is remembered as the doctor who suppressed the gaze in the clinic by inventing psychoanalysis. Psychoanalysis as an "eyes wide shut clinic," if I may say, is the couch depriving the analyst and analysand of the other's gaze. This is part of the development of the clinic in the 20th century, a clinic without a gaze, heterogeneous to the Foucauldian theory exposed in *The Birth of the Clinic*.

The clinic in the 21st century

If there are conditions for the possibility of medical experience in modern times, why would there not be, in postmodern times, the 21st century, conditions for the impossibility of the medical clinic? After all, many conditions are met. First, doctors no longer have the time for clinical observation. Their mission has changed in response to economic and managerial factors. Doctors are no longer clinicians; the clinic is no longer what is expected of them. Consulting 60, 80, 100 patients a day does not allow the time necessary for clinical observation. The doctor, therefore, becomes the user's health manager: He controls the arms of health workers and makes decisions based on data collected by machines or computers. This is an illustration of what I call the subordination of disciplinary (medical) power to biopower (health).

The 20th century marked acute clinical observations of symptoms as the source of diagnostic accuracy and, with the rise of medical power, helped establish the authority of physicians. Today, however, accurate symptom observation is no longer enough because symptoms and the gaze are misleading; symptoms and the imprecise human eye are a source of diagnostic error. The authority of doctors no longer relies on the quality of their clinical observation, the exercise of the medical gaze. The doctor's authority is based on his ability to assist himself with machines connected to the organism. It is necessary to "make speak" genes, molecules, cells, circuits, physiology (RDoC). These are the many units of analysis that make it possible to identify clusters, x, y, or z, new labels originating from precision and computational medicine for pathologies that clinicians used to identify with the naked eye. Medical power as a variant of disciplinary power has, therefore, not disappeared, but the postmodern era exposes its subordination to biopower. What the patient shows or hides, the clinic as a school, as a pedagogy, all of this continues and will continue to exist, albeit to a lesser extent, because what is becoming generalized is direct access to the body's data without recourse to the doctor's human gaze.

Data is collected without the human gaze, and in many situations, it is now possible for the doctor to have no physical contact with the sick. This is demonstrated by the so-called boom in telemedicine and health apps (self-help on smartphones), so much so that it is easy to imagine that hospitals will receive fewer and fewer patients and that these patients, in one way or another, and above all, for economic reasons, will mainly be treated at home. We continue to use the word patient, but the patient has become no more than the shadow of the user. Doctors will simply intervene to verify data produced by machines and applications, manage cheap human arms, and make appropriate decisions concerning the user. The idea is, above all, to reduce seemingly unnecessary health costs, i.e., infrastructure, and workforce.

Reducing costs would also be made possible by artificial intelligence. One, therefore, promotes artificial intelligence in the health field. One imagines that the intervention of a human being, the doctor, is neither useful nor necessary and that treatment should mostly be automated for a simple reason: Humans make more mistakes than machines. What is more, in the field of disorders, is the diagnosis not produced at the end of an algorithm? However, machines or computers have more computing power than humans. Machines are faster and make fewer mistakes than humans, if at all. Frankly, who would trust a human rather than artificial intelligence?

More than 20 years ago, Kandel (1998: 464) wrote, "The basis of the new intellectual framework for psychiatry is that all mental processes are biological, and therefore any alteration in those processes is necessarily organic." As we have seen with Thomas Insel, Joshua Gordon, and others, this has nothing to do with a new intellectual framework. For there is nothing fundamentally new here, on the contrary: It is simply a *renouveau* of naturalistic reductionism in psychiatry. Certainly, some tools are new, impressive, and colorful, but daily applications of the aforementioned principle in scientific research often fall into an observational bias known as streetlight effect, i.e., searching where the light is.

The times of the end of the clinic might mean a great deal for global health policy. In this respect, I share Arthur Kleinman's opinion:

> Academic psychiatry has become more or less irrelevant to clinical practice and to the major developments in the mental health field. After decades of investment in biological psychiatric research, there are

many intriguing and potentially significant findings, yet still not a single biological test that can be routinely used in the clinic to determine whether someone has a particular mental disorder. Brain science has advanced impressively for neurological conditions, and for our general knowledge of how the brain works, but it has not determined what causes schizophrenia, depressive disorder or anxiety diseases (…) we still do not understand the pathophysiology of these mental illnesses or of other psychiatric conditions, from eating disorders to autism.

(Kleinman 2012: 421)

He also distinguished academic psychiatry from clinical psychiatry and pondered how we could save psychiatry:

If by, say, 2030 we still have no clinically useful biological test for mental disorders and little in the way of new therapeutic agents, academic psychiatry will, I believe, be consigned to irrelevancy that will be ruinous to the profession (…). By 2030, there definitely will be a profession of clinical and community psychiatry, but perhaps there will no longer be many academic researchers in psychiatry (Kleinman 2012: 422).

These considerations might seem pessimistic in the sense that Kleinman believes that academic psychiatry will disappear. However, the statement that clinical psychiatry will survive is clearly optimistic. I would like to share this optimism and wager that there is still hope for clinical psychiatry, though it might already be too late. Health and welfare ministries around the world have for decades failed to solve many issues, including depression, schizophrenia, homelessness, and social isolation. Our societies would benefit from less costly and less bureaucratic apparatuses dedicated to "loneliness," which is at the intersection of the distress implied by many conditions, including depression, schizophrenia, homelessness, and social isolation. A ministry of loneliness, which has been attempted in the United Kingdom, might seem naïve to some, but it might also be a possibility for the restoration of dignity, which the parties concerned lost over decades. This cannot be done without an overhaul of health ministries, systems, and psychiatric authorities. It is a challenge that implies agents in the field of global mental health, if we follow Kleinman's reflections, and I would add that it also implies a global thought about the appropriate and bearable balance between disciplinary power and biopower in health policies.

Finally, intellectual history has proven to be extremely valuable in questions of whether psychiatry can determine an objective norm for madness (Castel 2009). By getting rid of psychiatric categories, contemporary biomedical research has tried to avoid the question of norms of madness established by psychiatry. This consideration deals with a much broader biomedical problem, which was addressed by Georges Canguilhem decades ago through the concept of biological normativity (Canguilhem 1966) and the norms defining health.

> Human diseases are not only limitations on his physical power, they are tragedies in his history. Human life is an existence, a being there for an unordered becoming, in the dread of its end. Man is therefore open to illness not by condemnation or by destiny but by his mere presence in the world. In this respect, health is by no means an economic require-ment to be asserted in the context of legislation, it is the spontaneous unity of the conditions of life.
>
> *(Canguilhem 2002: 89)*

> Let us harden the Kantian statement: there is no health science. Let us admit it for now. Health is not a scientific concept, it is a vulgar concept. This does not mean trivial, but simply common, within everyone's reach.
>
> *(Canguilhem 2002: 52)*

The end of the clinic, the return of unreason and hikikomori as the new abnormal

The shut-in, the recluse, the person who finds himself or herself in a sit-uation of social isolation for a long period of time is, in the Foucauldian sense, the new abnormal, and I interpret it as a sign of the return of unrea-son in the 21st century. It exposes, with many other phenomena, what I call the end of the clinic. We are currently experiencing the end of the clinic, a logical consequence of the rise of the biopower–neoliberalism couple: *hikikomori*, the new abnormal, is one of its features.

Hikikomori phenomenon, far from being homogeneous, appears as the history of a myriad of singular subjects: The colorful crowd (*la foule bariolée*) described by Foucault has been mutating from embarkation (*The Ship of Fools*), then confinement (17–18th century), hospitalization (19–20th century) to social isolation (21st century). Social withdrawal is a symptom that can be found in many mental disorders. It is transnosographic, meaning that many different people with disabilities, disorders, or illnesses are socially isolated. There is a diversity, and simultaneously the social perception of a unity: A social sensitivity recognizes that *hikikomori* cannot be reduced to a mental disorder or disability. *Hikikomori* is unique, it is a resurgence of unreason. Unreason has never ceased to exist: It has been hidden, and it finally found a new idiom. *Hikikomori* is unique and multiple. There is a perception of a unicity of *hikikomori* and, simultaneously, shouting evidence of a multiplicity of the torn presence of unreason.

One could think that the rise of social isolation is coextensive of the achievement of deinstitutionalization. However, *hikikomori* is born in Japan, where institutionalization is still very strong. Indeed, almost a fifth of psychiatric beds worldwide are in Japan: precisely 334,258 according to the Ministry of Health Labour and Welfare (MHLW) (2017). One could also think that the achievement of deinstitutionalization would mean the return of the patients to their family. In other words, that one would find a psychiatric bed in every single home; or, in countries where homelessness is extremely strong, that some streets transform into anarchic psychiatric wards. Although these statements are not completely inaccurate, what I would argue here is that we must fully consider that a fundamental change has already occurred: The doctor–patient relationship has completely collapsed. *Hikikomori* exposes it. In Japan, the vast majority of *hikikomori* individuals are not hospitalized, they do not fall into doctor's hands. It is not only that *hikikomori* individuals do not recognize themselves as patients, but it is also that doctors do not see them as patients. As I wrote repeatedly, *hikikomori* is not a medical condition, it is not a mental disorder, and speaking about comorbidity simply misses the point: *hikikomori* is a psychosocial condition.

Hikikomori is a deeply subjective and eminently social idiom, not limited to Japan and not solely related to Japanese culture. *Hikikomori* resists medicalization and does not meet coherent and consistent criteria for being described as a spectrum in the psychiatric sense (i.e., what I would call "Hikikomori Spectrum Disorder, HSD"). My insistence in writing that it resists medicalization and also means that it resists medical gaze, it fails to fall under the medical gaze, and I interpret it as a sign among many others that we are experiencing the end of the clinic.

It is obvious that most *hikikomori* subjects have a history of absenteeism or dropping out of school and are most likely to be male (Yong and Nomura 2019). In this respect, they could belong to the Foucauldian category of the individual to be corrected, the delinquent, though I find it is misleading. Support initiatives in Japan are trying to send them back to work, but they are overwhelmingly failing to achieve this goal. Moreover, I maintain that female *hikikomori* do exist, but it is underreported or reported in other categories such as an affinity group (59.3% women are in the affinity group in the 2016's Cabinet Office survey). Such a lack of recognition is to be understood through the prism of gender inequalities (see, for instance, Lock 1995, Holloway 2010, Kitanaka 2012, Nakamura 2013, Gender Equality Bureau 2020) and gender studies.

As we have seen in Chapters 4, 6, and 7, excessive use of the Internet among the *hikikomori* population is largely an inaccurate stereotype: Within the 15–39 age group, there is simply no significant difference between the proportion of individuals who used the internet in the hikikomori group (59.2%) and in the general group (59.6%). Note: individuals in the *hikikomori* group age 40–64 used the Internet less often than those in the general group [Cabinet Office of the Government of Japan (Director-General for Policy on Cohesive Society) 2019: 43].

Hikikomori subjects are simultaneously pressured by society and their families, and at the same time abandoned in a situation that I would call "homeless at home." Instead of being active or surfing the Internet, they are abandoned in a state of extreme passivity, mostly watching television. This passivity also leads them to not refuse consciously to go to school, university, or work: Not participating is not refusing to participate.

That is how I would portray *hikikomori*: a pervasive social phenomenon in Japan that spreads abroad, for sure; and also a passive and socially isolated subject that has ceased being a patient, for he does not consider himself or herself one, and is not considered by others and doctors as such. A surge of unreason in the 21st century, the new abnormal that is the *hikikomori* person exemplifies what I call the end of the clinic.

Perspectives

Some of the readers might still question what I am introducing here: Are we really witnessing the end of the clinic? Let me answer in a more nuanced fashion. Certainly yes, and possibly no. Yes in the sense that "the end of the clinic" is what is promoted by the biopower–neoliberalism couple in a formidable and very effective way: close the maximum number of public establishments, employ the minimum number of personnel under the pretext of saving health-care costs, and reject supposedly outdated systems. All these work to the death of the clinic and the closure of spaces that care for human pathology. As we have seen in the Covid-19 pandemic that spread in 2019 and 2020, suppression of hospital beds and decades of cuts in funding for health systems contributed to tragic consequences for millions of people around the globe.

The answer is in the affirmative in another sense. The cases of conversational robots or of individuals who self-diagnose (e.g., *hikikomori*, aspies, borderline) also represent a transfer of authority. Psychiatrists, psychologists, and psychoanalysts – i.e., those who have training and legitimacy to establish a diagnosis – no longer have the authority to do so. It is not exactly that the diagnosis no longer belongs to them; the diagnosis of a professional is often needed. Rather, authority has been transferred to the person concerned (*tōjisha*). The sovereignty of the person concerned (biopower) is claimed in defiance of the knowledge of clinicians (psychiatric power). It goes without saying that this sovereignty of the person concerned does not come from disciplinary power but, rather, from a biopower, which aims neither to "make live" nor "to let die," but "to make survive." It is clear that clinicians, if they still have the knowledge to confirm or disconfirm a diagnosis, no longer have the authority to disconfirm a diagnosis. The assertion of the identity of the person concerned is sovereign. The clinician can only confirm – or affirm it.

The answer is also in the affirmative when applied to *hikikomori*. If the birth of the clinic can be embodied by the coupled doctor–hysteric of disciplinary power, the end of the clinic is illustrated by the *hikikomori* individual whose partner is assigned to be nothing more than the shadow of the other (*une ombre d'homme baclée à la six-quatre-deux* to quote French translation of Schreber). If we obviously do not observe a return to a premodern unreason free from physicians' gaze, physicians, psychiatrists, and society as a whole face a return of unreason. *Hikikomori* came to tell us that unreason is back and that we are experiencing "the times of the end of the clinic." In truth, *hikikomori* is a form of passive aggression that meets the normative standards of neoliberal societies and is one of their by-products. Moreover, the shut-in obeys the imperative of biopower: survival. While Foucault (2004) defined a group of abnormal individuals made of three elements – the human monster, the individual to be corrected, the onanist – my investigations contribute to the argument that the postmodern shut-in is a fourth element of Foucault's theory of the abnormal. *Hikikomori*, the new abnormal, embodies the return of unreason in 21st century Japan, and beyond.

Yet, simultaneously, the *hikikomori* phenomenon can be seen as a struggle inside the home, outside social institutions, and against current mental health practices. And there is a space here where psychoanalysis, anthropology, and social isolation meet.

Notwithstanding, the other answer to the question – are we really witnessing the end of the clinic – is no, at least to a certain extent. In a very modest and vulnerable way, if I dare say so, the clinic took refuge partly in anthropological and psychoanalytic terrains: anthropological because only anthropologists can subtly describe the complexity of what is at stake in the doctor–patient (Luhrman 2001) or analyst–analysand (Lézé 2010) relationship, both in hospitals and elsewhere; psychoanalytical because Freud will be remembered in history as the doctor who suppressed the gaze in the clinic while inventing psychoanalysis, the couch depriving the analyst and analysand from the gaze of the other. Besides, Freud would no doubt be surprised to find his practice transformed today, with many analysands needing the gaze of the other during sessions. Admittedly, it is no longer exactly the medical gaze, but it is a gaze, a certain gaze, for example, a presence that guards against sinking, or collapsing. From this point of view, there is no use denying that psychoanalysis is the daughter of disciplinary power, but it cannot be diluted in biopower. Psychoanalysis is not intended for those who do not question their unconscious: It can do nothing for those who are satisfied with a "conversation" with a robot. What can it do for a person who isolates himself in a *hikikomori* situation? If "*hikikomori*" is a master signifier found to order a person's life and spares him/her the recognition of a subjective division, then the answer might be nothing. What I have tried to show in this book, and especially with the case of Misaki, is that the psychoanalytic clinic, combined with anthropological methods, can contribute to the subjective formation of the speaking being (*parlêtre*). Subject formation is one of the objectives of psychoanalysis, and it is not expected in the relationship of the anthropologist with his/her object. In the case of socially withdrawn subjects, I hypothesize that psychoanalysis alone can do nothing and that it must be confronted with anthropological knowledge to have some effect. No doubt, I have only sketched its outlines, and I beg the reader who has come so far to forgive me.

To conclude, if I had to take a picture, it would be that of the entrance of Japanese homes: the *genkan*. The *hikikomori* person is trapped in a space-time between the interior and exterior, the pure and impure: In the Japanese imaginary, he remains at the gates of society without entering it. From an ethical point of view, there is no choice but to help him venture into society. When he finally enters, if I have to employ a fairly common metaphor, the train will have already passed by. It will be too late. There is no point denying it. Similarly, the psychoanalyst stepping outside the limits of his office would correspond to the *hikikomori* person stepping outside his home. However, the person who is gradually emerging from social withdrawal finds him/herself on a platform where trains no longer pass for him/her. The role of the psychoanalyst is to confront the subject with his/her own desire – *Che vuoi?* – and to indicate that the one who cannot take the highway can take minor roads (Lacan 1997: 293), provided that the ex-*hikikomori* subject consents to the company of a few small others. From this point of view, the person who escapes the *hikikomori* situation puts aside the "survival" imperative of biopower. Psychoanalysis, combined with certain aspects of the anthropological approach, can be seen as a resistance to biopower, a resistance the slogan of which could be: The clinic must be defended.

References

Agamben, Giorgio. 1999. *Remnants of Auschwitz. The Witness and the Archive.* New York: Zone Books.

Artières, Philippe, and Jean-François Bert. 2011. *Un succès philosophique. L'Histoire de la philosophie à l'âge classique de Michel Foucault.* Caen: Presses Universitaires de Caen.

Artières, et al. 2011. *Histoire de la philosophie à l'âge classique de Michel Foucault. Regards Critiques 1961-2011.* Caen: Presses Universitaires de Caen.

Barnhill, John W., et al. 2014. *DSM-5 Clinical Cases.* Washington DC: American Psychiatric Publishing.

Basso, Elisabetta. 2014. "Double Review-History of Madness." *Foucault Studies* 18: 279–286.

Cabinet Office of the Government of Japan (Director-General for Policy on Cohesive Society) 内閣府政策統括官 (共生社会政策担当). 2019. *Seikatsu Jōkyō ni Kansuru Chōsa* 生活状況に関する調査 (Survey on Living Conditions). https://www8.cao.go.jp/youth/kenkyu/life/h30/pdf-index.html.

Canguilhem, Georges. 1966. *Le normal et le pathologique.* Paris: Presses Universitaires de France, Quadrige.

Canguilhem, Georges. 2002. *Écrits sur la médecine.* Paris: Seuil.

Castel, Pierre-Henri. 2009. *L'esprit malade: Cerveaux, folies, individus.* Paris: Ithaque, collection "Philosophie, Anthropologie, Psychologie".

Castel, Pierre-Henri. 2012. *La Fin des coupables, suivi de Le Cas Paramord. vol. II: Obsessions et contrainte intérieure, de la psychanalyse aux neurosciences.* Paris: Ithaque. Collection: Philosophie, Anthropologie, Psychologie.

Clementz, Brett A., et al. 2016. "Identification of Distinct Psychosis Biotypes Using Brain-Based Biomarkers." *American Journal of Psychiatry* 173: 373–384.

Cuthbert, Bruce N., and Thomas R. Insel. 2013. "Toward the Future of Psychiatric Diagnosis: The Seven Pillars of RDoC." *BMC Medicine* 11 (1): 126.

Drysdale, et al. 2016. "Resting-State Connectivity Biomarkers Define Neurophysiological Subtypes of Depression." *Nature Medicine* 23: 28–38.

Dumouchel, Paul. 2006. "Qu'est-ce qu'une maladie? Pinel, aliéniste et nosographe." *Philosophiques* 33 (1): 19–35.

Ehrenberg, Alain. 2010. *La Société du malaise. Le mental et le social*. Paris: Odile Jacob.

Emanuel Ezekiel J., and Linda L. Emanuel. 1992. "Four Models of the Physician-Patient Relationship." *JAMA* 267 (16): 2221–2226.

Foucault, Michel. 1976. *The Birth of the Clinic*. London: Tavistock Publications.

Foucault, Michel. 2003. *Society Must be Defended: Lectures at the Collège de France (1975–76)*. New York: Picador.

Foucault, Michel. 2004. *Abnormal: Lectures at the Collège de France, 1974–1975*. New York: Picador.

Foucault, Michel. 2006a. *History of Madness*. Oxon, New York: Routledge.

Foucault, Michel. 2006b. *Psychiatric Power: Lectures at the Collège de France, 1973–1974*. New York: Palgrave MacMillan.

Foucault, Michel. 2015a. "Folie et Déraison. Histoire de la folie à l'âge classique." In *Œuvres I*. Paris: Gallimard, La Pléiade.

Foucault, Michel 2015b. "Chronologie." In *Œuvres II*. Paris: Gallimard, La Pléiade.

Gender Equality Bureau. 2020. *Women and Men in Japan 2020*. Tōkyō: Cabinet Office, Government of Japan. Available at: http://www.gender.go.jp/english_contents/pr_act/pub/pamphlet/women-and-men20/index.html.

Gordon, Joshua. 2017. *Outcome to causes and back*. Blog post. Available at: https://www.nimh.nih.gov/about/director/messages/2017/rdoc-outcomes-to-causes-and-back.shtml.

Holloway, Susan D. 2010. *Women and Family in Contemporary Japan*. Cambridge University Press.

Insel, Thomas R., and Bruce N. Cuthbert. 2015. "Brain Disorders? Precisely." *Science* 348 (6234): 499–500.

Insel, Thomas R. 2013. *Transforming diagnosis*. Blog post. Available at: https://www.nimh.nih.gov/about/directors/thomas-insel/blog/2013/transforming-diagnosis.shtml.

Kitanaka, Junko. 2012. *Depression in Japan, Psychiatric Cures for a Society in Distress*. Princeton, NJ: Princeton University Press.

Kleinman, Arthur. 2012. "Rebalancing Academic Psychiatry: Why It Needs to Happen – and Soon." *British Journal of Psychiatry* 201 (6): 421–422.

Kandel, Eric R. 1998. "A new Intellectual Framework for Psychiatry." *American Journal of Psychiatry* 155: 457–469.

Kitanaka, Junko. 2012. *Depression in Japan, Psychiatric Cures for a Society in Distress*. Princeton, NJ: Princeton University Press.

Lacan, Jacques. 1997. *The Seminar, Book III: The Psychoses (1955-1956)*. London, New York: W.W. Norton & Company.

Leblanc, Guillaume. 2014. "L'histoire de la folie à l'âge classique. Une histoire de la pauvreté." In *Usages de Foucault*. Edited by Hervé Oulc'hen, 65–81. Paris: Presses Universitaires de France, Pratiques Théoriques.

Leuret, François. 1834. *Fragmens psychologiques sur la folie.* Paris: Crochard.

Lézé, Samuel. 2010. *L'autorité des psychanalystes.* Paris: Presses Universitaires de France.

Lock, Margaret. 1995. *Encounters with Aging. Mythologies of Menopause in Japan and North America.* Berkeley, CA: University of California Press.

Luhrmann, Tania M. 2001. *Of Two Minds: An Anthropologist Looks at American Psychiatry.* New York: Vintage books.

Ministry of Health Labour and Welfare (MHLW) 厚生労働省. 2017. Handbook of Health and Welfare Statistics 2017, *Table 2-32.* Available at: https://www.mhlw.go.jp/english/database/db-hh/2-2.html.

Nakamura, Karen. 2013. *A Disability of the Soul: An Ethnography of Schizophrenia and Mental Illness in Contemporary Japan.* Ithaca: Cornell University Press.

Quétel, Claude. 2012. *Histoire de la folie de l'Antiquité à nos jours.* Paris: Tallandier/ Texto.

Rossner, Mike, and Kenneth Yamada. 2004. "What's in a Picture? The Temptation of Image Manipulation." *The Journal of cell biology* 166: 11–15.

Tajan, Nicolas (2017a). "Traumatic Dimensions of Hikikomori: A Foucauldian Note." *Asian Journal of Psychiatry* 27: 121–122.

Tajan, Nicolas (2017b). *Génération hikikomori.* Paris: L'Harmattan/Japon, études du fait japonais.

Williams, Leanne M. 2016. "Precision Psychiatry: A Neural Circuit Taxonomy for Depression and Anxiety." *The Lancet* 3 (5): 472–480.

Yong, Roseline, and Kyoko Nomura. 2019. "Hikikomori is Most Associated with Interpersonal Relationships, Followed by Suicide Risks: A Secondary Analysis of a National Cross-Sectional Study." *Frontiers in Psychiatry* 10: 247.

Index